Unusual and Rare Psychological Disorders

Unusual and Rare Psychological Disorders

A Handbook for Clinical Practice and Research

EDITED BY BRIAN A. SHARPLESS

OXFORD

UNIVERSITY PRESS

Oxford University Press is a department of the University of Oxford. It furthers
the University's objective of excellence in research, scholarship, and education
by publishing worldwide. Oxford is a registered trade mark of Oxford University
Press in the UK and certain other countries.

Published in the United States of America by Oxford University Press
198 Madison Avenue, New York, NY 10016, United States of America.

Library of Congress Cataloging-in-Publication Data
Names: Sharpless, Brian A., editor.
Title: Unusual and rare psychological disorders : a handbook for clinical
practice and research / edited by Brian A. Sharpless.
Description: Oxford ; New York : Oxford University Press, [2017] | Includes
bibliographical references and index.
Identifiers: LCCN 2016027899 (print) | LCCN 2016028870 (ebook) |
ISBN 9780190245863 | ISBN 9780190245870 (ebook)
Subjects: | MESH: Mental Disorders | Rare Diseases | Handbooks
Classification: LCC RC355 (print) | LCC RC355 (ebook) | NLM WM 34 |
DDC 616.8—dc23
LC record available at https://lccn.loc.gov/2016027899

9 8 7 6 5 4 3 2 1
Printed by WebCom, Inc., Canada

*I dedicate this book to Thomas Wachter, Jamie Weaver,
and Desmond Oathes: three rare and unusual people.*

CONTENTS

We are in an age when psychiatric diagnosis is under the spotlight—and all its unsightly blemishes are being revealed. Instead of smooth lines separating each condition we have jagged craters of uncertainty. Psychiatrists are accused of creating pathology where none exists, and, therefore, by implication exposing patients to dangerous treatments with all their adverse effects. As Allan Frances in his book *Saving Normal* (2013) writes:

> "In aggregate, the new disorders promoted so blithely by my friends would create tens of millions of new 'patients.' I pictured all these normal-enough people being captured in DSM-5's excessively wide diagnostic net, and I worried that many would be exposed to medication with possibly dangerous side effects . . ."

This case for restricting diagnosis to a minimum of conditions, for which we have firm and unassailable data, appears completely convincing. This could be called the minimalist or Hairshirt diagnostic approach.

But there is another argument to make, which is equally compelling. Time after time I have seen patients who, when I have explained a diagnosis, however imperfectly, smile in relief and say, "Good, I'm so relieved, I thought I must be the only person in the world to be like this." Even if the condition is improperly described, has no obvious links to any other form of pathology, or in colloquial terms is completely wacky, it has substance to the people who are suffering from it. This could be called the Validation diagnostic approach.

Brian Sharpless's new book trumpets the Validation approach loudly and convincingly. Whether we diagnose conditions imperfectly or not, we should not simply put them into the standard box called *Not Otherwise Specified*, an archaic and complete failure of diagnosis that can be summarized as *ANTEDILUVIAN* (A Notional Term Essentially Describing, In Language Unashamedly Vacuous, It's Absolutely Nothing).

When we come across something new in science we go through a set of questions: Is this genuinely new? Why hasn't it occurred or been recognized before? Is it replicable? How did it happen? What is its outcome? Of course, we cannot answer all these questions at once but in deciding whether a syndrome is new in psychiatry, we need first to know whether it occurs in others, and this is where the science of classification begins. Sorting into groups is all part of the scientific method, and frequently can lead to great advances—just remember Gregor Mendel and his apparently useless sorting of those silly wrinkled and round peas, now recognized as the birth of genetics.

So when you read about asphyxiophilia later on in this book, do so with an open mind. Here is a condition that may be extraordinarily common—we only come across it when it goes too far and people die—but because it is a secretive condition we have no idea whether thousands across the world are using it to achieve sexual satisfaction. Could this disorder be behind the effectiveness of Viagra, a drug that selectively reduces cortical blood supply with built-in safeguards to avoid asphyxiation, and which could be used to treat sexual offenders and others for whom we currently have no effective treatments? So, whatever you do, do not scoff at the Exploding Head Syndrome, *Taijin Kyofusho* (a major public health issue in Japan), or the Alice in Wonderland Syndrome, as unlike Alice we may not be running as fast as we can to stay in the same place. Rather, around the corner we may greet a major scientific advance.

The authors of the chapters in this book have probably all gone through the JBS Haldane tetrad, the four stages of advancement in science seen from the biased standpoint of academic competitors (i.e., those people who work in the same field and have a mixture of envy and annoyance when they read about what others are doing). JBS Haldane was a maverick and extraordinarily gifted physiologist, geneticist, and evolution writer who always had something important to say whenever he made any communication to the world, and he did so pretty frequently. JBS, as he was commonly called, said the process of acceptance of a new idea goes through four opinion stages of "sour peer expert review":

1. It is worthless nonsense.
2. It is an interesting, but perverse, point of view.
3. This is true, but quite unimportant.
4. I always said so.

Not many of the syndromes described in this book have completed all four of these stages. Hoarding disorder is an exception (see Chapter 20). It has gradually moved from Stage 1, when it started life as "senior squalor" (McMillan & Shaw, 1966), been saddled with other rather inappropriate labels such as the Diogenes syndrome, and is now currently accepted as the formal diagnosis of hoarding disorder in both DSM-5 and the forthcoming ICD-11 (Stein et al., 2016). But as we follow JBS's tetrad, we cannot claim this is new, so what is the fuss about?

I am not going to be outdone by the illustrious international polymath authors of this book, but I myself have long wanted to put into the public domain a condition called the "Limpet Syndrome." I have encountered this in several patients, seen at the hospital where Duncan MacMillan used to work, all of whom were male and had past histories of homelessness. When placed in any safe environment, be it a hospital, a hostel, or supported accommodation, they are inclined to stick. When I say stick, I mean stick—as firm as a limpet. When told that their time is up and they should be ready to move on to more appropriate accommodation, they procrastinate and delay, insist they are perfectly all right where they are, and resist all attempts to move them. Eventually they have to be literally manhandled away, but all the time are passive, never really putting up a fight. I suspect this should be placed among the obsessional disorders, but despite this I could find few other obsessional features in these people (I can sense the neuroscientists hovering).

So I invite you to read about all those conditions that you suspected existed but were too embarrassed to mention to your colleagues. After you have improved your self-confidence—and added to your lexicon of psychiatric terminology—you can at least comfort yourself with the idea that even if the knowledge you have gained is possibly "true, but quite unimportant," it will be a comfort to the sufferers of these conditions. They will be able to say when talking to their friends, "Nobody knew what it was until I met Dr X., and when I told him no one had believed me before, he just smiled and said quietly, 'I always said so.' So modest, and what a magnificent therapist."

REFERENCES

Frances, A. (2013). *Saving normal: an Insider's revolt against Out-of-Control Psychiatric Diagnosis, DSM-5, Big Pharma and the Medicalization of Ordinary Life.* New York, NY: William Morrow.

MacMillan, D., & Shaw, P. (1966). Senile breakdown in standards of personal care and environmental cleanliness. *British Medical Journal, 2,* 1030–1037.

Stein, D. J., Kogan, K. S., Atmaca, M., Fineberg, N. A., Fontenelle, L. F., Grant, J. E . . . . Reed, G. M. (2016). The classification of obsessive-compulsive and related disorders in the ICD-11. *Journal of Affective Disorders, 190,* 663–674.

Peter Tyrer
Professor of Community Psychiatry
Imperial College, London
March, 2016

ACKNOWLEDGMENTS

A number of people contributed to making this volume a reality. I would first like to express my gratitude to the amazing team of Sarah Harrington and Andrea Zekus at Oxford University Press. Next, I would like to thank all the chapter authors for taking the time to pour their esoteric knowledge onto these pages. All my friends and students at the American School of Professional Psychology, the University of Pennsylvania, Pennsylvania State University, and Washington State University (you know who you are) also deserve recognition. Last, but not least, Gary Sharpless, Linda Sharpless, Stefanie Allister, Rodney Ascher, Jason Baker, Jacques Barber, Thomas Borkovec, Jared Bruce, Dianne Chambless, Richard Christy, Mariana Dobre, Ellen Dougherty, Karl Doghramji, Chris French, the Kelleys James Martin, Kevin McCarthy, Barbara Milrod, F.Z. Moop, Niels Nielsen, Calvin Oathes, Matt Rothrock, Ayelet Ruscio, Deborah Seagull, Stacy Simon, Skeptics in the Pub UK, Howard Allan Stern, Sandra Testa, David Trost, Elizabeth Tusk, the Wachters, and Alissa Yamasaki all provided help, fun, and support over the years that will always be remembered.

ABOUT THE EDITOR

Brian A. Sharpless, PhD, is an associate professor of clinical psychology at The American School of Professional Psychology at Argosy University, Washington, DC. He has authored over 35 publications on various topics related to psychopathology, psychotherapy, and the history and philosophy of clinical psychology. His previous book, *Sleep Paralysis: Historical, Psychological, and Medical Perspectives*, co-authored with Karl Doghramji, MD, is also available through Oxford University Press.

CONTRIBUTORS

Shalini Andrews
Surrey Sexual Health Services
  and University of Surrey
Guilford, United Kingdom

Amy L. Balko
Institute for Graduate Clinical
  Psychology
Widener University
Chester, Pennsylvania

Jan Dirk Blom
Faculty of Social Sciences
University of Leiden
Leiden, the Netherlands

Brenda Bursch
David Geffen School of Medicine
  at UCLA
Los Angeles, California

Elena del Busto
Department of Psychiatry
University of Pennsylvania
Philadelphia, Pennsylvania

Jourdan S. Cruz
School of Social Policy
  and Practice
University of Pennsylvania
Philadelphia, Pennsylvania

Hans Debruyne
Dr. Guislain Psychiatric Hospital
Ghent, Belgium

Dan Denis
Department of Psychology
University of Sheffield
Sheffield, United Kingdom

Peter O. Ebigbo
Department of Psychological
  Medicine
University of Nigeria, Enugu Campus
Enugu, Nigeria

Chimezie Lekwas Elekwachi
International Federation for
  Psychotherapy Center
Enugu, Nigeria

Petra Garlipp
Department of Psychiatry, Social
  Psychiatry, and Psychotherapy
Hannover Medical School
Hannover, Germany

David Goldmeier
Imperial College and Imperial
  College NHS Healthcare
London, United Kingdom

Jessica Lynn Grom
Department of Psychology
Villanova University
Villanova, Pennsylvania

Robert Haskell
Private Practice
Los Angeles, California

Stephen Hucker
Department of Psychiatry
University of Toronto
Toronto, Canada

Moshe Kalian
Ministry of Health (retired)
Jerusalem, Israel

Sandra Kooji
Parnassia Psychiatric Institute
Institute of Mental Health
The Hague, the Netherlands

Roberto Lewis-Fernández
Department of Psychiatry
Columbia University
New York State Center of Excellence
  for Cultural Competence
New York State Psychiatric Institute
New York, New York

Irene López
Department of Psychology
Kenyon College
Gambier, Ohio

Rocio Martín-Santos
Department of Psychiatry and Clinical
  Psychobiology
Hospital Clinic, University of
  Barcelona, Faculty of Medicine
Centro de Investigación Bimédica en
  Red en Salud Mental
Barcelona, Spain

Richard McAnulty
Department of Psychology
University of North
  Carolina—Charlotte
Charlotte, North Carolina

Ricard Navinés
Department of Psychiatry and Clinical
  Psychobiology
Hospital Clinic, University of
  Barcelona, Faculty of Medicine
Centro de Investigación Bimédica en
  Red en Salud Mental
Barcelona, Spain

Marieke Niemantsverdriet
Department of Personality Disorders
Parnassia Psychiatric Institute
Institute of Mental Health
The Hague, the Netherlands

Felix Chukwunenyem Nweze
International Federation for
  Psychotherapy Center
Enugu, Nigeria

Brian O'Shea
Health Services Executive/Mental
  Health Commission
Newcastle Hospital
Newtownmountkennedy, Ireland

Phillip J. Resnick
Department of Psychiatry
Case Western Reserve University
  School of Medicine
Cleveland, Ohio

Anna Sedda
Department of Psychology
Heriot–Watt University,
  Edinburgh Campus
Edinburgh, Scotland

Brian A. Sharpless
Clinical Psychology Program
The American School of Professional
  Psychology at Argosy University,
  Washington DC
Arlington, Virginia

Arthur Sinkman
Department of Psychiatry
New York University School
  of Medicine
New York, New York

Anke Spuijbroek
Department of Psychiatry
Parnassia Psychiatric Institute
Institute of Mental Health
The Hague, the Netherlands

Frederick R. Stoddard II
Psychiatric Associates of Pennsylvania
Wynnewood, Pennsylvania

Manuel Valdés
Department of Psychiatry and Clinical
  Psychobiology
Hospital Clinic, University of
  Barcelona, Faculty of Medicine
Barcelona, Spain

Sara G. West
Department of Psychiatry
Case Western Reserve University
Northfield, Ohio

Eliezer Witztum
Beer-Sheva Mental Health
  Center
Division of Psychiatry
Ben-Gurion University
Beer Sheba, Israel

Jacob A. Zimmerman
Department of Psychology
Washington State University
Pullman, Washington

Unusual and Rare Psychological Disorders

Introduction

BRIAN A. SHARPLESS ■

Psychopathology is limited in that there can be no final analysis of human beings as such, since the more we reduce them to what is typical and norma-tive the more we realize there is something hidden in every human individ-ual which defies recognition. We have to be content with partial knowledge of an infinity which we cannot exhaust.

—KARL JASPERS, *1963*

There is something intrinsically fascinating about the unusual, odd, and some-times extreme variations found in human behavior. This fascination, in one way or another, is a main reason many of us entered the mental health fields. Regardless of whether we are primarily researchers or clinicians, we are all linked by a fundamental curiosity about human beings *qua* human beings and the many puzzling things they say and do.

This curiosity has a long history. Since at least the time of the ancient Greeks and Romans (e.g., Hippocrates, Celsus), and possibly far earlier, significant efforts have been made to catalogue, systematize, and understand both mental health complaints and maladaptive variants in human functioning. This drive for nosology is likely a small part of a more fundamental human conceptual activ-ity; namely, the capacity to formulate abstract concepts/categories for the pur-pose of understanding our environment, other people, and ourselves. Some, like Immanuel Kant (1996) would argue that acts of classification are an inevitable consequence of our innate capacities for organization. It is perhaps not surprising that psychological misery in all its myriad forms would become one focus of this human skill.

Efforts to classify and understand psychopathology intensified during the Enlightenment (e.g., Ernst von Feuchtersleben, William Cullen), and this trend continued to Modernity and beyond (e.g., Emil Kraepelin, the various editions of the *Diagnostic and Statistical Manual of Mental Disorders* [DSM] and *International Classification of Diseases* [ICD]). Some would say that the proliferation of categories over time has been a good thing, and is indicative of scientific progress. Others believe that the ethos of "splitting" psychopathology into various categories has gone too far. Instead, it might be better if these putatively discrete disorders were "lumped" together into more encompassing general categories (e.g., Andrews, 1996). Regardless, due to any number of philosophical, practical, political, or economic reasons, certain symptom sets were prioritized over others, and this fact is reflected in the two dominant diagnostic compendiums.

Such a prioritization is inevitable, of course, but may give the erroneous impression that the true range of psychopathology is exhausted by the table of contents in these respective manuals. This is obviously incorrect, and not an intention of the manuals' authors. If existing categories were naively accepted, however, and given a veracity that outstrips their actual empirical basis (viz., they became reified) instead of being viewed as potentially useful and all-too-human artifacts that ineluctably reflect the values of their creators, these classification systems may inadvertently blind well-meaning individuals to manifestations of psychopathology that fall *outside* of this limited range. For as with any paradigm, classifications provide a means of both seeing the world in a particular way and making orderly sense of it, but just as surely cast other "non-relevant" or "non-paradigmatic" phenomena to the periphery (Kuhn, 1996).

This would be a shame not only for patients, but also for basic science. Regarding the former, there are practical consequences for individuals who do not have conventionally accepted symptoms. First, these symptoms may never be identified by professionals if they are neither a routine part of clinical assessment nor well-known to assessors. Second, patients may have a difficult time explaining their symptoms to a professional and, at least in some cases (e.g., sleep paralysis, body identity integrity disorder), may feel too embarrassed to disclose them in the absence of direct prompts. At an even more practical level, insurance companies typically only cover approved diagnoses, and most of these have specific ICD/DSM codes. It is important, however, to note that those manifestations of psychopathology that fall outside of these volumes may still be categorized. For instance, patients could be given an *Other Specified* X diagnosis or *Unspecified* X diagnosis. This is obviously not the preferred state of affairs, given that two of the main purposes of diagnostic labelling are to make communication meaningful and more efficient (e.g., Blashfield, 1984) and to allow for patient comparisons (e.g., Ustun et al., 2002).

In the realm of basic science, the study of lesser-known symptoms and syndromes could lead to advances in our understanding of general psychopathological processes. Although having 21 chapters devoted to some of these lesser-known syndromes may seem like more (and potentially unnecessary) "splitting," I would argue that our knowledge of psychopathology might actually best progress through a dialectical process of *alternating* between lumping and splitting. Thus, the process of learning more about fairly discrete symptom sets and lesser-known disorders could lead to more encompassing and valid categories of psychopathology as opposed to an illusion of ontological discreteness and rampant levels of (artificial) comorbidity.

Along with the concerns mentioned above, this book is also intended to fill several gaps. First, because advanced courses in psychopathology usually follow one of the two main classification systems (i.e., DSM or ICD), most graduate and medical students are only exposed to a relatively small sampling of the disorders contained within. Consequently, few have had extensive training on other symptoms, syndromes, and classification systems. Second, with increased pressures to specialize, many researchers and practitioners may not know how to accurately diagnose (or even identify) many lesser-known conditions or be aware of available treatment options. As will be demonstrated, there are clinical resources available for many of these disorders, but these tools are often scattered widely across complex and heterogeneous literatures. Finally, and related to the initial part of this preface, we hope many readers will be intrigued by the prospect of learning about phenomena that they may never have directly encountered or about which they have never even heard.

AUTHORS

Chapter authors were selected because of their expertise in one or more of these esoteric topics of psychopathology. They are a truly international group of scientists and scholars who come from various theoretical orientations and intellectual backgrounds. Many have made substantial, and even formative, contributions to our current understandings of these clinical phenomena.

BOOK STRUCTURE

This book consists of chapters focused on a number of lesser-known disorders. For inclusion, each had to have some empirical literature base, clinical importance, and/or intrinsic level of interest. There is no presumption that any of the disorders discussed is truly a "discrete" diagnostic entity or is best conceptualized as a symptom, sign, syndrome, idiom of distress, or disease. After reviewing the theoretical and empirical literatures, some authors provided recommendations, and all were asked to discuss the role, if any, that their topic has (or should have) in the current diagnostic landscape. Authors were also encouraged to not just focus on the research basis for these phenomena, but to compile and suggest assessment and treatment options that would be useful for clinicians.

In order to make this edited volume more readable and consistent across different disorders and writing styles, authors were asked to adhere to the following 10-part chapter structure:

1. **Vignette** (i.e., a clinical vignette or firsthand narrative of a de-identified individual suffering from the disorder)
2. **Historical/Cultural Context** (e.g., a discussion of cultural implications of the disorder (if any); when, where, and how it was identified; and other important historical information)
3. **Role in Current Diagnostic Systems** (e.g., the symptom/disorder's role, if any, in ICD, DSM, and/or an indigenous diagnostic system)
4. **Symptomatology** (i.e., a description or list of diagnostic criteria/core features)
5. **Prevalence Rate and Associated Features** (e.g., comorbidity patterns, risk factors, medical implications, clinical impacts, age of onset, clinical course)
6. **Theories of Etiology** (i.e., discussion of the available etiological theories and relevant supporting data, if available)
7. **Assessment Options** (e.g., assessment procedures/measures and their evidence base/psychometric properties)
8. **Differential Diagnosis** (i.e., practical guidance for accurate differential diagnosis and/or a description of other conditions that may make accurate diagnosis difficult).
9. **Treatment Options** (i.e., available treatments [medical, psychological, indigenous, "folk," or otherwise] and their evidence base)
10. **Recommendations for Future Work** (i.e., what else might we need to know about the condition and/or promising directions for future research)

REFERENCES

Andrews, G. (1996). Comorbidity and the general neurotic syndrome. *British Journal of Psychiatry, 168(suppl. 30)*, 76–84.

Blashfield, (1984). *The classification of psychopathology.* New York: Plenum Press.

Jaspers, K. (1963). *General psychopathology* (J. Hoenig & M.W. Hamilton, Trans.). Chicago, IL: University of Chicago Press (Original work published 1923).

Kant, I. (1996). *Critique of pure reason* (W. S. Pluhar, Trans.). Indianapolis, IN: Hackett (Original work published 1781).

Kuhn, T.S (1996). *The structure of scientific revolutions* (3rd ed.). Chicago, IL: University of Chicago Press.

Ustun, T. B., Chatterjee, S., & Andrews, G. (2002). International classifications and the diagnosis of mental disorders: Strengths, limitations, and future directions. In M. Maj, W. Gaebel, J. Lopez-Ibor, and N. Sartorious's (Eds.), *Psychiatric diagnosis and classification* (pp. 25–46). New York: Wiley & Sons.

Sleep Disorders

Isolated Sleep Paralysis

BRIAN A. SHARPLESS AND DAN DENIS ∎

VIGNETTE

"At first you don't really know what's going on when you're paralyzed . . . you're kind of like "this is weird" and you're trying to figure it out, and so then it suddenly starts feeling really horrible. I feel like the fear increases as you're lying there on your back immobilized, and unable to speak. I can sense something there with me. I can't see it, but I know that there's something negative, like a force or entity, hovering over me, crushing my chest and suffocating me. It wants to take over my body. I also hear a mumbling sound from it. I don't know what that is and can't understand what it's saying, which is terrifying. That's when I try to wake myself completely up. I'm Catholic, and have found prayer can help it stop sometimes. I've tried to talk to people about it and everyone's kind of skeptical of the experience. When it happens, it's the worst feeling ever. It feels like you are about to die."

The narrative above is the description of an isolated sleep paralysis episode given by a 20-year-old Hispanic female interviewed by the first author. She was of average intelligence (IQ = 105), had intact reality-testing, and reported her overall health to be excellent. She denied taking any medications or illegal drugs. As for psychiatric symptoms, she reported a history of mild insomnia, night terrors, and relatively high levels of anxiety sensitivity. Interestingly, she also endorsed a number of anomalous beliefs. These included believing in the reality of witches, demons, and aliens, with a belief that the latter two entities can directly interact with humans. As will be shown below, many aspects of her narrative are fairly typical of the phenomenon of isolated sleep paralysis.

HISTORICAL AND CULTURAL CONTEXT

Sleep paralysis has a remarkably rich social and cultural history. It appears to be a universal phenomenon not bound to any particular place or time (Sharpless &

Doghramji, 2015). Accounts of sleep paralysis can be found in folklore (Hufford, 1982), works of art (e.g., Fuesli's 1781 painting, "The Nightmare," French & Santomauro, 2007), and early medical writings (e.g., Aegineta, 1844; Bond, 1753).

The characteristic experiences of sleep paralysis were often ascribed to supernatural causes. This is perhaps not surprising given the bizarre and terrifying nature of the episodes. In medieval Europe, for example, episodes were commonly believed to be actual nocturnal attacks by libidinal *incubi* (male demons) and *succubi* (female demons). During their attacks these entities would lie upon the victim's chest, crushing and immobilizing them (note: *incubus* derives from *incubare* or "to lie down upon"). The demon would then physically and/or sexually assault the victim.

Historical records imply that episodes of sleep paralysis may have been used as evidence in witch trials, with a widespread belief that sleep paralysis-like symptoms were the result of malevolent magic (Davies, 2003; Hufford, 1982). This can be seen not only in medieval witch hunting "manuals," such as the *Malleus Maleficarum* (i.e., "*Hammer of Witches*," Kramer & Sprenger, 1971), but also in the testimony of several individuals during the Salem Village witch trials of 1692 (Mather, 1862). For example, Robert Downer provided testimony against Susanna Martin and described how, "as he lay in his bed, there came in at the window, the likeness of a cat, which flew upon him, took fast hold of his throat, lay on him a considerable while, and almost killed him" (Mather, 1892, p. 142). Bernard Peache described a similar episode while testifying against Martin: "She took hold of this deponent's feet, and drawing his body into an heap, she lay upon him near two hours; in all which time he could neither speak nor stir" (Mather, 1892, p. 141).

What should be derived from these accounts are the clear similarities between the court testimony and typical symptoms of sleep paralysis. The conscious awareness, atonia, fear, presence of strange beings in the room, and feelings of oppression are all found in these descriptions. For additional discussion on sleep paralysis and witchcraft, readers are directed to Davies, 2003.

Supernatural attributions of sleep paralysis can also be found in contemporary folklore. For example, sleep paralysis may provide a naturalistic explanation for claims of nocturnal alien abductions. Belief in aliens is fairly widespread, with 67% of Americans believing in intelligent extraterrestrial life (RoperASW, 2002) and 52% of surveyed UK residents believing that UFO evidence has been covered up by government agencies (as cited in Kumar, 2012). Belief in actual alien abductions, however, is somewhat difficult to assess with available data.

In a nationwide survey carried out through the Roper organization by ufologists Hopkins, Jacobs, and Westrum (1992), 5,497 American adults were given a list of supposed "signs" of alien abduction. If respondents answered "yes" to four of these five signs, it was deemed "likely" that the individual had been abducted by aliens. A total of 119 (2% of the sample) individuals answered yes to four or five of the signs, leading the authors to extrapolate and claim that 3.7 million Americans had been abducted by aliens. Interestingly, most of these indicator signs are also paradigmatic sleep paralysis experiences (e.g., "Waking up paralyzed with a sense of a strange person or presence or something else in the room"; "Seeing unusual lights or balls of light in a room without knowing what was causing them, or where they came from").

A second survey, again carried out by the Roper organization for the Syfy television channel, found that 20% of the 1,021 people surveyed had experienced, "Waking up paralyzed with a sense of a strange person or presence or something else in the room," and 10% had experienced, "Seeing unusual lights or balls of light in a room without knowing what was causing them, or where they came from" (RoperASW, 2002). As will be shown below, these prevalence rates are not dissimilar to estimates of sleep paralysis.

Only a few of the supernatural understandings of sleep paralysis have been documented here. Sharpless and Doghramji (2015) collected 118 different indigenous terms for the phenomenon from multiple languages and cultures. What is remarkable about these accounts is their consistency on core features: waking and being unable to move, a presence being sensed or seen in the room, and pressure on the chest. What seems to differ most is the nature of the "presence" and the potential remedies that could be utilized.

In many cultures, these experiences have been worked into folklore. Whether a sleep paralysis hallucination was the original cause of a legend (e.g., vampires in Europe, ghosts in Asia), or whether preexisting beliefs shaped the particular manifestations of sleep paralysis hallucinations, is a difficult question to answer. Either way, sleep paralysis experiences have been an important component of the unique beliefs of many cultures.

One of the earliest descriptions of sleep paralysis in medicine was made by Dutch physician Isbrand van Diemerbroeck (1609–1674). In a case report, van Diemerbroeck (1694) described the case of a woman who, "when she was composing herself to sleep, sometimes she believed the devil lay upon her and held her down, sometimes that she was choked by a great dog or thief lying upon her breast, so that she could hardly speak or breath, and when she endeavoured to throw off the burthen, she was not able to stir her members" (p. 183).

[V]an Diemerbroeck diagnosed this condition as "Incubus" or the "Night-Mare," though it is clear from the description that we would now term it sleep paralysis. In contrast to the supernatural explanations listed above, doctors such as van Diemerbroeck (1694) believed the causes to be natural: "This affection . . . is an Intercepting of the Motion of the Voice and Respiration . . ." caused by "over-redundancy of blood in the whole body (p. 184)." He also suggested a natural course of treatment: "Keep her in a pure and moderate hot Air. Let her Diet be sparing, but of good Juice and easy Digestion" (p. 185). Thus, alongside of supernatural interpretations lay some attempts at medical understanding. Some doctors even recommended the use of physical treatments to alleviate the symptoms (e.g., venesection; altering the body's pH, as summarized in Sharpless & Doghramji, 2015).

ROLE IN CURRENT DIAGNOSTIC SYSTEMS

Diagnostic criteria for the Nightmare/isolated sleep paralysis have been formalized in some manner since Ernest Jones's writings (Jones, 1949) and have been informally discussed since ancient Rome (Aegineta, 1844; Sharpless, 2014a). Entry into medical nosology, however, only began in 2001 with the publication of the revised edition of the *International Classification of Sleep Disorders* (ICSD, American Academy of Sleep Medicine, 2001). Since that time, each subsequent edition of the ICSD has retained *recurrent isolated sleep paralysis* as a diagnostic category and continued to modify criteria over time. For instance, the ICSD-3 (American Academy of Sleep Medicine, 2014) added clinically significant distress as a requirement. Alternative diagnostic criteria have also been proposed that require more specific thresholds on frequency, presence of clinically significant fear/distress, and/or clinically significant impairment (e.g., recurrent fearful isolated sleep paralysis, as in Sharpless, McCarthy, Chambless, Milrod, Khalsa, & Barber, 2010).

At present, recognition of isolated sleep paralysis in the two major diagnostic systems is fairly limited. The 10th edition of the *International Classification of Diseases and Related Health Problems* (ICD-10, World Health Organization, 2008) allows for coding recurrent isolated sleep paralysis (i.e., G47.53) as a *Parasomnia Usually Associated with REM Sleep*. The current edition of the *Diagnostic and Statistical Manual of Mental Disorders* (DSM-5, American Psychiatric Association, 2013), however, does not have a corresponding category. The only way to capture isolated sleep paralysis in this system would be to code it as either an *Other Specified Sleep-Wake Disorder* (code 307.49) or an *Unspecified Sleep-Wake Disorder* (code 307.40). It should also be noted that DSM-5 removed sleep paralysis from the diagnostic criteria for narcolepsy.

SYMPTOMATOLOGY

It is customary to differentiate cases of sleep paralysis that are due to medical reasons (e.g., narcolepsy, substance use) from those that are not (i.e., *isolated* sleep paralysis). Isolated sleep paralysis episodes are characterized by atonia in the trunk and limbs of the body during sleep transitions. These episodes are usually of a short duration (i.e., seconds to minutes). In order to meet *International Classification of Sleep Disorders* (American Academy of Sleep Medicine, 2014, p. 254) criteria for the diagnostic entity of recurrent isolated sleep paralysis, multiple episodes of isolated sleep paralysis must occur in the context of clinically significant distress (e.g., fear of sleep, bedroom anxiety) and not be better explained by another condition or the effects of a substance. As is apparent, this definition is fairly broad and does not require any of the more specific symptoms common to the experience (e.g., hallucinations) to establish a diagnosis. It is important, however, to understand the core symptoms that occur during conscious awakening as well as the typical hallucinations.

Muscle Atonia

The atonia found in sleep paralysis is one of the best understood symptoms of the condition. Paralysis is characteristic of Rapid Eye Movement (REM) sleep. REM sleep is distinct from other stages in a number of important ways. First, brain activity during this period is similar to, if not greater than, when we are awake. Second, this stage of sleep is most closely associated with vivid dreaming. Finally, individuals are completely paralyzed during REM sleep (except for the respiratory system and eyes). This is presumably so we do not act out our dreams.

In sleep paralysis we become consciously aware of this state of muscle atonia, but it could be considered a dissociated state of sleep, as it represents a simultaneous mixture of wakefulness with aspects of REM sleep (Mahowald & Schenck, 2005). There is experimental evidence for this hypothesis, and Terzaghi, Ratti, Manni, and Manni (2012) described the case of a narcoleptic patient who suffered from severe sleep paralysis episodes. They found that brain activity during sleep paralysis closely resembled a combination of waking and REM sleep brain activity.

Hallucinations During Sleep Paralysis

Hallucinatory experiences are estimated to occur in at least 75% of individuals who experience sleep paralysis, and are even higher in clinical samples (Cheyne, Newby-Clark, & Rueffer, 1999; Sharpless et al., 2010). Cheyne et al. (1999) derived a tripartite factor structure of sleep paralysis hallucinations. These three factors have been named Intruder, Incubus, and Vestibular–Motor. Their characteristic symptoms and prevalence rates are found in Table 2.1.

INTRUDER HALLUCINATIONS
The sensed presence is a core component of the Intruder factor. It is the feeling of an "otherness" in the room that is not seen, but felt, and is typically believed to have malevolent intentions. This combination of an evil presence and no means to escape not surprisingly leads to feelings of extreme fear. Cheyne and Girard (2007) found that the sensed presence occurred in the early stages of sleep paralysis episodes. This is subsequently followed by intense fear, with multisensory hallucinations appearing later. These are hypothesized to be attempts to interpret the sensed presence. The forms these hallucinations take are often human (or humanoid), but animal forms and supernatural intruders often are reported.

Cultural and personal beliefs play an important role in driving what is "seen" during sleep paralysis. Widespread beliefs in the supernatural phenomena discussed earlier may have played a part in the frequency with which those same phenomena appeared in sleep paralysis episodes. Circumstances during waking life have also been shown to be important. In one study of Cambodian refugees with sleep paralysis, many reported hallucinations of soldiers wearing Khmer Rouge uniforms (Hinton, Pich, Chhean, & Pollack, 2005).

Auditory hallucinations also fall within the Intruder factor, and are experienced as coming from the external environment. Frequently heard sounds include speech (both clear and unintelligible), footsteps, scratching and scraping, doors slamming, and other general environmental noises. These auditory hallucinations, especially speech, are frequently accompanied by visual hallucinations of an intruder.

Table 2.1. ISOLATED SLEEP PARALYSIS HALLUCINATIONS AND PREVALENCE RATES
ACCORDING TO CHEYNE'S THREE-FACTOR STRUCTURE

	Prevalence in Nonclinical Samples[1]	Prevalence in Clinical Samples[2]
INTRUDER FACTOR		
Sensed presence	57%	50%
Visual hallucinations	47%	35%
Auditory hallucinations	58%	39%
Tactile feelings of being touched	–	23%
INCUBUS FACTOR		
Pressure on body/ chest/ smothering sensations	63%	58%
Choking	34%	–
Pain	51%	19%
Fear	78%	69%[3]
Thoughts of death/fear of death	49%	58%
VESTIBULAR-MOTOR FACTOR		
Unusual body movements/feeling that body has moved	–	39%
Out-of-body experiences/ autoscopy	–	31%
Bliss	–	–
Floating, flying, falling	37%	35%
Spinning		–

NOTE: [1] = content derived from either Cheyne, Newby-Clark, & Rueffer, or Cheyne, 2001 (overlapping samples); [2] = content derived from Sharpless et al., 2010.; [3] = this refers to the percentage of all of those with isolated sleep paralysis who endorsed *clinically significant* levels of fear.

INCUBUS HALLUCINATIONS

Like their namesake, incubus hallucinations consist mainly of a sense of pressure on the chest. This tactile hallucination of a heavy weight on the chest is then associated with physical pain and breathing difficulties. Again, incubus hallucinations are associated with fear. Women tend to experience more intense incubus experiences than men as judged by their subjective levels of fear (Cheyne & Girard, 2004).

It is likely that during an incubus hallucination the feeling of pressure on the chest is felt first. This crushing sensation then may lead to physical pain perceptions and breathing difficulties, possibly due to catastrophic misinterpretations of these sensations (Sharpless, McCarthy, Chambless, Milrod, Khalsa, & Barber, 2010). This likely leads to increased autonomic arousal and may make it more likely that subsequent hallucinations will be negatively valenced.

The intruder and incubus clusters of hallucinations are correlated with each other. This is an important finding, because together they paint a fairly vivid picture of sleep paralysis as experienced around the world. Thus, when these waking dreams are experienced with some degree of conscious awareness, it is easy to see how they could be misconstrued as actual nocturnal assaults.

VESTIBULAR–MOTOR HALLUCINATIONS

This third category of hallucination is not as strongly associated with fear, and some individuals experience these episodes as pleasurable. Symptoms associated with the V–M hallucination factor include sensations of floating and flying, out-of-body experiences, and bliss.

To conclude this section, the factor structure put forward by Cheyne et al. (1999) was found to correspond well with narrative reports of sleep paralysis experiences. Furthermore, this particular structure appeared consistently in two large samples. Whether the same consistency would emerge in a clinical sample, or when another measurement tool was used, remains to be seen.

PREVALENCE RATE AND ASSOCIATED FEATURES

It is difficult to secure accurate prevalence rates for isolated sleep paralysis. This is largely due to the lack of a standardized procedure for assessing the phenomenon, with the presentation of vignettes, self-report questionnaires, and clinical interviews all in use. To complicate matters further, it has been shown that the terminology used to describe the experience can alter reported prevalence (Fukuda, 1993). Finally, sleep paralysis is a known symptom of narcolepsy, which affects 0.02% of the population (Mahlios, Herran-Arita & Mignot, 2011). It is, therefore, important to rule out narcolepsy when researching isolated sleep paralysis. Such checks, however, were not always conducted.

Sharpless and Barber (2011) conducted a systematic literature review of lifetime rates of sleep paralysis. (It was impossible to determine isolated sleep paralysis rates due to the limitations noted previously.) They identified 35 suitable studies (N = 36,533 individuals). Lifetime episodes of sleep paralysis were found in 7.6% of the general population, with higher prevalence rates in psychiatric patients (31.9%) and students (28.3%). Possible reasons for this higher prevalence in these groups are discussed in the next section. Prevalence rates in non-Caucasians were slightly higher than Caucasians, though these differences were relatively small. The authors also found a slightly higher prevalence rate in females (18.8%) than males (15.7%), but this gender difference was inconsistent across individual studies.

Data on recurrent isolated sleep paralysis is likely unreliable, but suggests at least 2% of people may experience multiple isolated sleep paralysis episodes per week (Ohaeri, Awadalla, Maknjuola, & Ohaeri, 2004; O'Hanlon, Murphy, & Di Blasi, 2011; Ohayon, Zulley, Guilleminault, & Smirne, 1999).

Risk Factors Associated with Isolated Sleep Paralysis

A summary of high-risk groups and potential risk factors associated with iso-lated sleep paralysis can be found in Table 2.2. Sharpless and Barber's (2011) review found an increased prevalence rate of isolated sleep paralysis in psychiat-ric patients, and there is strong evidence that isolated sleep paralysis is associated with a number of psychiatric conditions, anxiety sensitivity (or the predisposi-tion to fear anxiety-related symptoms and sensations), and psychiatric comorbid-ity in general. Interestingly, to our knowledge there is no evidence for a higher prevalence rate of isolated sleep paralysis in psychotic disorders, and its relation to major depressive disorder is somewhat ambiguous.

Risk factors for nonclinical groups can also be found in Table 2.2. Nonclinical anxiety is a risk factor, with dysfunctional social imagery linked to the amount of distress caused by isolated sleep paralysis episodes (Solomonova et al., 2008). This was most notable for Intruder hallucinations, as examples of dysfunctional social imagery include incorrect feelings of being observed and extreme anxiety in nonthreatening situations. A similar finding was reported in individuals with high levels of social anxiety (Simard & Nielsen, 2005).

Denis et al. (2015) found, in a nonclinical sample, that self-reported levels of exposure to threatening events (such as death of a spouse), levels of anxiety, and subjective sleep quality were all independently associated with the presence of sleep paralysis. Experimental work has also shown that systematic disrup-tions to the sleep cycle can induce episodes of isolated sleep paralysis (Takeuchi, 1992; 2002). Poor sleep quality and disruption to the sleep cycle may be a rea-son why students and shift workers are more likely to experience isolated sleep paralysis, given that these are both groups where regular sleep patterns are often tenuous at best.

Recent evidence has shown genetics to constitute a risk factor for sleep paraly-sis. Using a twin study, Denis et al. (2015) found a moderate genetic influence on sleep paralysis, with 53% of variance of sleep paralysis scores explained by a genetic component. This supported earlier studies that showed sleep paralysis to be familial, but which could not identify whether this was due to genetic or envi-ronmental influences (Bell et al., 1986; Dahlitz & Parkes, 1993).

We have a reasonable understanding of a number of risk factors associated with sleep paralysis. However, with commonly experienced risks such as anxi-ety, subjective sleep quality, and stress it is important to note that it can often be difficult to disentangle cause and effect. In other words, does stress cause

Table 2.2. POTENTIAL RISK FACTORS FOR SLEEP PARALYSIS

Risk Factor	Key Reference(s)
DIAGNOSTIC RISK FACTORS	
Psychiatric patient status	(Sharpless & Barber, 2011)
Presence of psychiatric comorbidity	(Sharpless et al., 2010)
Diagnosis of panic disorder	(Otto et al., 2006; Sharpless et al., 2010; Friedman & Paradis, 2002; Yeung et al., 2005)
Diagnosis of post-traumatic stress disorder	(Gupta, 2012; Hinton et al., 2005; Ohayon & Shapiro, 2000; Sharpless et al., 2010; Yeung et al., 2005)
Diagnosis of generalized anxiety disorder	(Otto et al., 2006)
Diagnosis of social anxiety disorder	(Otto et al., 2006)
Diagnosis of exploding head syndrome	(Sharpless, 2015)
OTHER POTENTIAL RISK FACTORS	
Student status	(Sharpless & Barber, 2011)
Shift worker status	(Kotorii et al., 2001)
Presence of stress	(Mellman et al., 2008)
Exposure to threatening/traumatic events	(Mellman et al., 2008; Denis et al., 2015)
Anxiety symptoms	(Solomonova et al., 2008; Denis et al., 2015)
Anxiety sensitivity	(Ramsawh et al., 2008; Sharpless et al., 2010)
Social anxiety symptoms	(Simard & Nielsen, 2005)
Depressed mood	(Mellman et al., 2008)
Poor sleep quality/sleep disruption	(Takeuchi et al., 1992, 2002; Denis et al., 2015)
Genetic risk factors	(Denis et al., 2015)
Sleeping in a supine position	(Cheyne, 2002)
Bimodal timing distribution	(Cheyne, 2002)
Higher body mass index	(Sharpless et al., 2010)
Imaginativeness	(Spanos et al., 1995)
Belief in the paranormal/supernatural	(Ramhsawh et al., 2008)
Death anxiety/death distress	(Arikawa et al., 1999)

sleep paralysis, or does sleep paralysis, a highly stressful event in itself, elevate stress levels?

THEORIES OF ETIOLOGY

Sleep paralysis can be thought of as the juxtaposition of the muscle atonia and dream activity of REM sleep with waking consciousness. How this state arises is of primary concern when trying to understand the causes of sleep paralysis. We summarize some more specific theories below.

Typical Sleep Cycle

Sleep is highly complex, consisting of both REM and non-REM sleep. Non-REM sleep is further subdivided into three stages. These sleep stages were divided using a technique known as polysomnography, which consists of the recording of muscle tone through electromyography (EMG), eye movements through electro-oculography (EOG), and brain activity through electroencephalography (EEG) (American Academy of Sleep Medicine, 2014). A typical night's sleep consists of a progression from Stage 1 to Stage 3 non-REM sleep, before ascending back to Stage 1 again. After this ascension is completed, a period of REM sleep ensues. REM sleep is distinct in a number of important ways. First, cortical activity is very high during REM sleep, similar to waking consciousness. Second, it is the period of sleep most closely associated with vivid dreaming, and third, we experience complete paralysis during this stage of sleep (except for the eyes and respiratory system).

Sleep Neurobiology

On a neurobiological level, non-REM sleep can be characterized as the inhibition of the ascending arousal system. Inhibition of this system is crucial for the maintenance and consolidation of sleep (Fuller, Gooley, & Saper, 2006).

REM sleep is believed to be under the control of cholinergic neurons located in the pedunculopontine and laterodorsal tegmental (PPT/LDT) nuclei. Gamma-aminobutyric acid (GABA) and glycine are also important in the inhibition of motor neurons during REM sleep, and thus also contribute to the muscle atonia (Brooks & Peever, 2012). Working against this inhibition are monoamines such as NE and 5-HT, both of which increase muscle tone by directly exciting motor neurons. During wakefulness and non-REM sleep, REM-active cholinergic neurons are inhibited by 5-HT, NE, and HA. The interaction then between cholinergic and monoaminergic populations forms the basis of explaining the alternating between wakefulness, non-REM, and REM sleep states (Espana & Scammell, 2011).

Sleep Disruption

Disruption of REM sleep seems to be important (Takeuchi et al., 2002). Dysregulation of the sleep cycle may cause changes in the interactions between cholinergic and monoaminergic neurotransmitter systems. We speculate that the unique state of consciousness achieved during sleep paralysis could be due to partial suppression of the REM-inducing cholinergic system, which is enough to induce awareness, but not enough to cause a full awakening. This is, of course, merely speculative, and to our knowledge there is no empirical work supporting this view.

Genetics

Dysregulation of the sleep cycle may be due to genetic factors. Denis et al. (2015) presented preliminary evidence that a polymorphism in the *PER2* gene was linked with sleep paralysis. The *PER2* gene is one of several "clock" genes that govern circadian rhythms and act as regulators of the molecular clock. Polymorphisms in this set of genes are linked to a number of phenotypes such as sleep quality, sleep duration, and diurnal preferences (Parsons et al., 2014; Carpen et al., 2006; Lee et al., 2011). In gene knockout studies in mice of *PER* genes, the animals showed much shorter circadian periods. It is important to note that the rhythmic nature of the sleep cycle is lost when these genes are removed in animals (Bae et al., 2001). Relating this to sleep paralysis in humans, if different polymorphisms in circadian-expressed genes lead to some irregularity in the sleep cycle, then this could be expected to put such individuals at a higher risk of sleep paralysis, based on the experimental evidence linking sleep cycle disruptions to sleep paralysis. Again, however, this is purely theoretical with no direct evidence currently available to support it.

Biological Basis for Hallucinatory Symptoms

Cheyne et al. (1999; 2002) theorized that intruder hallucinations are caused by a Threat Activated Vigilance System (TAVS). The TAVS monitors environmental stimuli, and when a source of danger is identified the system searches an individual's surroundings for additional information and cues. In sleep paralysis, TAVS may activate as a result of the sensed presence. When no obvious danger is found, hallucinations may arise as a result of the brain trying to make sense of an ambiguous, unidentified threat. The amygdala is likely involved, due to its known role in fear processing and emotion regulation.

Incubus hallucinations may arise due to an awareness of REM respiration. During REM, the airways become constricted and breathing becomes shallow, which would likely lead to the feelings of suffocation and crushing commonly felt during sleep paralysis. Furthermore, breathing is reflexive during REM sleep, and regaining full conscious control over it during sleep paralysis would be difficult, if not impossible. This lack of control could further lead to feelings of suffocation (Cheyne et al., 1999).

Vestibular-motor hallucinations have been proposed to originate in the resolution of an impossible conflict between movement and nonmovement. When we are awake, medial and superior vestibular nuclei contribute to the coordination of head and eye movements. Vestibular nuclei located in the pontine brainstem are closely associated with pontine centers controlling the sleep-wake cycle. During sleep paralysis there is no movement, yet vestibular nuclei are activated. With no proprioceptive feedback, this vestibular activation gets interpreted as sensations of floating or flying. The out of body experience (OBE) occurs due to a mismatch between internal sensations of movement (vestibular activation that indicates movement) and external sensations of movement (the fact that there is no movement). Thus, in summary, there is a "splitting" of the phenomenal self and the physical body, leading to an OBE (Cheyne et al., 1999).

Psychological Causes

It is important to consider causal factors on the psychological level, especially as based on our current understanding of sleep paralysis phenomena. Such ideas will also likely be of more practical importance to clinicians.

As shown previously, high levels of stress and exposure to trauma likely play an important role in the genesis of sleep paralysis. This may be due to the general day/night hyperarousal and hypervigilance common to PTSD patients, with the ultra-high arousal making awakenings during REM more likely and the hypervigilance leading to a higher chance for intruder hallucinations. Individuals experiencing high levels of stress are then likely to be caught in a vicious circle. Assuming that stress and/or trauma initially triggered the sleep paralysis, suffering may keep increasing because the episodes themselves are typically highly stressful and traumatic. This is why identification of sleep paralysis episodes by clinicians during diagnostic intakes is important, as additional stress and anxiety may ensue after episodes of sleep paralysis that may, in effect, intensify other psychiatric conditions.

Finally, those who ascribe cultural/supernatural causes to their sleep paralysis have been shown to suffer post-episode distress (Cheyne & Pennycook, 2013). This is not surprising, given that it is likely much more stressful to think that one is being assaulted by a demon than thinking one is experiencing a relatively common sleep anomaly. This underscores the importance of educating the public on the nature of sleep paralysis.

ASSESSMENT OPTIONS

Unlike many disorders listed in this book, there is a plethora of instruments available to assess isolated sleep paralysis symptomatology. Sharpless and Doghramji

(2015) recently reviewed the literature and identified 38 measures. Most were in English, but nine other languages were represented. Regarding format, the majority ($N = 25$) were self-report, with the remainder being clinical interviews possessing varying levels of structure (i.e., completely structured questions to minimally structured ones). Whereas in many ways the diversity of measures is a positive attribute for the field (in that very specific research questions can be assessed), the current lack of a "gold standard" may make selecting measures and comparing data across studies difficult tasks.

Sharpless and Doghramji (2015) made recommendations for measure selection based upon symptom content, depth of coverage, and psychometric properties of the instruments. For very brief screenings, they recommended the *Munich Parasomnia Screening* (self-report, Fulda et al., 2008) and the isolated sleep paralysis module from the *Duke Structured Interview for Sleep Disorders* (Edinger et al., 2004). More in-depth assessments could be obtained through use of the *Waterloo Unusual Sleep Experiences Questionnaire* (self-report, Cheyne, Newby-Clark, & Rueffer, 1999), *Unusual Sleep Experiences Questionnaire* (self-report, Paradis et al., 2009), the *Isolated Sleep Paralysis Interview* (Ramsawh et al., 2008), or the *Fearful Isolated Sleep Paralysis Interview* (Sharpless et al., 2010; Sharpless & Doghramji, 2015).

DIFFERENTIAL DIAGNOSIS

In order to ensure accuracy of diagnosis, one must be able to clearly differentiate isolated sleep paralysis from other manifestations of psychopathology. Ideally, the assessment of sleep paralysis should be situated within a larger, more encompassing clinical interview such as the *Structured Clinical Interview for DSM-5 Disorders* (First, Williams, Karg, & Spitzer, 2015) or the *Anxiety and Related Disorders Interview Schedule* (Brown & Barlow, 2014). Even in these cases, however, many disorders relevant to differential diagnosis (e.g., nightmare disorder, hypokalemia) may not be sufficiently addressed. Thus, a thorough knowledge of ICD-10 (World Health Organization, 2008b), DSM-5 (American Psychiatric Association, 2013), and/or ICSD-3 (American Academy of Sleep Medicine, 2014) may be required. We provide several recommendations for differential diagnosis below.

Differential Diagnosis of Medical Conditions

In order to establish a diagnosis of *isolated* sleep paralysis, one must first eliminate medical conditions that also contain episodes of sleep paralysis as a core, associated, or probable feature. Depending upon one's clinical training, this may necessitate consultation with a specialist or the provision of a medical referral. Whenever a patient reports sleep paralysis episodes, it is important to eliminate narcolepsy as a possibility. Diagnosticians should, therefore, inquire into this disorder's core features (e.g., cataplexy, excessive daytime sleepiness). It is important to keep in mind that the paralysis of skeletal muscles in cataplexy is typically preceded by emotionally intense stimuli and also occurs in the context of wakefulness. In addition to narcolepsy, focal epileptic seizures, atonic seizures, transient compression neuropathies, and familial periodic paralysis (i.e., hypokalemic, hyperkalemic, Andersen-Tawil syndrome, and thyroxic) should also be eliminated. We will not go into additional detail for differential diagnosis of these medical conditions (the interested reader is referred to Sharpless & Doghramji, 2015 and Sharpless, 2016), but will instead focus more specifically on psychiatric conditions.

Differential Diagnosis of Psychiatric Conditions

Although the symptoms of isolated sleep paralysis can be quite dramatic, and in some ways almost unique, care must be taken in assessment or else mistakes can occur. Misdiagnoses (e.g., psychosis) may sometimes eventuate in severe clinical consequences (viz., prescribing pharmacological agents that may intensify their respective symptom sets). Diagnostic difficulties arise not only due to the breadth of symptoms possible during episodes (some of which overlap with better-known conditions), but can also result from idiosyncratic patient descriptions of episodes. The latter are often affected by distress, avoidance, and/or personal embarrassment, and can make the diagnostic picture murky. In general, we recommend focusing upon the following core isolated sleep paralysis features for differential diagnosis: (1) the degree of conscious awareness and alertness to surroundings, (2) the presence/nature of paralysis, (3) the duration of the paralysis, (4) and the presence/nature of REM activity/hallucinations.

Nightmare disorder, like sleep paralysis, also includes REM imagery, but can be distinguished from sleep paralysis on points 1, 2, and 4. Namely, individuals in sleep paralysis have conscious awareness (i.e., they are not completely asleep) and the ability to perceive their immediate surroundings. If hallucinations are present, those with sleep paralysis may have a more difficult time noting that they are indeed hallucinations, whereas there is a clearer cessation of REM activity when waking from a nightmare. Further, although dreams of paralysis obviously occur, actual atonia is always present in sleep paralysis. Finally, a minority of sleep paralysis sufferers have either no hallucinations or even pleasant ones, but this is not the case in nightmare disorder.

Apart from the fact that *sleep/night terrors* often include vocalizations that are not found in sleep paralysis, they also differ on points 1, 2, and 4. Often during sleep terrors, individuals are confused and only partially responsive when they awake. They also do not experience paralysis, and hallucinatory images, if present at all, are not usually remembered and fairly impoverished in their level of detail.

Nocturnal panic attacks must also be distinguished from sleep paralysis, and this can be done using points 1, 2, and 4. Unlike sleep paralysis, nocturnal panic attacks are unexpected paroxysms of intense fear, whereas the fear found in sleep paralysis is usually secondary to either the paralysis or REM hallucinations. Nocturnal panic attacks lack paralysis and dream imagery (as they appear to occur during non-REM sleep as in Mellman & Uhde, 1989), and care must be taken to ensure that cognitive appraisals of the panic (e.g., fear of death) are not misconstrued as hallucinations.

Post-traumatic stress disorder (PTSD), a common condition associated with isolated sleep paralysis (e.g., Sharpless et al., 2010), can also include subjective feelings of being paralyzed, vivid and intrusive imagistic flashbacks, and OBEs. It can be distinguished from sleep paralysis, however, using points 2, 3, and 4. Paralysis in sleep paralysis is not just a subjective feeling of being frozen or a misperception of motor capability, but is an actual atonia that only abates upon cessation of the episode. Hence, careful questioning of the patient with PTSD is required. The images found in PTSD flashbacks are always trauma-related, whereas this is not necessarily the case in sleep paralysis (though it can also occur, as in Hinton, Pich, Chhean, Pollack, & McNally, 2005). Flashbacks are often triggered by associations with trauma-related cues whereas sleep paralysis images only occur at sleep-wake transitions. The chronic hypervigilance found in PTSD is also usually absent in those suffering from sleep paralysis and, when present at all, occurs close to bedtime or in bedroom surroundings.

Exploding head syndrome (see Chapter 4) is another parasomnia that appears to be linked with sleep paralysis, possibly through activities of the reticular formation (e.g., Sharpless, 2014b; 2015), but can be differentiated from it using points 1, 2, and 4. In contrast to sleep paralysis, individuals with exploding head syndrome lack conscious awareness of their surroundings during episodes. Paralysis is not present, but auditory (and sometime visual) hallucinations are. In contrast to hallucinations during sleep paralysis, those found in exploding head syndrome are fairly nondifferentiated (e.g., bangs as opposed to articulate speech; visual static or light flashes as opposed to discernable figures). Episodes are also much briefer than sleep paralysis (one or more seconds), but can be similarly jarring.

Sleep paralysis can also be challenging to differentiate from *schizophrenia and other psychotic disorders*, especially when individuals are in acute post-episode distress. We recommend focusing on points 2 and 4. We should also note that it is possible to have both psychosis and sleep paralysis, and that hypnagogic/hypnopompic hallucinations are more common in psychotics in general (Plante & Winkelman, 2008). Paralysis is absent during the hallucinations of psychotic individuals, whereas this is the *sine qua non* of sleep paralysis. Further, those with psychotic disorders do not only experience hallucinations at sleep-wake transitions.

Conversion disorder (also known as *functional neurological symptom disorder*) may also consist of paralytic symptoms. In line with points 3 and 4, however, the paralysis seen in conversion disorder is usually more localized (e.g., one limb) and persists much longer than in sleep paralysis (viz., not only during the sleep transitions). Hallucinations are also not a core feature of conversion.

TREATMENT OPTIONS

Given the high levels of fear and general distress that typically accompany sleep paralysis, there have been many attempts made throughout history to prevent and disrupt episodes of it. Unfortunately, empirical documentation of their efficacy is currently lacking.

Folk Remedies

Traditional folk remedies range from the intuitive and likely helpful to the bizarre and potentially dangerous (summarized in Sharpless & Doghramji, 2015). Given the strong belief that sleep paralysis represented an actual attack from a malevolent entity, many "treatments" were oriented toward self-defense. These consisted of keeping knives and swords in the bedroom for physical defense, using bibles or other religious artifacts to ward off attacks, and uttering prayers for protection before bed or during the "attacks" (e.g., Hufford, 1982; Jalal, Simons-Rudolph, Jalal, & Hinton, 2014). Some of the more unusual defenses included throwing rice or millet on the floor in order to distract the attacker through obsessive counting and placing a towel covered with feces over one's body prior to sleep (Jones, 1949). Interestingly, some ancient defensive practices (e.g., use of salt, iron, magnets) used to ward off supernatural attackers are still in use today as a means of combatting alien abductions (e.g., see Druffel, 1998).

Sharpless and Grom (2016) investigated contemporary folk practices in college students suffering from isolated sleep paralysis and found that the majority attempted to disrupt episodes through various means, but less than 20% attempted to prevent them. Regarding disruption, the most effective techniques were attempting to move fingers and other extremities and making various attempts to "calm down." The most effective prevention strategies were changing sleeping patterns and positions (e.g., not sleeping on one's back) and using any number of relaxation techniques.

Psychological Approaches to Treatment

Although case studies of psychological treatments (e.g., psychoanalysis, hypnosis) can be found in the literature, large-scale clinical trials have yet to be conducted. Further, the majority of treatments have not been well-articulated (as reviewed in Sharpless & Doghramji, 2015).

Certain approaches derived from cognitive and behavioral approaches appear promising, however. Several research groups have applied numerous emblematic techniques to decrease sleep disturbances and anxiety symptoms in those suffering from chronic sleep paralysis (e.g., Hinton, Pich, Chhean, & Pollack, 2005; Hinton, Pich, Chhean, Pollack, & McNally, 2005; Ohaeri, Adelekan, Odejide, & Ikuesan, 1992; Stores, 1998). Sharpless and Doghramni (2015) recently published the first psychological (i.e., cognitive behavior therapy) manual to treat recurrent isolated sleep paralysis that builds upon these earlier approaches and incorporates techniques derived from both recent empirical findings (e.g., Cheyne & Girard, 2007; Sharpless & Grom, 2016) and already established treatments for insomnia (e.g., sleep hygiene specific to sleep paralysis). It consists of psychoeducation, sleep hygiene, episode prevention, direct episode disruption techniques, *in vivo* practice, and cognitive restructuring.

Psychopharmacology for Isolated Sleep Paralysis

As with psychological approaches, the use of medications to treat isolated sleep paralysis is in its relative infancy. When sleep paralysis occurs within the context of narcolepsy, it is generally thought that reduction in other symptoms (e.g., cataplexy) leads to reductions in sleep paralysis, but more data are needed.

Antidepressants of various types (e.g., tricyclic antidepressants, selective serotonin reuptake inhibitors, serotonin–norepinephrine reuptake inhibitors) appear promising. This is presumably due to their well-known REM-suppressing qualities (e.g., see Morgenthaler et al., 2007). More general guidance on medication utilization can be found in Sharpless and Doghramji (2015) and Sharpless (2016), but side-effect profiles and other comorbid psychiatric and medical conditions should obviously be taken into account before prescribing.

RECOMMENDATIONS FOR FUTURE WORK

Although in some ways sleep paralysis is a well-described condition, more empirical work on it is needed. This holds not only for basic psychopathology research, but for clinical work and even cultural and historical methods of analysis. We list some of what we believe to be the more promising recommendations below:

1. Assess isolated sleep paralysis more frequently and systematically in clinical and research settings in order to gain basic and applied information
2. Better determine the range and extent of clinical interference due to isolated sleep paralysis
3. Better determine not only the connections between isolated sleep paralysis and other medical/psychiatric conditions, but also better understand potential common pathways to development
4. Conduct more basic laboratory research to better understand the neurophysiology of sleep paralysis
5. Systematically test available treatment methods in efficacy and effectiveness trials
6. Utilize isolated sleep paralysis as a means to explore the causal links between anomalous experiences and anomalous beliefs

7. Use the hallucinatory content of isolated sleep paralysis as a means of better understanding cultural and historical differences in the context of how psychopathology may manifest.

REFERENCES

Aegineta, P. (1844). In F. Adams (Ed. & Trans.), *The seven books of Paulus Aegineta. Translated from the Greek with a commentary embracing a complete view of the knowledge possessed by the Greeks, Romans, and Arabians on all subjects connected with medicine and surgery.* London: Syndeham Society.

American Academy of Sleep Medicine. (2001). *International classification of sleep disorders.* Darien, IL: American Academy of Sleep Medicine.

American Academy of Sleep Medicine. (2014). *International classification of sleep disorders: Diagnostic and coding manual* (3rd ed.). Darien, IL: American Academy of Sleep Medicine.

American Psychiatric Association. (2013). *Diagnostic and statistical manual of mental disorders: DSM-V* (5th ed.). Arlington, VA: American Psychiatric Association.

Bae, K., Jin, X., Maywood, E.S., Hastings, M.H., Reppert, S.M., & Weaver, D.R. (2001). Differential features of mPer1, mPer2, and mPer3 in the SCN circadian clock. *Neuron, 30*, 525–536.

Bell, C.C., Dixie-Bell, D.D., & Thompson B. (1986). Further studies on the prevalence of isolated sleep paralysis in black subjects. *Journal of the National Medical Association, 78*(7), 649–659.

Bond, J. (1753). *An essay on the incubus, or night mare.* London: D. Wilson and T. Durham.

Brooks, P.L., & Peever, J.H. (2012). Identification of the transmitter and receptor mechanisms responsible for REM sleep paralysis. *The Journal of Neuroscience, 32*(29), 9785–9795.

Brown, T.A., & Barlow, D.H. (2014). *Anxiety and related disorders interview schedule for DSM-5: Lifetime version.* New York, NY: Oxford University Press.

Carpen, J.D., von Schantz, M., Smits, M., Skene, D.J., & Archer, S.N. (2006). A silent polymorphism in the PER1 gene associates with extreme diurnal preference in humans. *Journal of Human Genetics, 51*, 1122–1125.

Cheyne, J.A., (2001). The ominous numinous: Sensed presence and "other" hallucinations. *Journal of Consciousness Studies, 8*, 133–150.

Cheyne, J.A. (2002). Situational factors affecting sleep paralysis and associated hallucinations: Position and timing effects. *Journal of Sleep Research, 11*(2), 169–177.

Cheyne, J.A., & Girard, T.A. (2004). Spatial characteristics of hallucinations associated with sleep paralysis. *Cognitive Neuropsychiatry, 9*(4), 281–300. doi:http://dx.doi.org.ezaccess.libraries.psu.edu/10.1080/13546800344000264

Cheyne, J.A., Newby-Clark, I.R., & Rueffer, S.D. (1999). Relations among hypnagogic and hypnopompic experiences associated with sleep paralysis. *Journal of Sleep Research, 8*, 313–317.

Cheyne, J.A., & Girard, T.A. (2007). Paranoid delusions and threatening hallucinations: A prospective study of sleep paralysis experiences. *Consciousness and Cognition: An International Journal, 16*(4), 959–974.

Dahlitz, M., & Parkes, J. (1993). Sleep paralysis. *Lancet, 341*, 406–407.

Davies, O. (2003). The nightmare experience, sleep paralysis and witchcraft accusations. *Folklore, 114*(2), 181.

Denis, D., French, C.C., Rowe, R., Zavos, H.M.S., Nolan, P.M., Parsons, M.J., & Gregory, A.M. (2015) A twin and molecular genetics study of sleep paralysis and associated factors. *Journal of Sleep Research, 24*(4), 438–446. doi: 10.1111/jsr.12282

Druffel, A. (1998). *How to defend yourself against alien abduction.* New York: Rivers Press.

España, R.A., & Scammell, T.E. (2011). Sleep neurobiology from a clinical perspective. *Sleep, 34*(7), 845–858. doi:10.5665/SLEEP.1112

First, M.B., Williams, J.B.W., Karg, R.S., & Spitzer, R.L. (2015). *Structured clinical interview for DSM-5 disorders: Patient edition.* New York: Biometrics Research Department.

French, C.C., & Santomauro, J. (2007). Something wicked this way comes: Causes and interpretations of sleep paralysis. *Tall tales about the mind & brain: Separating fact from fiction* (pp. 380–398). New York, NY: Oxford University Press.

Fuller, P.M., Gooley, J.J., & Saper, C.B. (2006). Neurobiology of the sleep-wake cycle: Sleep architecture, circadian regulation, and regulatory feedback. *Journal of Biological Rhythms, 21*(6). 239–245.

Hinton, D.E., Pich, V., Chhean, D., & Pollack, M.H. (2005). The ghost pushes you down: Sleep paralysis-type panic attacks in a Khmer refugee population. *Transcultural Psychiatry, 42*(1), 46–77. doi:http://dx.doi.org.ezaccess.libraries.psu.edu/10.1177/1363461505050710

Hinton, D.E., Pich, V., Chhean, D., Pollack, M.H., & McNally, R.J. (2005). Sleep paralysis among Cambodian refugees: Association with PTSD diagnosis and severity. *Depression and Anxiety, 22*(2), 47–51. doi:http://dx.doi.org.ezaccess.libraries.psu.edu/10.1002/da.20084

Hopkins, B., Jacobs, D.M., & Westrum, R. (1992). *Unusual personal experiences: An analysis of data from three national surveys conducted by the Roper Organization.* Las Vegas, NV: Bigelow Holding Corporation.

Hufford, D. (1982). *The terror that comes in the night: An experience-centred study of supernatural assault traditions.* Philadelphia: University of Pennsylvania Press.

Jalal, B., Simons-Rudolph, J., Jalal, B., & Hinton, D.E. (2014). Explanations of sleep paralysis among Egyptian college students and the general population in Egypt and Denmark. *Transcultural Psychiatry, 51*(2), 158–175. doi:10.1177/1363461513503378

Jones, E. (1949). *On the nightmare* (2nd impression ed.). London, UK: Hogarth Press and the Institute of Psycho-analysis.

Kramer, H., & Sprenger, J. (1971). In M. Summers (Ed.) & M. Summers (Trans.), *The malleus maleficarum.* Mineola, NY: Dover Publications.

Kumar, A. (2012). More Brits believe in aliens than god, survey claims. *The Christian Post,* October 1, 2012.

Lee, H.J., Paik, J.W Kang, D.G., Yoon, H.K., Choi, J.E., Park., Y.M., Kim, S.J., & Kripke, D.F. (2011). PER2 variation is associated with diurnal preference in a Korean young population. *Behavior Genetics, 41*(2), 273–277.

Mahowald, M.W., & Schenck, C.H. (2005). Non-rapid eye movement sleep parasomnias. *Neurological Clinics, 23*, 1077–1106.

Mather, C. (1862). *The wonders of the invisible world.* London: John Russel Smith.

Mellman, T.A., & Uhde, T.W. (1989). Sleep panic attacks: New clinical findings and theoretical implications. *The American Journal of Psychiatry, 146*(9), 1204–1207.

Morgenthaler, T.I., Kapur, V.K., Brown, T., Swick, T.J., Alessi, C., Aurora, R.N., et al. (2007). Practice parameters for the treatment of narcolepsy and other hypersomnias of central origin: an American Academy of Sleep Medicine report. *Sleep, 30*(12), 1705.

Ohaeri, J.U., Adelekan, M.F., Odejide, A.O., & Ikuesan, B.A. (1992). The pattern of isolated sleep paralysis among Nigerian nursing students. *Journal of the National Medical Association, 84*(1), 67–70.

Parsons, M.J., Lester, K.J., Barclay, N.L., Archer, S.N., Nolan, P.M., Eley, T.C., & Gregory, A.M. (2014). Polymorphisms in the circadian expressed genes PER3 and ARNTL2 are associated with diurnal preference and GNβ3 with sleep measures. *Journal of Sleep Research, 23*(5), 595–604. doi 10.1111/jsr.12144.

Plante, D.T., & Winkelman, J.W. (2008). Parasomnia: Psychiatric considerations. *Sleep Medicine Clinics, 3*, 217–229.

RoperASW. (2002). UFOs & extraterrestrial life: Americans' beliefs and personal experiences. (No. C205-008232).

Sharpless, B.A. (2014a). Changing conceptions of the nightmare in medicine. *Hektoen International: A Journal of Medical Humanities (Moments in History Section).* Retrieved from http://www.hektoeninternational.org/index.php?option=com_content&view=article&id=841

Sharpless, B.A. (2014b). Exploding head syndrome. *Sleep Medicine Reviews, 18*(6), 489–493.

Sharpless, B.A. (2015). Exploding head syndrome is common in college students. *Journal of Sleep Research, 24*, 447–449.

Sharpless, B.A. (2016). A clinician's guide to recurrent isolated sleep paralysis. *Neuropsychiatric Disease and Treatment, 12*, 761–1767. doi 10.2147/NDT.S100307

Sharpless, B.A., & Doghramji, K. (2015). *Sleep paralysis: Historical, psychological, and medical perspectives.* New York, NY: Oxford University Press.

Sharpless, B.A., & Grom, J.L. (2016). Isolated sleep paralysis: Fear, prevention, and disruption. *Behavioral Sleep Medicine, 14*(2), 134–139.

Sharpless, B.A., McCarthy, K.S., Chambless, D.L., Milrod, B.L., Khalsa, S.R., & Barber, J.P. (2010). Isolated sleep paralysis and fearful isolated sleep paralysis in outpatients with panic attacks. *Journal of Clinical Psychology, 66*(12), 1292–1306. doi:10.1002/jclp.20724; 10.1002/jclp.20724

Stores, G. (1998). Sleep paralysis and hallucinosis. *Behavioural Neurology, 11*(2), 109–112.

Terzaghi, M., Ratti, P.L., Manni, F., & Manni, R. (2012). Sleep paralysis in narcolepsy: More than just a motor dissociative phenomenon? *Neurological Sciences, 33*(1), 169–172. doi:http://dx.doi.org.ezaccess.libraries.psu.edu/10.1007/s10072-011-0644-y

van Diemerbroeck, I. (1694). *The anatomy of human bodies, comprehending the most modern discoveries and curiosities in that art. To which is added a particular treatise of the small-pox and measles. Together with several practical observations and experienced cures.* (W. Salmom, Trans.). London: Whitwood.

World Health Organization. (2008). *International statistical classification of diseases and related health problems* (10th rev. ed.). Geneva, Switzerland: World Health Organization.

3

Sexual Behaviors in Sleep

ELENA DEL BUSTO, FREDERICK R. STODDARD II,
AND JOURDAN S. CRUZ ■

VIGNETTE

Mr. D is a thirty-eight-year-old white man with a past medical history of hypertension, diabetes, and morbid obesity. He was referred to a sleep lab by his primary care physician for evaluation of excessive day-time sleepiness. Mr. D presented to the office with his wife of five years who reported frequent, loud snoring, which resulted in several awakenings per night. Upon further questioning about his awakenings, the wife reported that, on a few occasions, he has gotten out of bed, walked around their room, and became extremely "frisky." When asked to clarify, his wife stated that he made groaning sexual sounds, masturbated in the corner, and even attempted to initiate coitus with her. On a few occasions she acquiesced to his behavioral, non-verbal requests and stated that intercourse was significantly "rougher," "more aggressive than usual," and "animalistic." Mrs. D admitted that initially she enjoyed it and thought Mr. D was exhibiting more passion, but she soon realized after discussions on the following mornings in question that he was not even aware of his actions. Mr. D denied any memory of these encounters.

Mr. D's sleep history included a brief period of frequent somnambulism as a teenager, which improved by the age of 18. He typically drank one to two beers a night prior to bed and took Zolpidem 5 mg QHS prn sleep. On occasion he was aware of his snoring but denied waking up gasping for breath. He experienced a 50-pound weight gain over the last two years. He reported that he always remembered being tired during the day, but that this had worsened recently to the point where he often felt unsafe driving and was concerned it would affect his work.

A wakeful electroencephalogram (EEG) yielded normal results, and a polysomnogram (PSG) showed muscle atonia during rapid eye movement (REM) sleep. He had a severe sleep apnea and underwent a split sleep study with continuous positive airway pressure (CPAP) titration. No leg movements were recorded. No sexual vocalizations or overt sexual acts were observed during the exam. Mr. D was given instruction to improve his sleep hygiene and to limit alcoholic beverages prior to sleep. Zolpidem

was further changed to Melatonin 3 mg QHS prn sleep. Interestingly, polysomnogram
also revealed three other abrupt wakeful periods from the deeper sleep stages.

Upon follow-up one month after the initial exam, Mr. D reported that he used the
CPAP nightly and that his sleep had improved substantially. He felt more refreshed
upon waking in the morning and, furthermore, he had had no further episodes of
somnambulism or sexual behavior during sleep.

HISTORICAL/CULTURAL CONTEXT

Sexual activity is a complex behavior that usually leads to a heightened sense of
both physical and psychological arousal. Because of the cognitive and physical
demands associated with the act, it seems difficult to believe that sex could be
initiated, sustained, and completed while in a sleep state or partial-sleep state. In
1897, however, Motet described the first forensic case of a man who was arrested
for indecent exposure but who was later acquitted because the acts were believed
to have occurred while he was asleep and not aware of his actions. Unfortunately,
it took almost one hundred years for the disorder to be described in more detail,
and not until 2003 was it formally conceptualized and named *sexual behavior in*
sleep (SBS) (Shapiro, Trajanovic, & Fedoroff, 2003).

The sentinel article describing sexsomnia was by the prominent forensic psychiatrist Dr. Albrecht Langeluddeke in 1955. He described two case studies and,
in the process, laid the groundwork for understanding the disorder. In both cases,
key similarities were used to describe the "typical" sexsomnia patient. Both patients
were young individuals with a history of somnambulism. Additionally, neither had
recollection of the events in question and the acts were significantly out of character.

It is also important to understand the broader conceptualization of parasomnias at the time. Through the latter part of the 1900s, it was largely accepted that
parasomnias were normal in childhood, but when they persisted into adulthood,
and especially when they were associated with violent behavior, it was a sign of
underlying psychopathology (Mahowald & Schenck, 1995; Shapiro et al., 2003).
Furthermore, it was believed that most activities that occurred during sleep were
a variant of sleepwalking and/or sleep terrors (*pavor nocturnus*).

A key step in understanding disorders of arousal occurred in 1979 when it
was first proposed that sleep and wake states could coexist (Niedermeyer et al.,
1979). Later in the 1990s researchers began to understand sleep disorders and
their characteristics better (Mahowald & Schenck, 1991; 1992; Schenck, Boyd, &
Mahowald, 1997). Parasomnias largely were broken down into non-REM sleep
behaviors, REM-sleep behavior disorders, and overlap disorders, which showed
features of each (Mahowald & Schenck, 1991; 1992; Schenck et al., 1997). It
became widely accepted that sleep and wakefulness were not necessarily mutually
exclusive states, but could coexist (Mahowald & Schenck, 1991; 1992).

It was not until 2003 that abnormal sexual behavior that occurred during sleep
was finally characterized and named SBS. A review of the literature reveals that
SBS was referred to by several names, including "sleep sex," "abnormal sexual
behavior in sleep," and "sexsomnia." Since then, increased exposure has led to

more reports and studies on SBS. The phenomenon is relatively rare, however, and it has been difficult to study in a clinical setting. Most studies have been limited to small *N* case reports (Arino, Iranzo, Gaig, & Santamaria, 2014; Guilleminault, Moscovitch, Yuen, & Poyares, 2002; Shapiro et al., 2003), reviews (Ingravallo et al., 2014; Organ & Fedoroff, 2015; Pressman, 2013), and surveys (Chung, Yegneswaran, Natarajan, Trajanovic, & Shapiro, 2010; Trajanovic, Mangan, & Shapiro, 2007). Unfortunately, it has proven difficult to observe SBS in a controlled clinical setting and only a few cases have been observed during a sleep study. Whereas self-reports and forensic cases with sleep studies have provided some insight into the phenomenon, our understanding of the pathophysiology and management remains incomplete.

ROLE IN CURRENT DIAGNOSTIC SYSTEMS

The incorporation of SBS into current diagnostic systems has proven difficult because there is still no clear consensus on the phenomenon. Although some consider SBS a distinct diagnosis (Shapiro et al., 2003), others claim it to be a variant of somnambulism (Ebrahim, 2006; Rosenfeld & Elhajjar, 1998), and still others a syndrome (Buchanan, 2011). In Shapiro et al.'s (2003) seminal article, the authors suggested that SBS be categorized as a non-REM parasomnia. When finally incorporated into the *International Classification of Sleep Disorders—Second Edition* (ICSD-2, American Academy of Sleep Medicine, 2005) SBS was included as a distinct NREM parasomnia under the category "disorders of arousal." Since that initial report, however, a few researchers have described SBS in the context of: (1) REM sleep behavior disorder; (2) parasomnia overlap disorder; and (3) sleep epilepsy. Because of the variants, some have argued that SBS is a syndrome common to many sleep disorders rather than a distinct disorder in and of itself.

Diagnostically, SBS is currently only recognized in the ICSD-3, which labels it a variant of confusional arousal (American Acadamy of Sleep Medicine, 2014). The *Diagnostic and Statistical Manual of Mental Disorders, Fifth Edition* (American Psychiatric Association, 2013) places sexsomnia as a specifier of the sleepwalking subtype of non-REM movement sleep arousal disorder. *The International Classification of Diseases-10* (World Health Organization [WHO], 2010) does not list sleep sex specifically, instead including nonorganic sleep disorder, specified and unspecified.

SYMPTOMATOLOGY

SBS can refer to a wide array of sexual or sexualized behaviors. These range from simple vocalizations such as moaning or "talking dirty" to sexual movements such as pelvic thrusts and even masturbation. In the presence of a partner (or unwilling participant nearby), it may include genital fondling, orogenital sex, and even sexual intercourse. Oftentimes these acts are reported to be "uncharacteristic" for the individual (more aggressive, more experimental, etc.). There have even been reported cases of heterosexual males performing homosexual acts (Langeluddeke, 1955). Perhaps most common in cases of SBS is the subject's complete amnesia for the events. Subjects are often shocked and surprised when informed of their activities without any recollection of what happened (Langeluddeke, 1955; Morrison, Rumbold, & Riha, 2014; Organ & Fedoroff, 2015; Trajanovic & Shapiro, 2013).

PREVALENCE RATE AND ASSOCIATED FEATURES

Lifetime prevalence of SBS is a difficult value to determine. It generally is accepted that SBS is largely underreported for a variety of reasons. Oftentimes, individuals are embarrassed or confused by their SBS and, therefore, do not bring it to the attention of treating physicians. Similarly, there is a general lack of understanding and questioning about SBS on the part of treating physicians who, therefore, rarely ask about SBS. As a result, it is uncommon for SBS to surface clinically. This is likely why, until relatively recently, most cases only came to light due to the legal consequences of the SBS.

In a recent retrospective chart review of sleep clinic patients ($N = 832$), Chung et al. (2010) found that 7.6% reported at least one episode of SBS. Interestingly, of the 63 subjects who reported SBS, only seven had been referred for a sleep study for parasomnia activity, and only two for actual SBS. Instead, 89% of the subjects reporting SBS were referred for reasons other than parasomnias. In other words, SBS was only identified because a questionnaire was administered. This study was limited due to the selection bias of the specific clinic population, as well as the inability to verify reports independently of the questionnaire; however, it clearly demonstrated how easy it is to underreport SBS and how important routine questioning is to a better understanding of this phenomenon. A large population-based telephone survey in Norway suggested a lifetime prevalence of 7.1%, with 2.7% having at least one episode in the last three months and 0.4% occurring at least weekly (Bjorvatn, Gronli, & Pallesen, 2010). However, without being able to validate the reports with clinical data, either thorough medical charts or PSG, a reliable prevalence rate has yet to be identified.

Several small clinical case studies (Guilleminault et al., 2002; Shapiro et al., 2003) or online surveys (Trajanovic et al., 2007) have helped to identify features associated with SBS. SBS is two to four times more common in men than women (Chung et al., 2010; Trajanovic et al., 2007). Precipitating factors are thought to include: sleep deprivation, obstructive sleep apnea, alcohol and drug use, other medication use, and any sort of physical contact from a bed partner (Trajanovic et al., 2007). Comorbid parasomnias (Chung et al., 2010) are extremely common (approximately 80%) and comorbid psychiatric illnesses have also been observed. Often, there is even a family history of parasomnia activity. It is important to note that SBS also has been associated with nocturnal epilepsy, and this should be considered in differential diagnosis.

THEORIES OF ETIOLOGY

Because there is a paucity of experimental data on SBS, there is little direct evidence for the etiology of this disorder. Psychological explanations largely have followed a Freudian approach. These suggest that SBS is closely tied to dreaming and its wish-fulfillment function. As such, deeply rooted sexual urges that may not be fulfilled physically are acted out in dreams. SBS then serves as a means to fulfill those sexual desired that are not satisfied while awake (Shapiro, Fedoroff, & Trajanovic, 1996).

Scientific explanations primarily are derived from studies on more general sleep disorders. Non-REM parasomnia disorders of arousal are by far the most common theoretical cause of SBS and will be the focus of this discussion. Others, such as REM-sleep behavior disorder (RBD) and sleep epilepsy will be discussed briefly.

Disorders of arousal are considered to be a subset of non-REM parasomnias. The general theory is that subjects have disturbed or immature mechanisms of arousal, which result in "partial" or "incomplete" arousals. Ultimately, while certain brain centers remain asleep, and the subject appears asleep, other brain centers have "awoken," allowing the subject to perform certain "automated" behaviors such as walking (somnambulism), eating, or sexual activity (SBS). These arousals usually occur from slow wave sleep N3 (Mahowald & Schenck, 2005), primarily during the early part of the night, but they can occur during any stage of non-REM sleep and at any point in the night (Naylor & Aldrich, 1991).

Physiologically, there is thought to be instability in both the mechanisms responsible for maintaining a stable sleep state and those responsible for transitioning from sleep to wakefulness. PSGs often observe incomplete arousal from slow wave sleep (SWS, Bruni et al., 2008). PSG may also identify a high frequency of "Cyclic Alternating Patterns," which are a marker for poor sleep stability (Terzano & Parrino, 2000). Increased sleep inertia is also thought to play a role in the development of non-REM parasomnias (Ohayon, Guilleminault, & Priest, 1999).

The pathogenesis of parasomnias is thought to involve three broad contributing factors: (1) genetic predisposition, (2) priming factors, and (3) provoking or trigger factors (Pressman, 2013). Studies have suggested a genetic link in the development of disorders of arousal and it is often found to run in families (Cao & Guilleminault, 2010; Hublin, Kaprio, Partinen, Heikkila, & Koskenvuo, 1997; Licis, Desruisseau, Yamada, Duntley, & Gurnett, 2011). However, specific genetic defects responsible for this have yet to be identified. Predisposing factors can accumulate over a short period of time up until sleep initiation, and thus may make an individual more susceptible to having a disorder of arousal. These can include sleep deprivation, stress, drug use, and alcohol use (Ohayon et al., 1999). These factors tend to extend SWS, may lead to REM rebound, or may fragment or make arousal from sleep difficult (Bruni et al., 2008; Pressman, 2007). Triggers are those events that occur *during* sleep that can cause an arousal. These may include internal factors such as sleep apnea and restless leg syndrome, or external factors such the touch of a bed partner or other arousing stimuli (phone, pager, television, etc.). The combination of factors that increase the pressure for slow wave sleep, along with factors that cause arousal, can result in the sleep state dissociation seen in SBS (Bruni et al., 2008).

RBD and nocturnal epilepsy also have been suggested as possible causes of SBS (Guilleminault et al., 2002). REM is characterized by vivid dreams and muscle atony, which prevents us from acting out our dreams. If muscle atony is lacking in RBD, then individuals end up acting out their dreams. When these dreams are violent, aggressive, or sexual in nature, they may be acted out with anyone in the dreamer's immediate proximity (Wu, Anees, & Thorpy, 2013). Given that REM happens with more frequency in the later part of the night, RBD is more common during this time (Schenck & Mahowald, 2005). SBS associated with nocturnal epilepsy tends to occur when the epileptic focus is in the right temporal region (Schenck, Arnulf, & Mahowald, 2007). When these seizures start later in life, there may be a concomitant increase in SBS that correlates with a change in personality and other sequelae of the seizures. Personal and family histories of parasomnias may not be present as is common with other parasomnias.

ASSESSMENT OPTIONS

In the absence of ulterior motives (e.g., certain forensic cases), a patient's description of SBS is usually taken at face value. The work-up and differential diagnosis is, therefore, geared toward understanding the causes of SBS rather than on the SBS itself. Identification of the causal or risk factors can help to guide treatment options as described below. Additionally, in cases that create distress in a relationship, therapeutic efforts can be made to help couples deal with SBS.

As of this writing, there has been one assessment measure of sexsomnia used in the literature (Trajanovic, Mangan, & Shapiro, 2007; Mangan & Reips, 2007). The *Sexsomnia Internet Questionnaire* contained 28 items to assess an individual's experience with sexsomnia, including any precipitating factors, as well as medical and legal information. It has not been psychometrically validated, however, or used in clinical studies.

Under most circumstances, a label of SBS is given based on a patient's, or a bedmate's, recount of sexual events taking place during sleep. Because this is often not the primary complaint (Chung et al., 2010), it is important that all patients who present with sleep disturbances be questioned about SBS as well as other parasomnias. Suggested questioning for SBS includes:

- Has your libido or sexual activity changed, either while awake, or falling asleep, or during your sleep (Schenck et al., 2007)?
- Has your bed partner observed any sexual vocalizations or sexual behaviors on your part while you are asleep (Schenck et al., 2007)?
- Have you ever initiated sexual activity with a bed partner while asleep (Chung et al., 2010)?

- Have you ever engaged in any sexually related behaviors while asleep (Chung et al., 2010)?
- Has your bed partner ever initiated sexual activity with you while she or he was asleep (Chung et al., 2010)?

The work-up for an individual with SBS is similar to the work-up for other parasomnias. A thorough medical and psychiatric history should be obtained. Key details of the history should include (1) the timing (early or late in the night) and frequency of events, (2) severity and quality of events (short vs. long, aggressive vs. not) as well as any similarities to wakeful sexual activities, (3) longitudinal course, (4) associated dreams and amnesia for events, (5) predisposing and precipitating factors (including medications, nocturnal routines, and overall sleep hygiene), and (6) psychosocial and physical consequences (Schenck & Hurwitz, 2012). Patients should be questioned about other parasomnias as well. Physical exam should include neurologic, cardiac, and respiratory systems including upper airway anatomy.

The patient's history should also include questions about the personal and possible legal ramifications of SBS. Even in consensual relationships, SBS has been shown to have adverse effects on both the patients (initiators) and their bed partners (recipients). Feelings often described by initiators include confusion, shame, guilt, embarrassment, frustration, and self-incrimination (Mangan, 2004; Schenck & Hurwitz, 2012). Feelings described by recipients include annoyance, fear, suspicion, lack of emotional intimacy, repulsion, and sexual abandonment (Mangan, 2004; Schenck & Hurwitz, 2012).

Overnight video-PSG should be performed to help diagnose parasomnic activity and other possible triggers. It is important to note that it is exceedingly rare to observe SBS during a sleep study and that this should not be the goal of the PSG. Findings such as abrupt arousal from slow wave sleep (Bruni et al., 2008), hypersynchronous δ waves (Guilleminault, 2006), δ wave clusters, and increased or abnormal cyclic alternating pattern rates (Bruni et al., 2008; Guilleminault, 2006) are all more commonly found in individuals with parasomnias. They are, however, common in other sleep disorders as well, and are, therefore, nonspecific findings (Pressman, 2004). As a result, in a forensic setting these are insufficient to diagnose SBS and cannot discern, post hoc, the cause of a putative sleep-related event (Pressman, 2004). Extended electromyogram (EMG) should be utilized when there is a consideration for REM sleep behavior disorder (RBD) (Buchanan, 2011). If sleep epilepsy is suspected, then extended EEG montage PSG monitoring is warranted (Buchanan, 2011).

DIFFERENTIAL DIAGNOSIS

Most cases of SBS fall into the category of a non-REM parasomnia, although REM-sleep behavior disorder has also been described. Special consideration should be taken, however, to identify cases of possible nocturnal seizures, because their work-up, management, and clinical implications differ substantially from other sleep disorders. Features suggestive of nocturnal seizures include (1) very short duration (i.e., minutes), (2) patient memory of the events, (3) witnessing a jerking of the body, (4) tongue or cheek biting, (5) occasional urinary incontinence, and (6) possible personality changes. Details suggestive of a RBD include episodes that occur later in the night and those associated with vivid dreaming. It is important for clinicians to be cognizant that our understanding of SBS is still in its infancy and, therefore, they should be open to other differential diagnostic considerations that have yet to be described in the literature.

A unique diagnostic approach is necessary in the SBS forensic arena. This is because malingering must always be *highly* considered. The DSM-IV describes malingering as "intentional and purposeful feigning [of] illness to achieve some recognizable goal." In the case of most lawsuits involving a claim of SBS, the goal is to receive a verdict of not guilty due to absence of *mens rea*. In other words, because the individual was asleep and not aware of his or her actions at the time, he or she cannot be held accountable for these actions. Under such circumstances, it is impossible to know the exact level of awareness of the defendant during a crime. Instead, the goal for the forensic evaluator is to determine whether the details of the case are consistent with the field's understanding of SBS or other sleep-related violent acts. This includes looking at risk factors for SBS (genetic, predisposing, and trigger factors), corroborative evidence of previous episodes of SBS, possible PSG evidence supporting the potential for SBS, and an account of the crime that is consistent with SBS. General guidelines for evaluating the possibility of a sleep-related violence case have been proposed by Mahowald and Schenck (1999, p. 658):

(1) There should be reason (by history or formal sleep laboratory evaluation) to suspect a bona fide sleep disorder. Similar episodes, with benign or morbid outcome, should have occurred previously.

(2) The duration of the action is usually brief (minutes).

(3) The behavior is usually abrupt, immediate, impulsive, and senseless—without apparent motivation. Although ostensibly purposeful, it is inappropriate to the total situation, out of (waking) character for the individual, and without evidence of premeditation.

(4) The victim is someone who merely happened to be present, and who may have been the stimulus for the arousal.

(5) Immediately following return of consciousness, there is perplexity or horror, without attempt to escape, conceal, or cover up the action. There is evidence of lack of awareness on the part of the individual during the event.

(6) There is usually some degree of amnesia for the event; however, this amnesia need not be complete.

(7) In the case of sleep terrors, sleepwalking, or sleep drunkenness, the act may (a) occur upon awakening (rarely, immediately upon falling asleep or, usually, at least one hour after sleep onset); (b) occur upon attempts to awaken the subject; or (c) have been potentiated by sedative-hypnotic administration or prior sleep deprivation.

The legal arguments for sleep-related violence are complicated not only by defendants claims of sleep, but also by their understanding of their disorder in general and to what extent they know that such acts are a possibility for them. SBS is usually a frequent occurrence for an individual who experiences it, and it may have certain triggers such as alcohol use. Therefore, if persons with previous episodes of SBS engage in activities known to induce such behavior (such as alcohol or sleep deprivation), and then allow themselves to fall asleep in an environment where there is a reasonable likelihood of such an event taking place, can they be held culpable for criminal events that might transpire? How about in the absence of alcohol: if defendants knew that they had engaged in SBS previously and then knowingly slept near a minor, resulting in a charge of sexual assault on a minor, are they also not culpable? Defendants may not have been conscious at the time of the assault, but they most likely were when they allowed themselves to be in a situation where such an outcome was possible.

TREATMENT OPTIONS

Treatment of SBS is directed toward management of the suspected underlying disorder or the clinical features that contribute to SBS. The most commonly used medical treatment for non-REM parasomnias and RBDs is clonazepam (Guilleminault et al., 2002). When sleep apnea or restless leg syndrome is a suspected trigger, then CPAP or dopamine agonists can be prescribed, respectively. Nonmedical management of predisposing factors may focus on improving overall sleep hygiene, such as avoiding drugs and alcohol prior to bed, improving sleep habits to avoid excessive sleep deprivation, and managing stress. Control of external triggers also can be managed to help decrease the incidence of SBS.

Particular importance should be given to individuals for whom sleep epilepsy is suspected. These individuals should be evaluated by a neurologist who can adequately manage and monitor epileptic behavior. Often, treatment of seizure activity that occurs primarily in sleep can be difficult because most antiseizure medications have side effects that disrupt normal sleep architecture (Bazil, 2003). This can result in poor sleep patterns; the subsequent sleep deprivation can, in turn, increase seizure activity. Gabapentin is a favorable alternative because it can improve sleep as well as help control seizures (Bazil, 2003).

Counseling individuals about lifestyle modifications should also be an important part of treatment to ensure that a safe sleep environment is maintained at all times. Avoiding alcohol, stress, and other predisposing factors can be tried in addition to the above. All individuals should be informed of the potential legal ramifications of their nighttime behaviors. Those who share sleeping space with these individuals also should be made aware of the condition. Avoiding situations that might result in an inadvertent criminal act is crucial. For example, these individuals should avoid sleeping near children. Additionally, when sleeping near others, care should be taken to avoid predisposing factors and triggers (Schenck et al., 2007). When the behavior causes interpersonal tension within a couple, couples therapy can be beneficial.

RECOMMENDATIONS FOR FUTURE WORK

Despite increased interest in SBS over the last decade, little is known about the disorder. Cases still surface largely in the forensic arena. The extreme biases such individuals possess, along with an increased likelihood for malingering, make it difficult to draw strong scientific conclusions about the disorder. Increased efforts are needed to identify patients with SBS in clinical settings so that the disorder can be validated and studied. Studies on a larger scale are needed to understand and identify its salient features and treatment management.

Another recommended step is bringing the disorder to the attention of primary care physicians as well as sleep experts. This will allow for more routine screening of parasomnias and sleep-related disorders. This is particular important for the sleep clinics in which most of the patients who have SBS present with other sleep disorders. Therefore, presenting symptoms cannot be assumed to be the only sleep issues present; other parasomnias and sleep disorders such as SBS should be part of routine sleep histories.

Increased public awareness is also important. It is frequently the case that individuals are confused and embarrassed by their SBS and avoid discussing it with others. Increased public awareness of parasomnias will be important in making people feel more comfortable about discussing these disorders with their treatment providers.

REFERENCES

American Academy of Sleep Medicine. (2005). *International classification of sleep disorders* (3rd ed.). Darien, IL: American Academy of Sleep Medicine.

American Psychiatric Association. (2013). *Diagnostic and statistical manual of mental disorders: DSM-5*. Washington, DC: American Psychiatric Association.

Arino, H., Iranzo, A., Gaig, C., & Santamaria, J. (2014). Sexsomnia: parasomnia associated with sexual behaviour during sleep. *Neurologia, 29*(3), 146–152.

Bazil, C.W. (2003). Effects of antiepileptic drugs on sleep structure: are all drugs equal? *CNS Drugs, 17*(10), 719–728.

Bjorvatn, B., Gronli, J., & Pallesen, S. (2010). Prevalence of different parasomnias in the general population. *Sleep Med, 11*(10), 1031–1034.

Bruni, O., Ferri, R., Novelli, L., Finotti, E., Miano, S., & Guilleminault, C. (2008). NREM sleep instability in children with sleep terrors: the role of slow wave activity interruptions. *Clinical Neurophysiology, 119*(5), 985–992.

Buchanan, P.R. (2011). Sleep sex. *Sleep Medicine Clinics, 6*, 417–428.

Cao, M., & Guilleminault, C. (2010). Families with sleepwalking. *Sleep Medicine, 11*(7), 726–734.

Chung, S.A., Yegneswaran, B., Natarajan, A., Trajanovic, N.N., & Shapiro, C.M. (2010). *Sexsomnia in a sleep clinic population: frequency and association with other sleep and psychiatric reports.* Presented at SLEEP 2010, the 24th annual meeting of the Associated Professional Sleep Societies.

Ebrahim, I.O. (2006). Somnambulistic sexual behaviour (sexsomnia). *Journal of Clinical Forensic Medicine, 13*(4), 219–224.

Guilleminault, C. (2006). Hypersynchronous slow delta, cyclic alternating pattern and sleepwalking. *Sleep, 29*(1), 14–15.

Guilleminault, C., Moscovitch, A., Yuen, K., & Poyares, D. (2002). Atypical sexual behavior during sleep. *Psychosomatic Medicine, 64*(2), 328–336.

Hublin, C., Kaprio, J., Partinen, M., Heikkila, K., & Koskenvuo, M. (1997). Prevalence and genetics of sleepwalking: a population-based twin study. *Neurology, 48*(1), 177–181.

Ingravallo, F., Poli, F., Gilmore, E.V., Pizza, F., Vignatelli, L., Schenck, C.H., & Plazzi, G. (2014). Sleep-related violence and sexual behavior in sleep: a systematic review of medical-legal case reports. *Journal of Clinical Sleep Medicine, 10*(8), 927–935.

Langeluddeke, A. (1955). Delikte in Schlafzustanden. *Der Nervenarzt, 26*(1), 28–30.

Licis, A.K., Desruisseau, D.M., Yamada, K.A., Duntley, S.P., & Gurnett, C.A. (2011). Novel genetic findings in an extended family pedigree with sleepwalking. *Neurology, 76*(1), 49–52.

Mahowald, M.W., & Schenck, C.H. (1991). Status dissociates—a perspective on states of being. *Sleep, 14*(1), 69–79.

Mahowald, M.W., & Schenck, C.H. (1992). Dissociated states of wakefulness and sleep. *Neurology, 42*(7 Suppl 6), 44–51; discussion 52.

Mahowald, M.W., & Schenck, C.H. (1995). Complex motor behavior arising during the sleep period: forensic science implications. *Sleep, 18*(9), 724–727.

Mahowald, M.W., & Schenck, C.H. (1999). Sleep-related violence—forensic medicine issues. In S. Chokroverty (Ed.), *Sleep disorders medicine: basic science, technical considerations, and clinical aspects* (pp. 729–739). Boston, MA: Butterworth-Heinemann.

Mahowald, M.W., & Schenck, C.H. (2005). Non-rapid eye movement sleep parasomnias. *Neurologic Clinics, 23*(4), 1077–1106, vii.

Mangan, M.A. (2004). A phenomenology of problematic sexual behavior occurring in sleep. *Archives of Sexual Behavior, 33*(3), 287–293.

Mangan. M.A., & Reips, U.D. (2007), Sleep, sex and the Web: Surveying the difficult-to-reach clinical population suffering from sexsomnia. *Behavior Research Methods, 39*(2), 233–236.

Trajanovic, N.N., Mangan, M.A., & Shapiro, C. M. (2007). Sexual behaviour in sleep: An internet survey. *Social Psychiatry and Psychiatric Epidemiology, 42*(12), 1024–1031.

Morrison, I., Rumbold, J.M., & Riha, R.L. (2014). Medicolegal aspects of complex behaviours arising from the sleep period: a review and guide for the practising sleep physician. *Sleep Medicine Reviews, 18*(3), 249–260.

Naylor, M.W., & Aldrich, M.S. (1991). The distribution of confusional arousals across sleep stages and time of night in children and adolescents with sleep terrors. *Sleep Research, 20*(308).

Niedermeyer, E., Singer, H.S., Folstein, S.E., Allen, R.P., Miranda, F., Fineyre, F., & Bird, B.L. (1979). Hypersomnia with simultaneous waking and sleep patterns in the electroencephalogram. A case report with neurotransmitter studies. *Journal of Neurology, 221*(1), 1–13.

Ohayon, M.M., Guilleminault, C., & Priest, R.G. (1999). Night terrors, sleepwalking, and confusional arousals in the general population: their frequency and relationship to other sleep and mental disorders. *Journal of Clinical Psychiatry, 60*(4), 268–276; quiz 277.

Organ, A., & Fedoroff, J.P. (2015). Sexsomnia: sleep sex research and its legal implications. *Current Psychiatry Reports, 17*(5), 568.

Pressman, M.R. (2004). Hypersynchronous delta sleep EEG activity and sudden arousals from slow-wave sleep in adults without a history of parasomnias: clinical and forensic implications. *Sleep, 27*(4), 706–710.

Pressman, M.R. (2007). Factors that predispose, prime and precipitate NREM parasomnias in adults: clinical and forensic implications. *Sleep Medicine Reviews, 11*(1), 5–30; discussion 31–33.

Pressman, M.R. (2013). Classification of parasomnias and diagnostic criteria. In C.A. Kushida (Ed.), *The encyclopedia of sleep* (1st ed.). London, UK: Academic Press.

Rosenfeld, I.O., & Elhajjar, A. (1998). Sleepsex: A variant of sleepwalking. *Archives of Sexual Behavior, 27*, 269–278.

Schenck, C.H., Arnulf, I., & Mahowald, M.W. (2007). Sleep and sex: what can go wrong? A review of the literature on sleep related disorders and abnormal sexual behaviors and experiences. *Sleep, 30*(6), 683–702.

Schenck, C.H., Boyd, J.L., & Mahowald, M.W. (1997). A parasomnia overlap disorder involving sleepwalking, sleep terrors, and REM sleep behavior disorder in 33 polysomnographically confirmed cases. *Sleep, 20*(11), 972–981.

Schenck, C.H., & Hurwitz, T.D. (2012). Other parasomnias in adults: sexsomnia, sleep-related dissociative disorder, catathrenia, sleep-related hallucinations, and sleep talking. In T.J. Barkoukis, J.K. Matheson, R. Ferber, K. Doghramji, & J.L. Blumer (Eds.), *Therapy in sleep medicine* (1st ed., pp. 573–582). Philadelphia, PA: Elsevier Health Sciences.

Schenck, C.H., & Mahowald, M.W. (2005). Rapid eye movement sleep parasomnias. *Neurologic Clinics, 23*(4), 1107–1126.

Shapiro, C.M., Fedoroff, J.P., & Trajanovic, N.N. (1996). Sexual behavior in sleep: A newly described parasomnia. *Sleep Research, 25*, 367.

Shapiro, C.M., Trajanovic, N.N., & Fedoroff, J.P. (2003). Sexsomnia—a new parasomnia? *Canadian Journal of Psychiatry, 48*(5), 311–317.

Terzano, M.G., & Parrino, L. (2000). Origin and significance of the Cyclic Alternating Pattern (CAP). *Sleep Medicine Reviews, 4*(1), 101–123.

Trajanovic, N.N., Mangan, M., & Shapiro, C.M. (2007). Sexual behaviour in sleep: an internet survey. *Social Psychiatry and Psychiatric Epidemiology, 42*(12), 1024–1031.

Trajanovic, N.N., & Shapiro, C.M. (2013). Sexsomnia. In C.A. Kushida (Ed.), *Encyclopedia of sleep* (1st ed., pp. 248–253). London, UK: Academic Press.

WHO (World Health Organization). (2010). *International statistical classification of disease and related health problems: ICD-10* (10th ed.). Geneva, Switzerland: WHO.

Wu, W.P., Anees, S., & Thorpy, M.J. (2013). Pathophysiology, associations, and consequences of parasomnias. In C.A. Kushida (Ed.), *Encyclopedia of sleep*. London, UK, Academic Press.

4

Exploding Head Syndrome

BRIAN A. SHARPLESS AND JACOB A. ZIMMERMAN ■

VIGNETTE

Presented below is the account of a 21-year-old Caucasian female with exploding head syndrome. It is worth noting that the interviewee was found to also experience episodes of isolated sleep paralysis (see Chapter 2). Her level of typical anxiety symptoms was very low and unremarkable according to her responses on a battery of self-report measures. Her scores on the Insomnia Severity Index (Morin, 1993), however, fell within the "clinical insomnia" (i.e., moderate severity) range. Her case is noteworthy because her distress during episodes was severe per clinical interview. The frequency of episodes was also fairly high (i.e., 20 in the past year). However, much of the symptomatology presented in this account could be considered fairly typical, especially when considering the more severe cases. The following is her narrative:

"They started about a year ago when I was 20 years old. Last week was the last time it happened, and that sound is still very fresh in my memory. It happens more often when I'm on my back and always right as I'm just about to fall asleep. Then boom! It sounds like a bomb going off and my stomach drops. I'm awoken immediately when it happens, but the noise only lasts a second. I can't really pinpoint where the sound is coming from, but most likely from above. Every time this happens I wake up, my muscles jerk, and I have to force myself to breathe again. It's almost like I forgot how, and I'm left shaking. To me, the level of fear is severe. Once I'm awake I realize that I've broken out in sweat. It's not a lot of sweat, but more than normal. At first I was nervous for my health, and I always figured it had something to do with my dreams, but maybe not? Just in the past year I've dealt with about twenty of these. They started out as regular, but now they're random. I don't know how to stop it. After I have one, my sleep is really disrupted and I'm always really tired during the day."

HISTORICAL/CULTURAL CONTEXT

Although exploding head syndrome was only formally named in 1988 (Pearce, 1988), descriptions of this phenomenon can be traced back at least as far as the centennial celebration of the United States. The earliest reference we are aware of comes from the Philadelphia physician Silas Weir Mitchell (1876). He termed these episodes "sensory discharges" (Mitchell, 1876, pp. 778–780). Mitchell's descriptions of this phenomenon capture many of the defining characteristics of exploding head syndrome (American Academy of Sleep Medicine, 2014, p. 254). This early depiction was based on the case studies of two male patients who experienced anomalous explosive sounds during sleep transitions (e.g., pistol shots and loud bells, Mitchell, 1876). Mitchell hypothesized that this phenomenon likely had behavioral (e.g., excessive mental labor) and substance-induced (e.g., tobacco use) etiologies (Mitchell, 1876).

Other early clinical descriptions can be documented. Armstrong-Jones (1920) vividly termed these symptoms a "snapping of the brain" (Armstrong-Jones, 1920, p. 720). He noted that episodes tended to precede the development of other illnesses. For example, a snapping of the brain could precede the development of melancholia. In fact, more recent research implies that exploding head syndrome may act as a more proximal "aura" that precedes the experience of other parasomnias (e.g., isolated sleep paralysis as in Evans, 2006).

Interestingly, and in spite of the fact that a scientific literature base for exploding head syndrome has been recently forming, other nonscientific explanations have been proposed. For example, exploding head syndrome phenomena appear to have been worked into various conspiracy theories. More specifically, some individuals may interpret that the fright and auditory hallucinations so characteristic of exploding head syndrome are not natural events, but are the result of targeted harassment by nefarious government agents. A belief in so-called "gang stalking," which is the term used by alleged victims of psychological attacks/harassment (Kershaw, 2008), appears to be growing, as evidenced by thousands of websites, videos, and organized events centered on these alleged phenomena (CBS, 2014).

There seems to be a great deal of variety in the putative forms of attack and harassment attributed to the perpetrators of gang stalking (i.e., both physical and psychological). However, a major concern within the community of alleged "targeted individuals" is *electronic* harassment (CBS, 2014). This is believed to involve the use of directed energy weapons (e.g., microwave radiation generators) that can be used to inflict various forms of torture on the minds and bodies of targeted individuals (*Foundation Stop Electronic Weapons Stop Gang Stalking* [STOPEG], 2015).

This belief in directed energy weapons may be the primary link between gang-stalking conspiracies and symptoms of exploding head syndrome. Namely, one purported use of directed energy weapons is to prevent or disrupt sleep, sometimes through the use of a singular sound, of short duration, at night (Foundation STOPEG, 2015). Additionally, microwave radiation is thought to be projected through walls and directly at the body (especially the head) of the targeted individual. This radiation is believed to produce auditory effects that are unexpected and frightening to the sleeper, resulting in sudden awakenings with a racing heart and acute confusion (Foundation STOPEG, 2015) as well as sensations that can feel like electric shocks (Oliver, 2010). Along with the paroxysms of sound, directed energy weapons are thought to cause the victim to see lights and experience myoclonic jerks (e.g., Oliver, 2010).

Although many individuals have relatively isolated "pockets" of unusual beliefs in the presence of otherwise intact reality-testing (e.g., beliefs in psychic abilities or Bigfoot), the gang stalking community has been characterized by some psychiatrists as perhaps reinforcing the delusions of others and, in effect, intensifying these beliefs through social media and other means (Kershaw, 2008). Some have speculated that individuals involved with this community could, in fact, be psychotic throughout their waking life in addition to experiencing regular hypnagogic/hypnopompic hallucinations (Kershaw, 2008). Regardless, the phenomenology of exploding head syndrome appears consistent with the complaints of some of these "targeted individuals," who report otherwise inexplicable loud noises at night during sleep transitions. On a perhaps related note, one online survey ($N =$ 108) found a significant and positive association between anomalous beliefs and symptoms of exploding head syndrome (Sherwood, 1999). Anomalous beliefs in this survey included a range of experiences, including beliefs in extrasensory perception (ESP), psychokinesis, out-of-body events, and extraterrestrial experiences (Sherwood, 1999). Significant associations occurred between symptoms of exploding head syndrome and incidents of both childhood and adulthood anomalous beliefs, current levels of anomalous beliefs, as well as childhood fantasy proneness, which has been associated with reports of paranormal experiences. It is possible that such childhood (and adulthood) anomalous experiences and beliefs may lead to misinterpretations of exploding head syndrome symptoms (Sherwood, 1999). The possibility also exists that the frightening experiences in exploding head syndrome may lead some individuals to gravitate toward anomalous beliefs as a means of understanding these otherwise inexplicable phenomena.

ROLE IN CURRENT DIAGNOSTIC SYSTEMS

Exploding head syndrome is not specifically recognized in the current editions of either the *International Statistical Classification of Diseases and Related Health Problems—10th Edition Revised* (ICD-10; World Health Organization, 2008) or the *Diagnostic and Statistical Manual of Mental Disorders—5th Edition* (DSM-5; American Psychiatric Association, 2013). However, symptoms can be subsumed under the labels, "other specified sleep-wake disorder" or "unspecified sleep-wake disorder" (780.59, G47.8; American Psychiatric Association, 2013).

The diagnosis has been formalized in more domain-specific diagnostic systems. For example, exploding head syndrome made its first appearance as a formal diagnosis in the *International Classification of Sleep Disorders—2nd Edition* (ICSD-2). The more recent ICSD-3 (American Academy of Sleep Medicine, 2014) continues to include exploding head syndrome. Within both the ICSD-2 and ICSD-3, it is conceptualized as a sensory parasomnia.

SYMPTOMATOLOGY

There are three primary criteria for a diagnosis of exploding head syndrome per ICSD-3 (American Academy of Sleep Medicine, 2014, p. 264). These include (a) the perception of a loud noise or sense of explosion in the head, which occurs suddenly at wake–sleep transitions, (b) abrupt arousal from the noises, and (c) a lack of significant pain. As is likely apparent, the noises of exploding head syndrome and the subsequent arousal from sleep are usually associated with high levels of fear and sometimes with anticipatory anxiety as well. The specific sounds reported during episodes of exploding head syndrome are quite variable and can include perceptions of fireworks, lightening cracks, or nondescript screaming (see Box 4.1). Episodes are generally painless and, in the case of the ICSD-3 criteria, necessarily so. The careful questioning of a reported pain experience usually reveals it to have been a misinterpretation of shock (Pearce, 1988).

There is a lack of consensus at present regarding the specific locations where the auditory disturbances of exploding head syndrome are "heard." Some individuals report that the noises take place within both ears simultaneously (Jacome, 2001),

---

Box 4.1

SOUNDS REPORTED DURING EXPLODING HEAD SYNDROME

Violent explosions	Fireworks
Noise like electric current	Soughing sound (as if by fire)
Enormous roar	Cars driving by
Beep	Whiplash
Door slam	Someone yelling
Crashing waves	Clash of cymbals
Bangs on a tin tray	Metallic noise
Electric "jolt"	Lightning crack
Loud twang like a breaking guitar string	Nearby thunder
Buzzing	Electric short circuit
Crash of noise (something giving way in the brain)	Snap like a Christmas cracker
Clap	Blow to the head
Video static	A bell struck once
Pistol or shotgun	

Note: From "Exploding head syndrome," by B. Sharpless, 2014, Sleep Medicine Reviews, 18, p. 490. Copyright 2014 by Elsevier. Reprinted with permission.

---

whereas others hear the sounds on only one side of the head (Ganguly, Mridha, Khan, & Rison, 2013). It is possible that perceptual differences among individuals could indicate distinct subtypes of exploding head syndrome, etiological variations, or simply individual differences.

In addition to the paradigmatic sounds, there are other common symptoms, which, although associated with the syndrome are not outlined in the ICSD-3. For example, nondescript visual perceptions (e.g., flashes of light or visual static) have been found to occur in roughly 10% of exploding head syndrome cases (Pearce, 1989). Additionally, sensations of intense heat as well as strange feelings in the upper central region of the abdomen have been reported in some individuals. Interestingly, electrical sensations flowing from the torso to the head may sometimes immediately precede the auditory explosions (Bowen, 1993). It is perhaps noteworthy that themes related to electricity in general can be found in descriptions of exploding head syndrome auditory content; for example, electric "jolts" have been reported, as have the sounds of electric currents and short circuits (e.g., see Box 4.1).

PREVALENCE RATE AND ASSOCIATED FEATURES

Prevalence rates for exploding head syndrome are currently difficult to ascertain for several reasons. Perhaps the most salient is the paucity of empirical investigations that employed non-case study designs. Some have hypothesized that exploding head syndrome is a rare condition (e.g., Ganguly et al., 2013), and the perceived rarity of exploding head syndrome appeared to be the norm until fairly recently. There are likely two primary reasons for this belief. The first is that the number of individuals presenting for treatment of exploding head syndrome symptoms *alone* is quite rare (Pearce, 1988). Although exploding head syndrome symptoms are associated with fear and distress within the confines of any one particular *episode*, significant levels of clinical interference are relatively uncommon, although they do indeed occur (Sharpless, 2015). A second reason for the perceived rarity could simply be that individuals are reluctant or ashamed to report such experiences to others (especially medical professionals) for fear of embarrassment. The vast majority of patients are also unlikely to ever be *directly* asked about the specific symptoms of exploding head syndrome, and it stands to reason that spontaneous reports of such "unusual" perceptual experiences (especially if such experiences were not causing pervasive distress and/or impairment) would lead to underestimates of the true prevalence rate.

Perceptions aside, the existent literature and at least one recent large-scale study suggest that exploding head syndrome is more common than initially thought. For example, in one investigation involving 180 total participants, it was found that 13.8% of psychiatric patients, 10% of patients with a sleep disorder, and 10.7% of healthy control subjects reported exploding head syndrome symptoms on a self-report measure (Fulda et al., 2008). In an attempt to assess the validity of the self-report measure used, a randomly selected subset (n = 36) of this group engaged in a clinical interview where the exploding head syndrome rate remained at 11.1% (Fulda et al., 2008). An additional examination, which involved a self-report questionnaire employed on the Internet, found a lifetime prevalence rate of 50%, although certain methodological issues, such as unclear language within the question, were acknowledged by the author (Sherwood, 1999).

A recent study utilized a semistructured diagnostic interview and trained raters in order to assess exploding head syndrome prevalence rates among college students (Sharpless, 2015). A total of 211 undergraduate students participated in the study. The sample was young ($M = 19.7$ years old), ethnically diverse (40.5% identified as non-Caucasian), and primarily female (70.6%). Of note, participants who endorsed experiences consistent with isolated sleep paralysis were oversampled in the study. Results of the clinical interview (i.e., the *Exploding Head Syndrome Interview* described below) indicated that 18.0% of the sample had experienced at least one episode of exploding head syndrome; the vast majority of these individuals experienced recurrent cases of the syndrome (i.e., 16.6% of the sample). Consistent with study hypotheses, those diagnosed with isolated sleep paralysis episodes evidenced higher rates of exploding head syndrome (36.6%). When participants with isolated sleep paralysis were eliminated, the exploding head syndrome prevalence rate reduced to 13.5%, which was still higher than expected.

In terms of potential gender differences in exploding head syndrome, initial evidence suggested a greater proportion of females. Sharpless (2014) aggregated all published cases of exploding head syndrome from 1988 to 2014 in which gender was known ($N = 112$). The results of this analysis produced a 1.55–1 female-to-male ratio. Another review of the exploding head syndrome literature was conducted using slightly different search criteria (total $N = 76$), which also found the female-to-male ratio to be approximately 1.5–1 (Frese, Summ, & Evers, 2014). It is important to note that although this second review of the exploding head syndrome literature may have differed in terms of the search engines and inclusion criteria used, there was likely a high degree of overlap between the samples in these two reviews. The above-mentioned student study found that exploding head syndrome was not more common in young adult females than males (Sharpless, 2015). However, the possibility remains that the frequency of exploding head syndrome episodes may increase with age according to sex.

THEORIES OF ETIOLOGY

A variety of etiological theories exist for exploding head syndrome (see Sharpless, 2014, for a review) but the most popular of these implicates neuronal dysfunctions within the brainstem during sleep-wake transitions (e.g., Chakravarty, 2007). The normal transition from wakefulness to sleep involves the reduction of activity within the reticular formation. This reduced activity results in the temporary shutdown of areas associated with auditory, visual, and motor experience. It has been proposed that the perceptual experiences in exploding head syndrome are the result of a partial dysfunction in this overall "switching off" process (i.e., in the form of delays). These delays may, in turn, give rise to abnormal surges of neuronal activity which are perceived as the loud and startling nondescript sounds (and occasional visual experiences) found in exploding head syndrome.

Despite the popularity of the brainstem dysfunction hypothesis, several other proposed etiologies for exploding head syndrome have been put forth. Some have conceptualized exploding head syndrome as a side effect of rapid withdrawal from selective serotonin reuptake inhibitors (SSRIs) or benzodiazepines. Interestingly, electric-shock-like sensations in the scalp and "whooshing" noises in the ears have been noted as characteristics of the SSRI discontinuation syndrome (Haddad & Dursun, 2008). Further, such "electric" features (Sharpless, 2014) are perhaps similar to those experienced by individuals with exploding head syndrome. The last, and perhaps the most intuitively appealing, of the proposed etiologies of exploding head syndrome involve a host of possible ear dysfunctions. Examples include the sudden perturbation of components within the middle ear or Eustachian tube (Armstrong-Jones, 1920), labyrinthine membrane ruptures (in particular of the round window), and perilymph fistulas (Gordon, 1988).

ASSESSMENT OPTIONS

Until very recently there were few formal assessment options. The *Duke Structured Clinical Interview for Sleep Disorders* (Edinger et al., 2004) contains prompts specifically designed to assess for the ICSD-2 diagnostic criteria of exploding head syndrome. Although these prompts are not comprehensive if one wants to assess both the severity of exploding head syndrome episodes and associated features (e.g., specific symptoms), they are clear and concise for use in clinical settings.

A self-report measure titled the *Munich Parasomnia Screening* (Fulda et al., 2008) contains a single item on past and present exploding head syndrome episodes. If a current episode is endorsed, participants are further prompted to complete a five-point-frequency scale ranging from "very seldom" to "almost every night." The psychometric properties of this exploding head syndrome item appear to be good (Fulda et al., 2008). Thus, Fulda et al.'s (2008) measure is likely a very useful screening measure, but additional information may be needed to answer other research questions. Brevity, particularly in self-report measures, may sacrifice diagnostic accuracy, given that more specific questions relevant to differential diagnosis are likely needed with exploding head syndrome and other lesser-known disorders.

Situating the assessment of exploding head syndrome within a broader medical/psychiatric/sleep disorder assessment would likely not only lead to more valid diagnoses, but might further elucidate the particular relations between exploding head syndrome and other conditions. Such considerations led to the development of the *Exploding Head Syndrome Interview* (EHSI; Sharpless, 2015). The EHSI is a semistructured diagnostic interview specifically designed to assess for exploding head syndrome according to ICSD-3 criteria. The clinical interview was modeled after modules of the *Anxiety and Related Disorders*

Interview Schedule for DSM-5 (ADIS-5; Brown & Barlow, 2014). Thus, the EHSI allows for an assessment of the frequency of exploding head syndrome episodes, dimensional ratings of individual symptom severities, and overall ratings of distress and interference. Importantly, the interview includes a variety of items relevant for differential diagnosis (e.g., migraine headaches and seizure disorders). The EHSI is intended to be administered by trained clinicians with general diagnostic acumen and a specific knowledge of exploding head syndrome.

DIFFERENTIAL DIAGNOSIS

Misdiagnosis can occur with exploding head syndrome for a variety of reasons. Perhaps the most fundamental is the simple fact that it is so rarely assessed in clinical settings. Although exploding head syndrome can produce significant levels of distress in some individuals (Sharpless, 2015), it is rarely the *primary* presenting concern for patients seeking healthcare services. This does not represent a "misdiagnosis" in the traditional sense, but rather the *absence* of a diagnosis and an inability to receive potentially reassuring information regarding the syndrome (viz., that it is not dangerous). Further, when patients do spontaneously report exploding head syndrome symptoms to providers there is potential for misdiagnosis because some healthcare providers may be unfamiliar with exploding head syndrome and ill-equipped to accurately distinguish its symptomatology from other conditions.

When exploding head syndrome is assessed, it is clearly important that the primary features be distinguished from other conditions. First, it is important to distinguish between exploding head syndrome and various manifestations of headache (e.g., thunderclap headaches, migraine cluster headaches). Exploration of four areas by clinicians may serve to distinguish these phenomena. Specifically, the *duration* of episodes, the *timing* of episodes, the lateralization of symptoms, and the issue of *pain* should be considered. Exploding head syndrome episodes are brief in duration (i.e., one or more seconds), occur in the transition from wakefulness to sleep or sleep to wakefulness, and are generally (though not always) described as occurring in the "whole head" (as opposed to a specific localized area). Further, the issue of pain can help to reduce misdiagnosis substantially. Pain in exploding head syndrome, if present, is mild and transient. If it is more severe, one should look toward other conditions (e.g., subarachnoid hemorrhages). The many headache syndromes, in contrast, can be characterized as producing both severe and persistent pain. These features would clearly distinguish them from exploding head syndrome.

Two additional areas of differential diagnosis worth elaborating upon are nightmare disorder and post-traumatic stress disorder (especially flashbacks involving gunfire and/or explosions). Importantly, the loud noises sometimes experienced by individuals with these conditions occur within the context of dreams and flashbacks. In this sense, the content of the loud noises in these two disorders is more elaborate and thematic than that which is typically found in exploding head syndrome (i.e., the sounds represent content that is consistent with the broader dream/flashback). In contrast, the sounds of exploding head syndrome appear to be fairly undifferentiated. For example, in the earliest known description of the syndrome by Mitchell, one of his patients named "Mr. V," experienced, "... a sense of a pistol shot ..." while at other times he noted "... the sound of a bell, which has been struck once ... or else I hear a loud noise, which is most like that of a guitar string, rudely struck, and which breaks with a twang" (Mitchell, 1876, p. 780). These exploding head syndrome sounds are not representative of other perceptions, dream-like or otherwise, but appear in isolation and are very short in duration.

TREATMENT OPTIONS

As noted previously, case studies represent the bulk of the exploding head syndrome literature, and no clinical trials have yet been conducted. Several promising attempts, however, have been made to treat exploding head syndrome with pharmacological agents. The tricyclic antidepressant clomipramine, administered at doses of 50 milligrams and taken at night, was helpful in at least three documented patients with exploding head syndrome (Sachs & Svanborg, 1991). More recently, amitriptyline has been utilized with somewhat mixed results (Frese et al., 2014). In one case, the drug had no significant effect on a patient's exploding head syndrome; however, another patient with episodes occurring up to several times each night found that it significantly decreased the frequency of episodes. A third case study found that amitriptyline administered in the evening was associated with a near complete remission of episodes (Frese et al., 2014). Of note, the dosage in these three cases ranged from 25 milligrams to 50 milligrams, and two of the three patients reported adverse side effects as a result of the medication.

Tricyclic antidepressants do not exhaust all attempted pharmacological interventions for exploding head syndrome. Responses to flunarizine at 10 milligrams a day and slow-release nifedipine at 90 milligrams a day suggest that calcium channel blockers may be useful in the treatment of exploding head syndrome (Chakravarty, 2007; Jacome, 2001). Both medications reduced exploding head syndrome in a total of three cases. The anticonvulsant topiramate at 200 milligrams a day lessened the intensity of exploding head syndrome episodes (i.e., it reduced the volume of the bangs to a low buzzing noise), but did not eliminate episodes in one patient (Palikh & Vaughn, 2010). The anticonvulsant carbamazepine prescribed within a range of 200 milligrams to 400 milligrams a day, produced positive results in three individuals (Declerck & Arends, 1994). A very recent case study found no therapeutic response from long-term treatment with carbamazepine even after titrating up to the maximum dose. Specific dosages, however, were not cited in the report (Feketeova, Buskova, Skorvanek, Mudra, & Gdovinova, 2014).

Nonpharmacological interventions may also be useful in treating exploding head syndrome. One case study found that the treatment of sleep apnea with an oral breathing device resulted in a remission of exploding head syndrome symptoms (Okura, Taniguchi, Muraki, Sugita, & Ohi, 2010). Additional indirect evidence for the role of comorbid sleep disorders can be seen in a recent case study wherein obstructive sleep apnea was diagnosed *prior* to the onset of exploding head syndrome (Frese et al., 2014), but further causal data would be helpful.

Finally, it is worth mentioning the most straightforward and least intrusive intervention for exploding head syndrome. Specifically, it is the contention of some researchers that simply *educating* individuals about exploding head syndrome, and reassuring them that it is a fairly benign condition may, in-and-of-itself, represent an effective treatment (Casucci, d'Onofrio, & Torelli, 2004; Sachs & Svanborg, 1991). In one report, reassurance resulted in the remission of exploding head syndrome episodes at a six-month follow-up (Ganguly et al., 2013). Further, regardless of its efficacy in terms of symptom reduction, it is important that healthcare providers (who are confident that exploding head syndrome is the actual concern) provide this information to their patients. Equipping patients with greater knowledge of exploding head syndrome may empower them to make more informed decisions regarding their own medical treatment (e.g., Spring, 2007). For example, in one case study, a patient with exploding head syndrome was being treated with amitriptyline but was experiencing aversive side effects (Frese et al., 2014). When informed of the relatively benign nature of exploding head syndrome by a medical professional, the patient was reported to have chosen to discontinue the medication and to not seek further treatment for the syndrome (Frese et al., 2014).

RECOMMENDATIONS FOR FUTURE WORK

There is undoubtedly much more to discover about exploding head syndrome. What could be viewed as a silver lining to this lack of knowledge is that future research endeavors need not be terribly complicated or resource-heavy in order to make substantial contributions to the field's understanding of this phenomenon. Although case studies and self-report measures are invaluable methods for exploring any phenomenon that is not well-understood, such designs are not without their limitations (e.g., the potential for false positive responding). Such limitations may be reduced, at least in part, through the use of clinical interviews.

Additional knowledge of prevalence rates is needed. Although one recent study found that it was surprisingly common, even in younger individuals (Sharpless, 2015), more specific data are needed for other ages and populations. Such research may begin to clarify the mixed findings regarding sex differences. Additionally, the associations between exploding head syndrome and other conditions represent a promising area for future inquiry. Research into risk factors (i.e., medical and behavioral) that could render some individuals more prone to exploding head syndrome episodes also may be fruitful. Additionally, the relationship between symptoms of exploding head syndrome and anomalous beliefs and fantasy-proneness appears to be an interesting avenue. This line of research could shed light on the variability across *interpretations* of exploding head syndrome symptoms and perhaps even on causal mechanism(s) among exploding head syndrome, anomalous experiences, and anomalous beliefs.

Within the clinical realm more specifically, assessing for exploding head syndrome in routine clinical settings is advisable given that (a) patients appear to rarely report this syndrome spontaneously and (b) psychoeducation alone may be an effective intervention. Prior to this reassurance, however, it is vital that practitioners utilize their clinical judgment and take the time necessary to eliminate possible competing diagnoses by noting symptoms that are not characteristically associated with exploding head syndrome (e.g., severe levels of pain). Perhaps the most important future work will be research into the clinical implications of exploding head syndrome (i.e., those individuals who experience clinically significant levels of distress and/or impairment) as well as the development of effective treatment options. As noted above, one study using clinical interviews found that approximately 2.80% of a relatively large sample experienced exploding head syndrome to such a degree that it met criteria for clinical significance (Sharpless, 2015).

The available literature on treatment options for exploding head syndrome is a rather scattered landscape of individual case studies across heterogeneous patients. Not surprisingly, this makes generalizations somewhat hazardous. Even with the limited positive responses to treatment, in the absence of good experimental controls it remains difficult to attribute remission or reduction of exploding head symptoms to the actual treatment. Thus, larger trials, open or (preferably) randomized, would be helpful supplements to the case study literature. Further, should reliable psychological factors be found to play an important role in the genesis or maintenance of exploding head syndrome, psychotherapeutic approaches should also be developed.

Finally, it may be useful to evaluate whether "exploding head syndrome" is the most appropriate name for this experience. Although vivid and certainly memorable, it is, at best, an incomplete description of this parasomnia. Goadsby and Sharpless (2016) recently proposed an alternative label (viz., episodic cranial sensory shock). They argue that this phrase is not only more accurate (given that there clearly are no "real" explosions in EHS), but that it also encompasses the nonauditory experiences (e.g., light flashes) and better attributes the phenomenon to Mitchell.

REFERENCES

American Academy of Sleep Medicine. (2014). *International classification of sleep disorders: Diagnostic and coding manual* (3rd ed.). Darien, IL: American Academy of Sleep Medicine.

American Psychiatric Association. (2013). *Diagnostic and statistical manual of mental disorders: DSM-V* (5th ed.). Arlington, VA: American Psychiatric Association.

Armstrong-Jones, R. (1920). Snapping of the brain. *Lancet, 196,* 720. doi:10.1016/
s0140-6736(01)19805-3

Bowen, J. (1993). More things that go bang in the night. *New England Journal of Medicine,*
328, 1570–1571. doi:10.1056/nejm199305273282116

Brown, T.A., & Barlow, D.H. (2014). *Anxiety and related disorders interview schedule for*
DSM-5: Lifetime version. New York, NY: Oxford University Press.

Casucci, G., d'Onofrio, F., & Torelli, P. (2004). Rare primary headaches: Clinical insights.
Neurological Sciences: Official Journal of the Italian Neurological Society and of the Italian
Society of Clinical Neurophysiology, 25, S77–S83. doi:10.1007/s10072-004-0258-8

CBS, Atlanta. (2014). 'Gang-stalking' and electronic mind control community spreads
online. Retrieved from http://atlanta.cbslocal.com/2014/05/17/gang-stalking-and-
electronic-mind-control-community-spreads-online/

Chakravarty, A. (2007). Exploding head syndrome: Report of two new cases.
Cephalalgia: An International Journal of Headache, 28, 399–400. doi:10.1111/
j.1468-2982.2007.01522.x

Declerck, A.C., & Arends, J.B. (1994). An exceptional case of parasomnia: The exploding
head syndrome. *Sleep-Wake Research in the Netherlands, 5,* 41–43.

Edinger, J.D., Bonnet, M.H., Bootzin, R.R., Doghramji, K., Dorsey, C.M., Espie, C. A., . . .
Stepanski, E.J. (2004). Derivation of research diagnostic criteria for insomnia: Report
of an American academy of sleep medicine work group. *Sleep, 27,* 1567–1596.

Evans, R.W. (2006). Case studies of uncommon headaches. *Neurologic Clinics, 24,* 347–
362. doi:10.1016/j.ncl.2006.01.006

Feketeova, E., Buskova, J., Skorvanek, M., Mudra, J., & Gdovinova, Z. (2014). Exploding
head syndrome—a rare parasomnia or a dissociative episode? *Sleep Medicine, 15,*
728–730. doi:10.1016/j.sleep.2014.02.011

Foundation Stop Electronic Weapons Stop Gang Stalking. (2015). Stop electronic weapons stop gang stalking. Retrieved from https://www.stopeg.com/

Frese, A., Summ, O., & Evers, S. (2014). Exploding head syndrome: Six new cases and
review of the literature. *Cephalalgia: An International Journal of Headache, 34,* 823–
827. doi:10.1177/0333102414536059

Fulda, S., Hornyak, M., Muller, K., Cerny, L., Beitinger, P.A., & Wetter, T.C. (2008).
Development and validation of the Munich parasomnia screening (MUPS): A questionnaire for parasomnias and nocturnal behaviors. *Somnologie, 12,* 56–65.
doi:10.1007/s11818-008-0336-x

Ganguly, G., Mridha, B., Khan, A., & Rison, R.A. (2013). Exploding head syndrome: A case report. *Case Reports in Neurology, 5,* 14–17. doi:10.1159/000346595

Goadsby, P., & Sharpless, B.A. (2016). Exploding head syndrome, snapping of the brain,
or episodic cranial sensory shock? *Journal of Neurology, Neurosurgery & Psychiatry.*
Advance online publication. doi:10.1136/jnnp-2015-312617

Gordon, A.G. (1988). Exploding head. *Lancet, 332,* 625–626. doi:10.1016/
s0140-6736(88)90658-7

Haddad, P.M., & Dursun, S.M. (2008). Neurological complications of psychiatric
drugs: Clinical features and management. *Human Psychopharmacology, 23(Suppl 1),*
15–26. doi:10.1002/hup.918

Jacome, D.E. (2001). Exploding head syndrome and idiopathic stabbing headache
relieved by nifedipine. *Cephalalgia: An International Journal of Headache, 21,* 617–
618. doi:10.1046/j.1468-2982.2001.00227.x

Kershaw, S. (2008). Sharing their demons on the web. *The New York Times*, p. E1. Retrieved from http://www.nytimes.com/2008/11/13/fashion/13psych.html?

Mitchell, S.W. (1876). On some of the disorders of sleep. *Virginia Medical Monthly*, 2, 769–781.

Morin, C.M. (1993). *Insomnia: Psychological assessment and management.* New York, NY: The Guilford Press.

Okura, M., Taniguchi, M., Muraki, H., Sugita, H., & Ohi, M. (2010). Case of exploding head syndrome. *Brain Nerve*, 62, 85–88.

Palikh, G.M., & Vaughn, B.V. (2010). Topiramate responsive exploding head syndrome. *Journal of Clinical Sleep Medicine: JCSM: Official Publication of the American Academy of Sleep Medicine*, 6, 382–383.

Pearce, J.M. (1988). Exploding head syndrome. *Lancet*, 2, 270–271. doi:10.1016/s0140-6736(88)92551-2

Pearce, J.M. (1989). Clinical features of the exploding head syndrome. *Journal of Neurology, Neurosurgery, and Psychiatry*, 52, 907–910. doi:10.1136/jnnp.52.7.907

Oliver, R.K. (2010). Directed energy weapons electronic harassment symptoms. Retrieved from http://satelliteterrorism3.blogspot.com/2010/12/dew-directed-energy-weapons.html

Sachs, C., & Svanborg, E. (1991). The exploding head syndrome: Polysomnographic recordings and therapeutic suggestions. *Sleep*, 14, 263–266.

Sharpless, B.A. (2014). Exploding head syndrome. *Sleep Medicine Reviews*, 18, 489–493. doi: 10.1016/j.smrv.2014.03.001

Sharpless, B.A. (2015). Exploding head syndrome is common in college students. *Journal of Sleep Research*, 24, 447–449. doi:10.1111/jsr.12292

Sherwood, S.J. (1999). Relationship between childhood hypnagogic, hypnopompic, and sleep experiences, childhood fantasy proneness, and anomalous experiences and beliefs: An exploratory WWW survey. *The Journal of the American Society for Psychical Research*, 93, 167–197.

Spring, B. (2007). Evidence-based practice in clinical psychology: What it is, why it matters; what you need to know. *Journal of Clinical Psychology*, 63, 611–631. doi:10.1002/jclp.20373

World Health Organization. (2008). *International statistical classification of diseases and related health problems* (10th ed.). Geneva, Switzerland: World Health Organization.

Variations of Psychosis

5

Capgras and Other
Misidentification Syndromes

ARTHUR SINKMAN ■

VIGNETTE

Alex's main complaint when brought to my office by his parents was that he was upset that he had not seen his family in over a year. Referring to his father, mother, and several siblings, Alex complained, "They're all missing." He called the family that he was living with "fakes." He believed that his real parents were in another country, and he wanted to travel there to see them. Alex missed his family, wanted them back, and was annoyed about what had happened.

It was not just his immediate family who were "fakes" but other relatives, neighbors, and some of his friends, including his minister. Alex said that the FBI was involved and that agents used security cameras to videotape him.

When interviewed, Alex had an odd stare and a strange demeanor. He was preoccupied with the substitution and was otherwise guarded, vague, and evasive. He did not show loose associations or a formal thought disorder and denied hearing voices.

Over the previous three years, Alex had experienced a steady deterioration in his functioning, with increasing social isolation and withdrawal. Several months prior to coming to my office Alex became anxious and compulsive. His appetite was poor and he lost weight. He had trouble sleeping. He subsequently had an aggressive outburst and was hospitalized on a psychiatric unit. He was given a full evaluation, including magnetic resonance imaging (MRI) and electroencephalography (EEG). Treated with olanzapine, he calmed down but his delusions did not improve.

The patient was started on perphenazine. This was effective in reversing the delusions. Unfortunately, Alex did not continue taking the medication. He became delusional again and was rehospitalized.

HISTORICAL AND CULTURAL CONTEXT

Alex suffered from the Capgras Syndrome. This is the delusional belief that the people around him are not who they seem to be but are look-alike impostors. These phonies are believed to be duplicates who have been substituted for the originals. The real/original person is believed to be somewhere else. The copy looks just like the original, although sometimes the patient notices minor imaginary differences between the original and the copy, differences that the patient cites as confirmation that the person in front of him is an impostor. The delusion concerns mis-identity, or more precisely, the denial or negation of a person's identity, and the substitution of one person for another.

The syndrome was named in honor of Joseph Capgras, the French psychiatrist who, along with his intern, Dr. Jean Reboul-Lachaux, published the first case description of a patient with this unusual condition in 1923.

Several years after Dr. Capgras's report appeared, two other French psychiatrists, Paul Courbon and G. Fail, reported another unusual case marked by delusional mis-identity and the substitution of one person for another. Their patient, a 27-year-old woman suffering from schizophrenia, believed that she was being pursued by two famous actresses who took on the forms of various people that the woman knew or met, often strangers. These tormentors harassed and controlled the patient, including taking over her thoughts and making her do things. They named her condition the Fregoli Syndrome.

Unlike the Capgras Syndrome (CS), the Fregoli Syndrome (FS) was not named in honor of the clinicians who reported the first case. Rather, it was named after Leopoldo Fregoli, a famous actor who was able to change his appearance and dress quickly during a performance and appear as many different characters. His performance was similar to the patient's delusional experience.

Although both FS and CS concern mis-identity and substitution, in a certain sense they are opposites. In FS, strangers are identified as familiar while in CS familiar people become strangers. A patient with FS hyper-identifies people, adding an identity, while someone with CS hypo-identifies people, negating someone's identity. In other words, in FS there is a delusion of positive doubles while in CS there is a delusion of negative doubles.

Five years after FS was first described another syndrome involving change in identity was reported: the Intermetamorphosis Syndrome. Patients with this condition believe someone they know has been transformed into another person. The transformed person changes both his appearance and his identity and actually becomes that other person.

Years later another syndrome of delusional misidentification was described, the Syndrome of Subjective Doubles, in which the patient believes that another person exists who is his duplicate (Christodoulou, 1978). A variant of this is the patient who believes that he himself is an impostor. This syndrome often occurs along with CS in the same patient (Kamanitz, 1989).

In 1981, Christodoulou lumped together the four misidentification syndromes, Capgras, Fregoli, Intermetamorphosis, and Subjective Doubles, and designated them the Delusional Misidentification Syndromes, or DMS. Christodoulou believed that all four DMS delusions should be considered "variants of the same basic condition" (Christodoulou & Malliara-Loulakaki, 1981, p.246). Of the four, CS is by far the most common and Intermetamorphosis the least. These various delusions can occur together in a single patient, and a patient can have different delusions at different times.

It is not only people who can be substituted. Some patients believe that certain inanimate objects are not the originals, but have been replaced by look-alike duplicates. This is a variant of the Capgras delusion (Anderson & Williams, 1994).

Related to DMS is a rare neurological condition, Reduplicative Paramnesia, first described by Arnold Pick in 1903, 20 years before Capgras. In this condition the patient believes that a place has been duplicated; it exists simultaneously in two or more locations. For instance, the patient has the idea that the building where he is located has a duplicate that is located elsewhere. This condition involves duplication but not substitution.

Clinicians frequently encounter patients with delusions concerning mis-identity that are not one of the four DMS (Mojtabai, 1998), such as the delusional belief that multiple copies ("clones") of a single person exist. Clinicians have struggled to name and classify these various conditions (Markova, 1994; Banov et al., 1993; Rossner, 2002). Another tactic would be to consider these various delusions as more similar than different and part of a large group of misidentification delusions, thereby eschewing the need for separate classification. This was the approach in Germany for many years, in contrast to the French tradition of naming syndromes such as Capgras and Fregoli (Mojtabai, 1998).

ROLE IN CURRENT DIAGNOSTIC SYSTEMS

Initially, CS was considered to be a unique syndrome. It soon became apparent, however, that all patients who had this condition also were suffering from a major mental illness, most commonly schizophrenia. Other diagnoses included schizoaffective disorder, bipolar disorder, major depression, schizophreniform disorder, and delusional disorder (Forstl, 1991; Salvatore, 2014). A consensus developed that CS was not a condition in its own right, but rather a symptom of another mental illness. Thus, entries on CS are not found in current editions of either the *Diagnostic and Statistical Manual of Mental Disorders* (American Psychiatric Association, 2013) or the *International Classification of Mental and Behavioral Disorders* (WHO, 1993).

For many years it was believed that CS only developed in functional psychoses such as schizophrenia and not in patients with a brain injury. A "clear sensorium" was considered a hallmark of CS (Enoch et al., 1967, p.7). It is now recognized, however, that CS commonly occurs in patients with brain conditions. Most often seen in degenerative diseases of the brain, CS also has been reported in cerebrovascular disease, traumatic conditions, epilepsy, and other neurological illnesses, as well as in delirium and toxic metabolic conditions (Josephs, 2007).

SYMPTOMATOLOGY

The diagnosis of CS rests on confirming the presence of a delusion of substitution, that is, the fixed delusional belief that someone has been replaced by a look-alike impostor. The other DMS are likewise each diagnosed by observing in the patient the specific misidentification delusion that has been described for that condition.

PREVALENCE RATE AND ASSOCIATED FEATURES

For many years CS was considered so rare that individual cases or small series were reported in the scientific literature. Only 46 cases of CS were reported in the English literature in the half century that followed its initial description in 1923 (Merrin, 1976). Studies showed the incidence of CS was a small fraction of 1% (Fishbain, 1987). Other reports, however, began to show that the incidence was far higher, up to 5.3% of all psychiatric admissions and 15% of all admitted schizophrenic patients (Dohn & Crews, 1986).

In the next decade several well-designed and large prospective studies in various settings showed that the incidence of DMS in psychiatric admissions was in the range of 1.3% to 4.1 % (Kirov, 1994; Huang, 1999; Tamam, 2003; Joseph, 1994). More recently, two excellent studies reported a much higher incidence of 14% and 28%, respectively (Salvatore, 2014; Odom-White, 1995). The 28% figure appeared in a study of chronic treatment-resistant patients admitted to a clozapine unit. This is similar to my own clinical experience of seeing a high incidence of misidentification delusions in patients with chronic, treatment-resistant schizophrenia. In fact, a misidentification delusion is often a marker for severe schizophrenia.

There is also a significant incidence of misidentification delusions in patients suffering from Alzheimer's Disease, 7%–10% (Harwood, 1999; Mizrahi, 2006). Of note is the frequent occurrence of all types of delusions in Alzheimer's patients, 40% (Mizrahi, 2006; Mega, 1996; Murray, 2014). Given that the number of people suffering from Alzheimer's is enormous (estimated at five million in the United States) a rate of 7%–10% means that the total number of Alzheimer's patients with misidentification delusions is very large. In Dementia with Lewy Bodies, the incidence of CS is 20%, which is higher than it is in Alzheimer's (Josephs, 2007; Thaipisuttikul, 2013). This is similarly the case with of all types of delusions (Del Ser et al., 2000).

This significant incidence of DMS in schizophrenia along with its common occurrence in patients with Alzheimer's and Dementia with Lewy Bodies, as well as in other cases of brain injury, tells us that CS and the other DMS should no longer be considered rare or unusual, just very interesting.

It is important to note that CS can be either a primary condition (i.e., when it is part of a "primary mental illness," an illness without a clearly identifiable cause such as schizophrenia), or it can be a secondary condition when it is the direct result of an organic disease of the brain. The primary and secondary versions differ significantly in their presentation (Malloy, 1992; Madoz-Gurpide, 2010). When it is a primary condition CS is often associated with other delusions, particularly paranoia, which often precedes it. This is not the case when it is a secondary condition. In addition, when it is a primary condition the patient is more likely to be angry or violent toward the substituted person, whereas those with an underlying brain disease tend to respond to the substitution with a calm, indifferent, or puzzled manner.

This propensity to violence in primary cases is understandable given the tendency of those with CS to view the misidentified person with suspicion and hostility (Klein, 2014). An infamous case of this appeared in my hometown. A dismembered body, stuffed into a suitcase and two cardboard boxes, was found floating in the local marina and a nearby river. Walter Carlaftes was arrested for the murder and dismemberment of his sister, Maria Caputo. Carlaftes had a long history of paranoid schizophrenia. For many years he believed that his family had been replaced by alien clones. At his trial he denied that the murder victim was his sister (Gray, 1992).

There are other differences between primary and secondary cases. The former are more likely to have a gradual symptom onset before age 40 years. Reduplication of place is more common in secondary DMS, whereas self-misidentification is more common in primary cases (Forstl, 1991). In secondary cases, the impostors do not change over time (Feinberg et al., 2005) This is unlike the situation in schizophrenia where the delusions can vary.

These differences have led some observers to conclude that the primary and secondary forms of CS are distinct from each other and have different causes. They consider CS a final common pathway (Malloy, 1992; Sinkman, 2008; Madoz-Gurpide, 2010). In contrast to this dichotomy, other experts minimize the difference between the primary and secondary versions. Instead, they believe that the cause of CS is the same in all conditions and that all such patients have an admixture of brain damage and paranoia that combines in various ways to cause the delusion (Fleminger, 1993; Breen et al., 2000). These doctors maintain that all patients with delusional misidentification are on a continuum from paranoia on one end to brain damage on the other end. Of course, it should not be forgotten that schizophrenia itself is a brain disease frequently marked by cognitive impairment. This is true whether or not DMS is present.

The traditional description of the Capgras delusion is that "the delusion of doubles assumes a central dominating role in the symptomatology" (Enoch, 1967, p.1). Oftentimes, however, the Capgras delusion is just one of many delusions and not the central feature of the psychosis (Sinkman, 2008). It can be fleeting and change form over time, particularly in severely ill patients suffering from chronic schizophrenia. In addition, misidentification delusions show a great degree of overlap and coexistence (Forstl, 1991; Klein, 2014; Weinstein, 1994).

A common assumption has been that the replacement delusion in CS always involves members of the patient's family. In a significant number of cases, however, the duplicated people have only a limited relationship with the patient or are strangers. In other cases the patient's delusion about impostors starts with his immediate family being duplicated and then slowly expands to include others. This is what happened to Mrs. M., the original patient described by Capgras. Her delusion began with her children being duplicated, expanded to include the rest of her family, including herself, and then spread further to include all those with whom she had contact. She eventually believed that thousands of people all over Paris had disappeared. They had been abducted and substituted, with many of them held prisoner under the streets of the city. One expert has labeled this "the delirium of doubles" (Todd, 1957).

Regarding Capgras's patient, it is important to note that she had other delusions. She believed that she was the victim of an elaborate persecutory conspiracy and was the daughter of a duke and heiress to a vast fortune. She claimed that she was a member of a royal family, "de Rio-Branco." She called herself Mrs. de Rio-Branco, instead of Mrs. M.

Mrs. M's delusion of wealth and lineage seems to be a grandiose delusion. However, it also involved Mrs. M. assuming a new identity and appeared to be part of her extensive system of identity delusions, which included the idea that she had been replaced and that she had a double.

Oftentimes what is labeled a grandiose delusion involves the patient assuming the identity of a famous or powerful person. What on the surface appears to be a grandiose delusion also can be understood as a mis-identity delusion. Typically, patients state that a person they know is not who they claim to be, but is actually a celebrity or historical figure (Mojtabi, 1998). An example is my patient with CS who in addition to believing that his mother was replaced by an identical impostor also believed that his sister was replaced by LaToya Jackson and that he was Michael Jackson.

Categorizing some grandiose delusions as misidentification delusions highlights the fact that misidentification delusions are more common than assumed. One expert, Cutting (1994), wrote that "no less than 40%" of the schizophrenics he treated had some form of delusional misidentification (p. 235). Likewise, in the German literature these delusions are more commonly recognized (Mojtabai, 1998).

A problem in recognizing the frequency of misidentification delusions is that clinicians have not been trained to look for them. Until recently, textbooks omitted misidentification delusions from their list of delusions, relegating CS to the category of unusual psychiatric syndromes. This also is the case with most rating scales. If one considers these conditions rare then one is not going to look for them or find them.

THEORIES OF ETIOLOGY

Neurology

There is convincing evidence that disorders of the brain can cause CS, the other DMS, and reduplicative paramnesia. These delusions are associated with damage to specific areas of the brain, most commonly the right hemisphere (Feinberg & Roanne, 2005; Fleminger, 1993). When the injury is on the right side the most common pattern is frontal damage along with a variable temporal and parietal component. It is extremely rare for DMS to develop when the injury is restricted to the left hemisphere.

Although damage to the right side of the brain is most common, DMS also develops in patients with bilateral damage (Joseph, 1999). These delusions commonly occur in patients with damage to both frontal lobes, whether or not there is damage to other areas of the right hemisphere (Malloy, 1992; Edelstyn, 1999; Devinsky, 2009). In a study of 29 DMS patients all but one had a lesion in one or both of the frontal lobes (Feinberg & Deluca, 2005).

Specific mental functions are subserved by different regions of the brain. The sense of identity is associated with the right side of the brain, particularly the right frontal lobe (Cutting, 1991; Feinberg & Roane, 2005). An injury to the frontal lobes, especially on the right side, can impair the ability to monitor the self (including ego boundaries) and damage memory and familiarity. These issues of identity and monitoring of the self are important in the development of delusions about identity.

If the left hemisphere remains undamaged it can create a false explanation to fill in the gaps left by the defective right hemisphere. This can include creating a delusional impostor to resolve conflicting information. "Delusions result from right hemisphere lesions. But it is the left hemisphere that is deluded." (Devinsky, 2009, p. 850).

Injuries to the right temporal lobe are also important in the development of DMS (Feinberg & Shapiro, 1989; Mattioli, 1999) as is the disconnection of a functioning temporal lobe from the rest of the right hemisphere (Politis, 2012; Staton, 1982), most particularly disconnection of the frontal lobes from the temporal lobes and the limbic system. The limbic system itself is an area of concern (Oyebode, 2008).

The frequency of temporal lobe injuries in DMS patients is high (Malloy, 1994). Neurocognitive research has confirmed this importance of the temporal lobe in DMS, focusing on the role it plays in generating feelings of familiarity toward a face (Gainotti, 2007).

Much of this information on the role of specific brain regions in the development of delusional misidentification is based on case reports of patients with focal brain injuries. Many patients who develop DMS, however, do not have a focal injury but rather a generalized diffuse impairment of brain functioning as occurs in delirium or dementia (Feinberg & Roane, 2005). The neurologic basis of delusions in these patients is unclear. Research on Alzheimer's has yielded some information. Alzheimer's patients with delusions have a more severe impairment in functioning in the frontal lobe, particularly on the right side compared with those without delusions, once again implicating the frontal lobes in the formation of delusions. However, this refers to delusions in general. Alzheimer's patients with misidentification delusions show particular impairment in the temporal lobe, association areas, and connections to the frontal lobes (Mentis, 1995; Ismail, 2012). These findings suggest that the cause of DMS may be a disruption in brain network connectivity rather than a defect in a specific brain region (Sultzer, 2003). This is consistent with theories about network disruption causing schizophrenia (Woodward, 2015).

An alternative explanation of DMS in patients with diffuse brain injuries is that the cause is impaired neurotransmitter function rather than a focal injury. The high incidence of these delusions in Dementia with Lewy Bodies and the role of dopamine dysfunction in that condition supports that idea (Josephs, 2007).

Emotional Conflicts and Psychodynamic Theories

For many years it was assumed that there was no organic basis to CS. Rather, it was considered "a functional illness and as such is explained on a psychodynamic basis" (Enoch, 1967, p.5). During that time psychodynamic explanations held sway. The most popular theory involved the belief that mixed, ambivalent emotions felt toward the significant other were the starting point for the development of the duplicative delusion. Because the patient was severely conflicted over angry feelings and feared the consequences of expressing these feelings, the delusion of doubles helped to resolve this conflict such that all positive (acceptable) feelings were expressed toward the missing original person while the hostile unacceptable thoughts and urges were felt toward the duplicate. This compromise helped the patient avoid guilt over angry feelings and resolve anxiety. It was based on the overuse of the ego defenses of denial and displacement.

Although this theory can explain the delusion that a close family member has been duplicated, it is unable to account for other manifestations of CS (Sinkman, 1983) such as the delusional belief that strangers have been duplicated. Nor can it explain the frequently encountered co-occurrence of CS with FS and the Delusion of Subjective Doubles. In addition, it cannot account for the other symptoms of psychosis.

I have outlined below a new psychodynamic explanation of the illness suffered by Capgras's original patient (Mrs. M.) that is distinct from the ambivalence theory. It is based on information in the original case report.

According to Capgras, Mrs. M.'s illness began "during a crisis point ... following the death of four of her own [children]" (Ellis et al., 1994, p.127). In her delusion she believed that the deceased children were not her own but were substitutes. According to the patient, "I was thus at the burial of a child who was not mine" (p.122). Her delusion focused on children being abducted: "Under her own house she can hear the voices of children calling out: Mother, I beg you, come and get us out" (p.123). She stated, "I am a woman who has been stripped of everything, from whom they embezzled funds and taken children (p.121)." She heard children moaning wherever she went.

It would seem that Mrs. M's delusion began as a response to the catastrophic death of her children. A psychotic solution to her terrible experience of loss and likely depression was for her to deny that her children had died. Mrs. M. believed that the dead children were duplicates and that her real children were alive and trapped underground, crying out to her to be rescued. The delusion afforded her emotional relief from feelings of loss.

This speculative formulation can explain the content of some of Mrs. M's delusions. It cannot, however, account for her other delusions; for example, that numerous other people were also duplicated, not just her children; that she was persecuted in various ways; and that she herself was duplicated. This speculative formulation is another demonstration that psychodynamic formulations are limited in their ability to explain CS.

Regression

The theme of doubles, metamorphoses, and dualisms is common in myth, primitive religion, and literature (Todd, 1957; Christodoulou, 1986). For instance, in Greek mythology Zeus repeatedly transformed himself into other forms. An explanation of CS is that a "Functional psychotic illness may bring about a regression to primitive modes of thought, with a revival of archaic conceptions concerning doubles and dualisms" (Todd, 1957, p. 264).

This explanation of CS is related to the observation that in patients with brain damage primitive thoughts emerge as higher neurological functioning dissolves. This process was first noted by the eminent neurologist John Hughlings Jackson (York, 2011).

There are other theories of regression as a cause of CS. First, and related to the ambivalence theory and the work of Melanie Klein (1975) is the concept that in CS there is a regression to an early stage of childhood that predates the establishment of object constancy when there is a splitting of people into either all good or all bad. The overuse of the defense of projection is a key element.

Second, schizophrenic patients with CS seem to manifest "a regression to the very primitive emotional state of early childhood . . . marked by a loss of identity and fusion of self and object-representations" (Sinkman, 1983, p.432–433). This loss of identity is a key factor in the development of these delusions about identity.

Depersonalization

Ever since CS was first described clinicians have observed the high incidence of depersonalization in such patients (Christodoulou, 1986). Initially, patients recognize that these feelings of strangeness are subjective. In time, however, these subjective feelings are projected onto the outside world and the patient begins to feel that the world around him, including people, seems unreal and strange. This evolves into the idea that the people *are* unreal because they have been replaced by look-alike impostors. In this theory CS is understood as a psychotic expression of these experiences of unreality.

Depersonalization and de-realization experiences are also common occurrences in the prodrome of schizophrenia. They occur along with feelings of puzzlement that may include confusing the self with others (the loss of ego boundaries). This emotional state precedes the development of delusions and is commonly known as delusional mood.

Loss of Ego Boundaries

The loss of ego boundaries (viz., knowing where the self ends and where other people and the environment begins) is central to the neurological explanations of DMS (Feinberg & Roane, 2005). This term was first used to explain CS in a paper I wrote in 1983 (Sinkman, 1983). According to this theory, patients who suffer a loss of ego boundaries and identity confusion develop the idea that others around them also have the same unstable identity. The patient thus projects the internal experiences onto others. The idea that others have changed eventually turns into the delusion that they have become unreal impostors.

According to Maher (1988), a delusion is a patient's attempt to describe and explain the bizarre experiences that he has been undergoing—the confused and fragmented sense of identity of himself and others along with anxiety and depersonalization. Maher maintained that the reasoning process that led to the delusion was a logical attempt to explain these anomalous experiences. The subjective experiences are strange while the thinking process is logical (Parnas, 2003).

Although Maher's ideas have been widely accepted some commentators believe that they are inadequate. These theorists focus on the patient's failure to recognize that the delusional explanation of the odd experiences is an illogical idea that should be rejected as a nonsensical thought. This failure of normal belief evaluation is a major defect in the patient's thinking that enables the delusion to persist. It is the second step in a two-step process of delusion formation (Langdon, 2000). It has been hypothesized that the belief evaluation system is located in the right frontal lobe and an injury there causes the delusion (Coltheart et al., 2007).

Deficits in Mental Representations

Mental representations are the mental images (ideas) that a person uses to describe and understand every place, object, and person (including themselves) that they know. DMS patients have difficulty evoking and using appropriate mental representations (de Bonis et al., 1994; Sinkman, 1983;2008). Flooded with inchoate mental images of themselves and others, patients search for an explanation of these confusing ideas and develop a delusional solution. The cause of this impairment in evoking mental representations is a defect in brain functioning that has not yet been identified.

A very similar explanation was offered by Cutting (1991), who proposed that "delusional misidentification derives from a failure to appreciate the actual identity or uniqueness of something . . . whether it is a person, place, event or object" (p.73). He stated that the cause was a disturbance of the brain function of identification that is located on the right side of the brain.

This concept was expanded by Margariti (2006), who posited a mental function that establishes the uniqueness of every person, place, or thing. She described a "device" in the brain whose function is the "integration of perceptual, personal and affective information . . . on the ground of uniqueness" (p.266). The DMS occur when there is a breakdown of this system of uniqueness.

This uniqueness concept and the mental representation concept both explain the DMS as arising from the patient's difficulty establishing identity of all people, places, and objects and not just the people who are duplicated in a misidentification delusion.

Prosopagnosia

An early speculation was that CS was related to prosopagnosia, the neurological illness in which a brain injury leaves the patient unable to identify familiar faces. A patient with CS, however, can correctly identify the face of his loved one. The problem is that he denies that this person is the original/real person.

Therefore, the prosopagnosia explanation of CS was modified. A theory was developed that ascribed two components to the process of facial recognition: the overt visual recognition of a familiar face and, separate from that, a process that attaches an appropriate emotional response to the recognized face. Each of these two processes was hypothesized to be located in different brain tracts: the overt recognition at the bottom of the brain (ventral) and emotional recognition on the top of the brain (dorsal). According to this theory, in prosopagnosia there is an injury in the ventral tract while in CS the injury is in the dorsal tract. This dorsal lesion leaves the CS patient unable to attach a feeling of familiarity to a face he recognizes. In an attempt to explain this lack of emotional familiarity and to deal with the dissonance between recognition and emotion, the CS patient develops a delusional explanation of replacement (Ellis & Young, 1990).

Although there is some evidence confirming this theory there are also problems with it. This explanation of CS is based on a difficulty identifying familiar faces. It cannot explain the fact that patients with CS can have replacement delusions involving strangers. Furthermore, CS often occurs together with FS and the Delusion of Subjective Doubles and these other delusions could not be explained by this theory.

Going beyond this prosopagnosia theory, cognitive neuroscientists have researched face processing in normal people and the deficits that occur in patients with DMS (Breen, 2000; Young, 2008; Langdon, 2000). Gainotti (2007) has studied the neural mechanisms involved in facial recognition. He confirmed the importance of the right hemisphere. In addition, he stressed the importance of the frontal and temporal lobes (particularly the right frontal). The initial automatic and emotional phase of recognition is mediated by the right side of the brain that connects in a lateral subcortical route to the limbic system.

The Relationships Between Delusional Misidentification Syndromes and Schizophrenia

Two aspects of the complex relationship between schizophrenia and DMS will be reviewed. The first issue will be highlighted by a case report.

> Carl had chronic schizophrenia for many years but was relatively stable until he stopped taking his medications several months ago. He had various delusions. He maintained grandiose ideas that he had vast wealth and powers. He believed that he was persecuted by "the World Church," which used a "cloning machine" that made artificial bodies and clones of various people including himself and family members. Carl saw the clones in his apartment wearing masks. The machine cut up his body, drained his organs, and took parts of his body to make artificial bodies. The machine controlled him by inserting thoughts into his mind. He felt pain in his side and rectum that he attributed to the machine, which used "swords and knives." At various times he said that the machine was attached to his body "like an IV that drains blood and tissues" and at other times that his body was inside the machine. An evaluation included a negative noncontrast head CT.

Carl's mis-identity delusions and bizarre somatic delusions were manifestations of an underlying schizophrenic process involving the loss of ego boundaries and an inability to maintain stable images of self and other (e.g., Andreasen, 1999; Parnas, 2003). His presentation was consistent with the idea that schizophrenia is a disorder of the self (Nordgaard, 2014). Carl's mis-identity delusion about clones was not the focus of his psychosis nor did it stand out from the other delusions but seemed to be part of the process of schizophrenia. This suggests that in certain cases like Carl's there is nothing unique or specific about a mis-identity delusion. It is just one manifestation of schizophrenia. Taking this idea one step further leads to the idea that schizophrenia with mis-identity delusions is not distinct from schizophrenia without such delusions.

Two research studies have attempted to determine whether the presence of a mis-identity delusion makes a case of schizophrenia unique and different from other cases of the illness. Both studies compared the neuropsychological functioning of schizophrenic patients with and without DMS. One study found differences while the other did not, leaving the question unanswered and a topic for further research (Papageorgiou, 2005; Lykouras, 2008).

The second issue in the relationship between schizophrenia and DMS is the fact that the brain areas implicated in schizophrenia are the very same areas damaged in focal neurologic cases of DMS: the frontal lobes (especially on the right side), the temporal lobes, and the limbic system. Of particular note is that the right hemisphere and the frontal lobes of the brain, especially the right prefrontal lobe, are essential for the formation of a coherent image of the self, including ego boundaries (Keenan, 2003). The loss of ego boundaries that occurs in both schizophrenia and DMS appears to be related to these shared lesions in the frontal lobes.

The idea that the mis-identity delusions that occur in both schizophrenia and in brain injury share a common cause—damage to the frontal lobes of the brain—is an intriguing theory. Some data, however, present challenges to this theory. First, DMS commonly occurs in patients with diffuse brain disease where clear evidence of significant frontal deficits may be lacking. Second, so-called "hypo-frontality," or defective functioning of the frontal lobes in schizophrenia, was a central understanding of the syndrome 30 years ago. These ideas have evolved, however, and schizophrenia is now understood to be much more than just impaired neuronal functioning associated with gray matter reductions in the frontal lobes. Other brain defects identified in schizophrenia (e.g., dopamine dysregulation) could be crucial factors in the development of these delusions. Third, impaired functioning of the frontal lobes in schizophrenia is usually associated with the loss of initiative and other negative symptoms whereas delusions and other positive symptoms are correlated with impairments in other brain areas, the striatum, and limbic system (Lahti, 2006).

ASSESSMENT OPTIONS

At present, no validated questionnaires or clinical interviews focus on CS. In the absence of standardized tools, it is important to pay close attention to what patients describe and to pick up on any clues to CS symptomatology and impaired reality testing. Ask patients to explain what they mean and to give details. Misidentification delusions are not as rare as previously thought, so it is important to keep them in mind as a possibility and to pursue any leads. It is important to focus on comments that the patient makes about others' identities as well as changes that were noticed in the environment in regard to self or others. If a patient has any delusions, explore the content of them carefully and ascertain if aspects should be classified in the broad spectrum of misidentification delusions.

There is also a need to be concerned about the patient's propensity for violence and to evaluate for it thoroughly. A helpful question to ask the patient is, "How do you feel about what has happened to you, that people have been substituted?" It is important to determine if the patient is angry at the phonies and if he has plans to hurt them.

DIFFERENTIAL DIAGNOSIS

It is important to rule out the presence of brain disease in every patient with a misidentification delusion. Toward that end a complete mental status examination as well as thorough testing of cognition is essential. Neuropsychological testing and neuroimaging often are indicated. Once that has been done the next step is to clarify the nature of the underlying psychiatric illness.

TREATMENT OPTIONS

The correct approach to treating a patient with DMS is to treat the underlying condition. A review found a significant response to treatment with neuroleptics (63%–68%), with electroconvulsive therapy (ECT) and mood stabilizers also having a place in treatment (Silva, 1996).

In patients with Dementia with Lewy Bodies the treatment of delusions is difficult because of the significant adverse reaction to neuroleptics. Low dose quetiapine has been the treatment of choice, starting at 12.5 milligrams daily. Recent studies, however, have shown that there is no evidence that quetiapine is effective (Shotbolt, 2010). Clozapine is an option. There is some evidence for the efficacy of cholinesterase inhibitors (Weintraub, 2007), but further reviews have raised doubts. A new medication, pimavanserin, has just been approved for the treatment of delusions in Parkinson's disease psychosis (Cummings et al., 2014).

Recent research has demonstrated the efficacy of citalopram in treating delusions in patients with Alzheimer's Disease (Leonpacher et al. (2016).

Many of the schizophrenic patients with CS are severely ill and require high doses of neuroleptics or clozapine. There is a still a significant role for the use of first-generation typical neuroleptics such as perphenazine.

As for psychotherapy, there is little evidence for the efficacy of this treatment apart from one case. The successful psychotherapy of a 12-year-old boy with CS based on the ambivalence theory was reported by Moskowitz (1972). The delusion emerged within the context of disturbed family relationships. The therapist helped the patient learn that he conjured up doubles as way to deal with angry feelings toward his parents. The patient grew to understand that "feeling states might produce psychic phenomena of misperception and misidentification" (p. 55).

RECOMMENDATIONS FOR FUTURE WORK

- Rating scales for psychosis should include delusional misidentification among the symptoms to be evaluated.
- For patients with DMS, there needs to be a valid and reliable assessment tool to evaluate details and overall severity.

- Several questions about DMS need to be addressed: (1) Given that misidentification delusions are so common in Dementia with Lewy Bodies, what can that disease teach us about the cause of DMS? (2) Is primary DMS different from secondary DMS or are they just separate points on a continuum? (3) What is the mechanism causing DMS in patients with diffuse brain disease who do not have a focal lesion?

REFERENCES

Anderson, D.N., & Williams, E. (1994). The delusion of inanimate doubles. *Psychopathology*, 27, 220–225.

Andreasen, N.C. (1999). A unitary model of schizophrenia. *Archives of General Psychiatry*, 56, 781–787.

Banov, M.D., Kulick, A.R., Oepen, G., & Pope, H.G. (1993). A new identity for misidentification syndromes. *Comprehensive Psychiatry*, 34, 414–417.

Breen, N., Caine, D., Coltheart, M., & Hendy, J. (2000). Towards an understanding of delusions of misidentification: four case studies. *Mind & Language*, 15, 74–110.

Christodoulou, G.N. (1978). Syndrome of subjective doubles. *American Journal of Psychiatry*, 135, 249–251.

Christodoulou, G.N. (1986). The origin of the concept of doubles. *Bibliotheca Psychiatrica*, 164, 1–8.

Christodoulou, G.N., & Malliara-Loulakaki, S. (1981). Delusional misidentification syndromes and cerebral dysrhythmia. *Psychiatrica Clinica*, 14, 245–251.

Coltheart, M., Langdon, R., & McCay, R. (2007). Schizophrenia and monothematic delusions. *Schizophrenia Bulletin*, 33, 642–647.

Cummings, J., Isaacson, S., Mills, R., Williams, H., Chi-Burns, K., Dhall, R., & Ballard, C. (2014). Pimavanserin for patients with Parkinson's psychosis. *Lancet*, 383, 533–540.

Cutting, J. (1991). Delusional misidentification and the role of the right hemisphere in the appreciation of identity. *British Journal of Psychiatry*, 159(Suppl14), 70–75.

Cutting, J.C. (1994). Evidence for right hemisphere dysfunction in schizophrenia. In J.C. Cutting and A. David (Eds.), *The neuropsychology of schizophrenia* (pp. 231–244). Hove, UK: Lawrence Erlbaum.

deBonis, M., De Boeck, P., Lida-Pulik, H., Bazin, N., Masure, M-C., & Feline, A. (1994). Person identification and self-concept in the delusional misidentification syndrome. *Psychopathology*, 27, 48–57.

Del Ser, T., McKeith, I., Anand, R., Cicin-Sain, A., Ferrara, R., & Spiegel, R. (2000). Dementia with Lewy bodies: findings from an international multicenter study. *International Journal of Geriatric Psychiatry*, 15, 1034–1045.

Devinsky, O. (2009). Delusional misidentifications and duplications. *Neurology*, 72, 80–87.

Dohn, H.L., & Crews, E.L. (1986). Capgras syndrome: a literature review and case series. *Hillside Journal of Clinical Psychiatry*, 8, 56–74.

Ellis, H.D., Whitley, J., & Luaute, J.-P. (1994). Delusional misidentification. *History of Psychiatry*, V, 117–146.

Ellis, H.D., & Young, A.W. (1990). Accounting for delusional misidentifications. *British Journal of Psychiatry*, 157, 239–248.

Enoch, M.D., Trethowan, W. H., & Barker, J.C. (1967). *Some uncommon psychiatric syndromes.* Bristol, UK: John Wright & Sons.

Feinberg, T.E., Deluca, J., Giacino, J.T., Roane, D.M., & Solms, M. (2005). Right-hemisphere pathology and self: delusional misidentification and reduplication. In T.E. Feinberg & J.P. Keenan (Eds.), *The lost self, pathologies of the brain and identity* (pp. 100–130). New York, NY: Oxford University Press.

Feinberg, T.E., & Roane, D. (2005). Delusional misidentification. *Psychiatric Clinics of North America, 28,* 665–683.

Fishbain, D.A. (1987). The frequency of Capgras delusions in a psychiatric emergency service. *Psychopathology, 20,* 42–47.

Fleminger, S., & Burns, A. (1993). The delusional misidentification syndromes in patients with and without evidence of organic cerebral disorder. *Biological Psychiatry, 33,* 22–32.

Forstl, H., Almeida, O.P., Owen, A.M., Burns, A., & Howard, R. (1991). Psychiatric, neurological and medical aspects of misidentification syndromes: a review of 260 cases. *Psychological Medicine, 21,* 905–910.

Gainotti, G. (2007). Face familiarity feelings, the right temporal lobe and the possible underlying neural mechanisms. *Brain Research Reviews, 56,* 214–235.

Gray, K. (1992, May 5), Potential juror breaks down. *The Standard Star,* 18A.

Harwood, D.G., Barker, W.W., Ownby, R.L., & Duara, R. (1999). Prevalence and correlates of Capgras syndrome in Alzheimer's disease. *International Journal of Geriatric Psychiatry, 14,* 415–420.

Huang, T-L., Liu, C-Y., & Yang, Y-Y. (1999). Capgras syndrome: analysis of nine cases. *Psychiatry and Clinical Neurosciences, 53,* 455–460.

Ismail, Z., Nguyen, M-Q., Fischer, C.E., Schweizer, T.A., & Mulsant, B.H. (2012). Neuroimaging of delusions in Alzheimer's disease. *Psychiatry Research: Neuroimaging, 202,* 89–95.

Joseph, A.B. (1994). Observations on the epidemiology of the delusional misidentification syndromes. *Psychopathology 27,* 150–153.

Joseph, A.B., O'Leary, D.H., Kurland, R., & Ellis, H.D. (1999). Bilateral anterior cortical atrophy and subcortical atrophy in reduplicative paramnesia: a case-controlled study of computed tomography in 10 patients. *Canadian Journal of Psychiatry, 44,* 685–689.

Josephs, K.A. (2007). Capgras syndrome and its relationship to neurodegenerative disease. *Archives of Neurology, 64,* 1762–1766.

Kamanitz, J.R., El-Mallakh, R.S., & Tasman, A. (1989), Delusional misidentification involving the self. *The Journal of Nervous and Mental Disease, 177,* 695–698.

Keenan, J.P., & Wheeler, M.A. (2003). The neural correlates of self awareness. In T. Kirchner & A. David (Eds.), *The self in neuroscience and psychiatry* (pp. 166–179). Cambridge: Cambridge University Press

Kirov, G., Jones, P., & Lewis, S.W. (1994). Prevalence of delusional misidentification syndromes. *Psychopathology, 27,* 148–149.

Klein, C.A., & Hirachan, S. (2014). The masks of identities: Who's who? Delusional misidentification syndromes. *Journal of the American Academy of Psychiatry and Law, 42,* 369–378.

Klein, M. (1975). Some theoretical conclusions regarding the emotional life of the infant. In M. Klein (Ed.), *Envy and gratitude and other works 1946–1963* (pp. 61–93). New York, NY: The Free Press.

Lahti, A.C., Weiler, M.A., Holcomb, H.H., Tamminga, C.A., Carpenter, W.T., & McMahon, R. (2006). Correlations between rCBF and symptoms in two independent cohorts of drug-free patients with schizophrenia. *Neuropsychopharmacology, 31,* 221–230.

Langdon, R., & Coltheart, M. (2000). The cognitive neuropsychology of delusions. *Mind & Language, 15,* 184–218.

Leonpacher, A.K., Peters, M.E., Drye, L.T., Makino, K.M., Newell, J.A., Devanand, D.P., Frangakis, C. (2016).Effects of Citalopram on Neuropsychiatric Symptoms in Alzheimer's Dementia: Evidence From the CitAD Study. *Am J Psychiatry 173,*473–480.

Lykouras, L., Typaldou, M., Mourtzouchou, P., Oulis, P., Koutsaftis, C., Dokianaki, F., ... Christodoulo, C. (2008). Neuropsychological relationships in paranoid delusional misidentification syndromes. A comparative study. *Progress in Neuro-Psychopharmacology & Biological Psychiatry, 32,* 1445–1448.

Madoz-Gurpide, A., & Hillers-Rodriguez, R. (2010). Delerio de Capgras: una revision de las teorias etiologicas. *Revista Neurologica, 50,* 420–430.

Maher, B.A. (1988). Anomalous experience and delusional thinking: The logic of explanations. In T.F. Oltmanns and B.A. Maher (Eds.), *Delusional beliefs* (pp. 15–33). New York: Wiley.

Malloy, P., Cimino, C., & Westlake, R. (1992). Differential diagnosis of primary and secondary Capgras delusions. *Neuropsychiatry, Neuropsychology, and Behavioral Neurology, 5,* 83–96.

Malloy, P.F., & Richardson, E.D. (1994). The frontal lobes and content-specific delusions. *The Journal of Neuropsychiatry and Clinical Neurosciences, 6,* 455–466.

Margariti, M.M., & Kontaxakis, V.P. (2006). Approaching delusional misidentification syndromes as a disorder of the sense of uniqueness. *Psychopathology, 39,* 261–268.

Markova, I.S., & Berrios, G.E. (1994). Delusional misidentifications: facts and fancies. *Psychopathology, 27,* 136–143.

Mattioli, F., Miozzo, A., & Vignolo, L.A. (1999). Confabulation and delusional misidentification: a four-year follow-up study. *Cortex, 35,* 413–422.

Mega, M.S., Cummings, J.L., Fiorello, T., & Gornbein, J. (1996). The spectrum of behavioral changes in Alzheimer's disease. *Neurology, 46,* 130–135.

Mentis, M.J., Weinstein, E.A., Horwitz, B., McIntosh, A.R., Pietrini, P., Alexander, G.E., ... Murphy, D. (1995). Abnormal brain glucose metabolism in the delusional misidentification syndromes: a positron emission tomography study in Alzheimer disease. *Biological Psychiatry, 38,* 438–439.

Merrin, E.L., & Silberfarb, P.M. (1976). The Capgras phenomenon. *Archives of General Psychiatry, 33,* 965–968.

Mizrahi, R., Starkstein, S.E., Jorge, R., & Robinson, R.G. (2006). Phenomenology and clinical correlates of delusions in Alzheimer disease. *American Journal of Geriatric Psychiatry, 14,* 573–581.

Mojtabai, R. (1998). Identifying misidentifications: a phenomenological study. *Psychopathology, 31,* 90–95.

Moskowitz, J.A. (1972), Capgras' syndrome in modern dress. *International Journal of Child Psychotherapy, 1,* 45–64.

Murray, P.S., Kumar, S., DeMichele-Sweet, M.A., & Sweet, R. (2014). Psychosis in Alzheimer's disease. *Biological Psychiatry, 75,* 542–552.

Nordgaard, J., & Parnas, J. (2014). Self-disorders and the schizophrenia spectrum: a study of 100 first hospital admissions. *Schizophrenia Bulletin, 40,* 1300–1307.

Odom-White, A., deLeon, J., Stanilla, J., Cloud, B.S., & Simpson, G.M. (1995). Misidentification syndromes in schizophrenia: case reviews and implications for the classification and prevalence. *Australian and New Zealand Journal of Psychiatry, 29,* 63–68.

Oyebode, F. (2008). The neurology of psychosis. *Medicine Principles and Practice,* 17, 263–269.

Papageorgiou, C., Lykouras, L., Alevizos, B., Ventouras, E., Mourtzouchou, P., Uzunoglu, N., Christodoulou, G.N., & Rabavilas, A. (2005), Psychophysiological differences in schizophrenics with and without delusional misidentification syndromes; A P300 study. *Progress in Neuro-Psychopharmacology & Biological Psychiatry, 29,* 593–601.

Parnas, J., & Handest, P. (2003). Phenomenology of anomalous self-experience in early schizophrenia. *Comprehensive Psychiatry, 44,* 121–134.

Pick, A. (1903). On reduplicative paramnesia. *Brain, 26,* 242–267.

Politis, M., & Loane, C. (2012). Reduplicative paramnesia: a review. *Psychopathology, 45,* 337–343.

Rahman T., & Cole E.F. (2014). Capgras syndrome in homocystinuria. *Biologic Psychiatry, 76,* e11–12.

Rossner, V. (2002). A new classification of the delusional misidentification syndromes. *Psychopathology, 35,* 3–7.

Salvatore, P., Bhuvaneswar, C., Tohen, M., Khalsa, H-M. K., Maggini, C., & Baldessarini, R.J. (2014). Capgras syndrome in first-episode psychotic disorders. *Psychopathology, 47,* 261–269.

Shotbolt, P., Samuel, M., & David, A. (2010). Quetiapine in the treatment of psychosis in Parkinson's disease. *Therapeutic Advances in Neurologic Disorders, 3,* 339–350.

Silva, J.A., Leong, G.B., & Miller, A.L. (1996). Delusional misidentification syndromes—drug treatment options. *CNS Drugs, 5,* 89–102.

Sinkman, A. (1983). The Capgras delusion: a critique of its psychodynamic theories. *American Journal of Psychotherapy,* 37, 428–438.

Sinkman, A. (2008). The syndrome of Capgras. *Psychiatry, 71,* 371–378.

Staton, R.D., Brumback, R.A., & Wilson, H. (1982). Reduplicative paramnesia: a disconnection syndrome of memory. *Cortex, 18,* 23–35.

Sultzer, D.L., Brown, C.V., Mandelkern, M.A., Mahler, M.E., Mendez, M.F., ... Cummings, J.L. (2003). Delusional thoughts and regional frontal/temporal cortex metabolism in Alzheimer's disease. *American Journal of Psychiatry, 160,* 341–349.

Tamam, L., Karatas, G., Zeren, T., & Ozpoyraz, N. (2003). The prevalence of Capgras syndrome in a university hospital setting. *Acta Neuropsychiatrica, 15,* 290–295.

Thaipisuttikul, P., Lobach, I., Zweig, Y., Gurnani, A., & Galvin, J.E. (2013). Capgras syndrome in dementia with Lewy bodies. *International Psychogeriatrics, 25,* 843–849.

Todd, J. (1957), The syndrome of Capgras. *The Psychiatric Quarterly, 31,* 250–265.

Weinstein, E.A. (1994). The classification of delusional misidentification syndromes. *Psychopathology, 27,* 130–135.

Weintraub, D., & Hurtig, H.I. (2007). Presentation and management of psychosis in Parkinson's disease and dementia with Lewy bodies. *American Journal of Psychiatry*, *164*, 1491–1498.

Woodward, N.D., & Cascio, C.J. (2015). Resting-state functional connectivity in psychiatric disorders. *JAMA Psychiatry*, *72*, 743–744.

York, G.K., & Steinberg, D.A. (2011), Hughlings Jackson's neurological ideas. *Brain*, *134*, 3106–3113.

Young, G. (2008). Capgras delusion: An interactionist model. *Consciousness and Cognition*, *17*, 863–876.

6

Attention Deficit
Disorder Psychosis

JAN DIRK BLOM, MARIEKE NIEMANTSVERDRIET,
ANKE SPUIJBROEK, AND SANDRA KOOJI ∎

VIGNETTE

A 34-year-old music teacher[1] with a history of amphetamine and alcohol abuse was admitted to a psychiatric hospital because of formal thought disorder, delusions, and tactile as well as visual hallucinations. He was diagnosed with schizophrenia and comorbid substance abuse, treated effectively with the classic antipsychotic haloperidol, and advised to remain abstinent from illicit substances. Within a year, he was admitted a second time. Because of resistance to haloperidol, he was switched to the atypical antipsychotic clozapine. He recovered within a few weeks and was again discharged. When he was admitted for a third time several years later, once again due to severe psychosis, he reported that he kept using amphetamines the entire time because they helped him to stay focused and carry out his job and daily activities. Further diagnostic testing indicated that, apart from the above-mentioned diagnoses, he also fulfilled criteria for attention-deficit/hyperactivity disorder (ADHD). Although attention-deficit disorder psychosis (ADD psychosis) is not a diagnosis formally recognized in major publications such as the Diagnostic and Statistical Manual of Mental Disorders *(DSM-5, American Psychiatric Association [APA], 2013), his psychiatrist suggested that he might be suffering from this rare condition. His provider continued the clozapine, and added 10 milligrams of the stimulant drug methylphenidate. This initially provoked anxiety and a severe headache, but within a few days these adverse effects faded away and the patient stabilized. In accordance with the patient's clinical picture, the dose of methylphenidate was gradually*

---

1. This patient was described before in the Dutch scientific journal *Tijdschrift voor Psychiatrie* (Blom & Kooij 2012).

increased to 60 milligrams per day, and after a few weeks he improved so much that he was discharged to his home. When he later presented at the outpatient clinic for follow-up care, his psychiatric symptoms were closely monitored. At his request, the dose of methylphenidate was increased further until an optimal result was obtained with no more than 50 milligrams of clozapine and an unusually high dose of 220 milligrams of methylphenidate per day. With the aid of this combination treatment the patient was able to remain stable for eight consecutive years. Attempts to lower the dose of methylphenidate led to a rebound of his ADHD symptoms. Thus, no further attempts at reduction were made. Annual check-ups of blood pressure, pulse, and liver enzymes were normal and, apart from some weight loss, there were no significant side effects from the prolonged methylphenidate use.

A second patient did not have such a favorable outcome as the first. She was a 44-year-old woman with a history of alcohol, cannabis, cocaine, and amphetamine abuse who was admitted to an addiction treatment center because of severe restlessness, insomnia, and agitation. She reported suffering from mood swings, impulsivity, restlessness, and disorganization since childhood. She had been easily distracted, repeated the third grade twice, and eventually dropped out of high school. She later worked in the catering industry and as a prostitute, and had been in contact with the police several times due to minor infractions. At the addiction treatment center she was diagnosed with childhood-onset and persistent ADHD, and, accordingly, treated with short-acting methylphenidate. At a dose of 80 milligrams per day and while remaining abstinent from illicit substances, she obtained a significant decrease in all her symptoms. Upon discharge, however, she relapsed. Not only did she return to cocaine use, but also began abusing methylphenidate. She was readmitted and treated with methylphenidate 60 milligrams per day, but went on to develop formal thought disorders, delusions, and auditory hallucinations. The diagnosis was changed to ADD psychosis, and the atypical antipsychotic olanzapine was added at a dosage of 20 milligrams per day. After two weeks of unabated psychosis, the methylphenidate was tapered off. The psychotic symptoms diminished within a few days and the patient was discharged using only olanzapine. During the years that followed, she was admitted multiple times and treated with several combinations of antipsychotics and stimulants. Three years later she consulted the outpatient clinic due to the presence of formal thought disorders, delusions, auditory hallucinations, panic attacks, and agoraphobia. She insisted that she had remained abstinent from illicit substances. After the dose of long-acting methylphenidate was lowered to 50 milligrams per day, she discontinued all of her medications. However, because of her persistent anxiety and psychosis she was then treated with the atypical antipsychotic aripiprazole. Shortly thereafter she discharged herself from treatment and was lost to further follow-up.

HISTORICAL AND CULTURAL CONTEXT

Attention-deficit disorder psychosis (ADD psychosis) is a little-known diagnostic category that is currently enjoying a modest revival of scientific attention (Levy,

Traicu, Iyer, Malla, & Joober, 2015; Pallanti & Salerno, 2015). The concept was introduced in 1985 by Leopold Bellak (1916–2000), an Austrian-American psychiatrist, psychoanalyst, and professor of psychology who was best known for his myriad publications on minimal brain dysfunction (MBD), attention-deficit disorder (ADD), attention-deficit/hyperactivity disorder (ADHD), and psychosis. He also had a role in founding the *Center for Studies of Schizophrenia* (Bellak, 1979). Starting from the hypothesis that schizophrenia is probably best conceptualized as a syndrome comprising different disorders, and referring to it accordingly as "the schizophrenic syndrome" (Bellak, 1948), Bellak had long sought to identify phenomenologically and pathogenetically homogeneous categories that might help to prove this case. As a prelude to his subsequent concept of ADD psychosis, his work in the 1970s focused on possible relationships between the schizophrenic syndrome and MBD, the conceptual predecessor of AD(H)D (Bellak, 1976; 1977). It was not until 1985, however, that he felt he had collected sufficient evidence to justify the formal introduction of his ADD psychosis concept. As he and his group maintained,

> *We have previously argued that a diagnostic entity is heuristically useful if its intragroup similarities as well as intergroup differences are great, thus providing convergent and discriminant validation. These criteria are met in the designation of ADD psychosis by virtue of its having more unique features of its own—including special symptomatology, anamnesis, therapeutics, and prognosis—than in common with affective, schizophrenic, or schizophreniform psychosis, even though features often resembling these other conditions may lead to misclassification of the principal disorder* (Bellak, Kay, & Opler, 1987).

In the absence of any biological markers, Bellak and his group had to rely on clinical parameters to validate their concept (Kay & Bellak, 1986; Bellak & Opler, 1994). As indicated by the passage above, they also sought to do so by means of pharmacological dissection (i.e., by assessing the effects of psychostimulants and antipsychotics on patients with different combinations of symptoms). As Bellak maintained in his original paper on the subject, clinical and psychopharmacological observations led him to believe that ADD psychosis deserved to be considered a diagnostic category in its own right, characterized by psychotic symptoms that evolve from ADD or ADHD rather than from any type of schizophrenic or affective psychotic disorder (Bellak, 1985). On the basis of his clinical experience, he suggested that some 10% of all cases of schizophrenia (and perhaps also affective psychosis) should meet the diagnostic criteria of his new category.

Since then, however, cases of ADD psychosis have rarely been reported in the international literature (Blom & Kooij, 2012). What has emerged instead is a significant body of literature on the co-occurrence of psychotic symptoms and AD(H)D symptoms, which, in at least some cases, is attributed to a shared genetic vulnerability for both groups of symptoms (Hamshere et al., 2013). In addition, a number of studies have been published on the pros and cons of prescribing methylphenidate in these comorbid patients (as was advocated by Bellak). What has remained to this day, however, is the conceptual issue as to whether ADD psychosis deserves the status of an independent diagnostic category.

ROLE IN CURRENT DIAGNOSTIC SYSTEMS

The architects of the DSM-5 (American Psychiatric Association, 2013), ICD-10 (World Health Organization, 1993), and other major psychiatric classifications do not seem to think so. None of these classifications mention the concept of ADD psychosis or even list it as a preliminary category for possible inclusion in future editions. The reason for this omission is unknown, but it might be attributable to the conservative nature of these classifications, which does not allow their contributors to alter existing diagnostic constructs or to introduce any new ones in the absence of convincing empirical support and an elaborate review and approval process (Regier, Kuhl, & Kupfer, 2013).

In addition, there are likely other, more practical reasons. One of them might be that the possibility of a comorbid or dual diagnosis (of schizophrenia spectrum disorder *and* AD(H)D) is generally considered sufficiently convenient for clinical purposes. Moreover, a certain reluctance to grant ADD psychosis the status of an autonomous diagnostic category may stem from a fear of implicitly encouraging the prescription of psychostimulants, which are traditionally recognized as important risk factors for psychosis (Lieberman, Kane, & Alvir, 1987; Bulut, Kaynar, & Sabuncuoglu, 2013). The obvious downside of this is that withholding these drugs in designated cases may leave a substantial number of affected individuals undertreated (Bellak, 1985). Finally, the ADD psychosis concept may not have been included in psychiatric classifications because of the often-reported comorbid use of illicit substances, and the inclination to designate any psychotic symptoms experienced in that context as substance-induced.

SYMPTOMATOLOGY

The symptoms that Bellak and his group deemed characteristic of ADD psychosis are listed in Table 6.1 and Figure 6.1. For ease of reference, the differences between ADD psychosis and schizophrenia are also included in the table.

Judging by the differences listed in Table 6.1, Bellak and his group considered "schizophrenic symptoms" to be rather bizarre in nature, as opposed to the "simpler" or "reactive" symptoms of ADD psychosis. Another striking difference is the patient response to psychostimulants (i.e., favorable in cases of ADD psychosis and usually unfavorable in cases of schizophrenia) as well as to antipsychotics (favorable in schizophrenia, and neutral or unfavorable in ADD psychosis).

Table 6.1. CRITERIA FOR DIFFERENTIATION BETWEEN ADD
PSYCHOSIS AND SCHIZOPHRENIA

Area of Distinction	ADD Psychosis	Schizophrenia
Symptomatology	Rare or no hallucinations; if present, they are simple and brief	Frequent and often complex hallucinations
	Delusions, if present, are not well systematized and are transparently compensatory for a low self-esteem	Involved and often systematized delusions, which may take on a bizarre quality
	Intermittently poor reality testing due to poor object relations, poor impulse control, and impaired judgment	Poor reality testing; bizarre ideation
	Aggressive distortion of object relations	Poor object relations
	Concrete thinking with little disorganization of thought	Magical thinking, loose associations, overideation, and symbolization
	Little or no social withdrawal	Significant social withdrawal, often of a passive and apathetic nature
	Loss of impulse control, which is clearly reactive, yet not bizarre	Loss of impulse control under inappropriate circumstances; bizarre behavior
	Low stimulus barrier for light and sound, and other sensory overloads	Catatonic or other grossly disorganized behavior
	Soft neurological signs; frequent left-handedness; poor eye-hand coordination; aphasia-like difficulties	Differentiated from organic mental syndrome; ritualistic behavior; depersonalization; de-realization
Associated features	Increased mood lability; low frustration tolerance; temper outbursts; mischievous behavior	Apathetic immobility; affect flat or incongruous with thoughts; dysphoric mood
	Obstinacy, stubbornness; bossiness, bullying	Dishevelled, eccentrically groomed; poverty of speech
Anamnesis	Difficult delivery; hyperkinetic infancy; poor sleep	Unresponsive in infancy

(continued)

Table 6.1. CONTINUED

Area of Distinction	ADD Psychosis	Schizophrenia
	Later learning difficulties; short attention span, dyslexia, dysgraphia, strephosymbolia; neurological soft signs; EEG is normal or minimally and diffusely disturbed; physical awkwardness and clumsiness	Shy and withdrawn in school; daydreaming; neuropsychological findings not always positive; motor coordination not evidently impaired
	Conduct problems at school; impulsive behavior and ostracism by other children; devalued self-concept	Shy and withdrawn in school; daydreaming; becomes more disturbed around age 12 years
	Frequent job changes; alcohol and drug abuse as attempts at self-medication; excessive sensitivity to street drugs	Poor social and sexual relationships; occasional bizarre behavior; idiosyncratic thinking
Family history	Dyslexia and other learning disabilities are virtually always present; "explosive" and labile personalities; epilepsy; probable cases of ADD misdiagnosed as schizophrenia and affective disorder	Sometimes a history of schizophrenia or severely schizoid family members
Sex ratio	Ten times more common in males	Equal male to female ratio
Therapeutics	Lack of response to, or worsening by, neuroleptics	Favorable response to neuroleptics
	Favorable response to amphetamine-like drugs, tricyclics, which produce tranquility	Usually unfavorable response to psychostimulants
Prognosis	Short-term prognosis good, without deterioration	Prognosis variable, often with residual cognitive and social deficits despite recovery
	Long-term prognosis includes social pathology, such as alcoholism, criminality, job loss, and self-discharge or elopement from hospital; recurrence of brief episodes	Unrelieved chronicity with deterioration in a substantial percentage and residual deficits

NOTE: Table compiled by the author, based on Bellak, Kay, & Opler, 1987.
EEG = electroencephalogram.

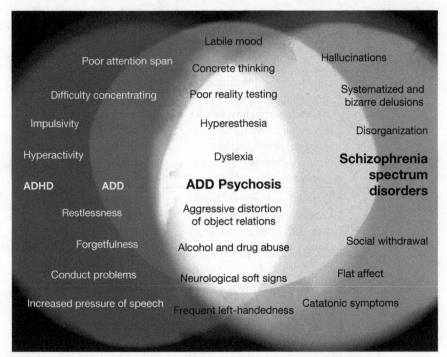

Figure 6.1 Continuum model of ADHD, ADD, ADD psychosis, and schizophrenia spectrum disorders.

PREVALENCE RATE AND ASSOCIATED FEATURES

Epidemiological surveys and clinical prevalence studies of ADD psychosis have not yet been carried out. Therefore, for the purposes of the present chapter, we conducted a systematic search for case reports and case series of patients aged 18–65 years in Pubmed and the Ovid database (until August 2015), using the search terms "attention-deficit disorder psychosis" and "ADD psychosis." We included papers that made explicit reference to Bellak's ADD psychosis concept and were written in English, German, Dutch, French, or Spanish. Reports that refrained from conceptualizing co-occurring psychotic and AD(H)D-like symptoms in terms of a unitary diagnostic entity were excluded.

Our search yielded 409 papers on AD(H)D and psychosis, including 13 clinical reports that described a total number of 31 patients who had been diagnosed with ADD psychosis. Among these patients, 13 stemmed from Bellak and his group. Upon closer inspection, however, the latter subgroup appeared to comprise four actual patients, three of whom were described four times in four different contexts (Bellak, 1976; Bellak & Charles, 1979; Bellak, Kay, & Opler, 1987; Opler, Frank, & Ramirez, 2001). Because we chose to include these patients only once, Table 6.2 provides an overview of 23 original case descriptions, including the two presented above (one of which was described previously by our own group in Blom & Kooij, 2012).

The 23 patients listed in Table 6.2 had a mean age of about 33 years (in two cases the exact age was unknown). Eight of them (35%) were females. Most patients had a history of more than 10 years of psychiatric care, pharmacological treatment, and intermittent hospitalization. Moreover, they suffered from widely varying and multiple psychiatric symptoms, many of which were in conformity with the diagnostic constructs of AD(H)D and/or schizophrenia spectrum disorder. In addition, eight patients (35%) suffered from comorbid substance abuse. For 16 patients (70%) the pharmacological treatment regimen was detailed in the original papers; in 38% of those cases, this involved the combined use of psychostimulants and antipsychotics. All patients who received pharmacological treatment experienced a remission of their symptoms, although many of them relapsed after periods of nonadherence and/or substance abuse. The duration of follow-up was registered for only seven patients (30%), and ranged from four months to eight years (with a median of 18 months).

We also found a clinical study that was designed specifically to test Bellak's diagnostic criteria (Benjumea Pino & Mojarro Práxedes, 1996). In this study, 41 patients diagnosed with schizophrenia or mood disorder were carefully re-examined with the aid of Bellak's criteria, standardized questionnaires such as the *Positive and Negative Syndrome Scale* (PANSS), a diagnostic tool developed by Bellak's colleagues Kay, Fiszbein, and Opler (1987), and the *Wender Adult Questionnaire–Childhood Characteristics* (ACQQ, Ward, Wender, & Reimherr, 1993), as well as various other neuropsychological assessment tools. Among these patients, the authors found only a single one who fulfilled "some of Bellak's criteria."

By and large, it would seem reasonable to argue that reported cases of ADD psychosis are rare. The real question to be answered, however, is whether this is due to the rarity of the disorder itself (or even the spurious identification of "patients" in the absence of any "real" disorder) or whether it is due to underreporting. On the one hand, the limited number of case reports contrasts sharply with the lifetime prevalence of AD(H)D in adults (3.4%) (Fayyad et al., 2007), the finding that 5% of all ADHD patients experience comorbid psychotic symptoms (Pine, Klein, Lindy, & Marshall, 1993; Stahlberg, Soderstrom, Rastam, & Gillberg, 2004), and the related finding that schizophrenia is preceded by ADHD symptoms during childhood in 17% of cases (Peralta et al., 2010). On the basis of these figures alone, AD(H)D and psychosis should be expected to co-occur quite frequently, and, hence, should justify a higher prevalence rate of the diagnostic category of ADD psychosis.

On the other hand, it remains uncertain whether Bellak's estimated prevalence figure of 10% of all psychotic disorders is in any way realistic. Taking into account that schizophrenia has a lifetime prevalence of around 1%, Bellak's conjecture that 10% of all psychoses deserve to be relabeled as ADD psychoses would mean that roughly one in a thousand individuals worldwide should be diagnosed as such. This figure would be even higher if we would take into account the lifetime prevalence of all psychotic disorders (i.e., including the affective psychoses), which has been found to be 3.06% (Perälä et al., 2007).

Table 6.2. REPORTED CASES OF ADD PSYCHOSIS IN THE LITERATURE

Case Number	Sex and Age	Symptoms	Treatment	Outcome	Duration of Follow-up	References
1	F 20 years	Learning difficulties, pressured speech, concrete thinking, motor signs, periodic explosive behavior, suicide attempt	methylphenidate hydrochloride 5 mg t.i.d, imipramine hydrochloride 75 mg h.s., lithium carbonate 300 mg t.i.d.	Full remission	–	Bellak, 1976; Bellak & Charles, 1979; Bellak et al., 1987; Opler et al., 2001
2	F 40 years	Thought disorder, concrete thinking, limited attention span, poor reality testing, dyslexia, problems in geographic orientation, soft neurological signs, sensitivity to noise and bright lights, migraine headaches	imipramine hydrochloride 10 mg h.s., psychotherapy	Remission	–	Bellak, 1976; Bellak & Charles, 1979; Bellak et al., 1987; Opler et al., 2001
3	M ±25 years	Irritability, grandiose delusions, clang associations, letter reversals, mirror writing, sensitivity to alcohol	methylphenidate 10 mg h.s.	Remission	–	Bellak, 1976; Bellak & Charles, 1979; Bellak et al., 1987; Opler et al., 2001
4	M 23 years	Concentration deficits, hyperactivity, motoric restlessness, poor coordination, impulsiveness, temper tantrums, aggression, confusion, delusions of reference, auditory hallucinations	methylphenidate 25 mg	Remission	4 months	Huey et al, 1978

5	F middle-aged	Neurotic difficulties, word-finding problems, poor impulse control, problems with geographical orientation	–	–	–	Bellak & Charles, 1979
6	F 39 years	Distractibility, limited attention span, hyperactivity, inattentiveness, impulsivity, mood lability, temper outbursts, aggression, automutilation, suicidality, anhedonia, insomnia, paranoid delusions	dextroamphetamine 40 mg	Full remission	10 months	Pine et al., 1993
7	M 31 years	Distractibility, inattentiveness, impulsivity, moderately pressured speech, insomnia, weight loss, paranoid and grandiose delusions, roaming way of life	methylphenidate 30 mg, desipramine 150 mg, lithium (no dose stated)	Remission	–	Pine et al., 1993
8	F 26 years	Hyperactivity, impulsivity, concentration deficits, paranoid delusions	methylphenidate 30 mg, antipsychotic medication (type and dose unknown)	Remission	-	Vergouwen & Gorissen, 2001
9	M 25 years	–	–	–	–	Stahlberg et al., 2004
10	M 31 years	–	–	–	–	Stahlberg et al., 2004
11	M 35 years	–	–	–	–	Stahlberg et al., 2004
12	M 36 years	–	–	–	–	Stahlberg et al., 2004
13	M 38 years	–	–	–	–	Stahlberg et al., 2004

(continued)

Table 6.2. CONTINUED

Case Number	Sex and Age	Symptoms	Treatment	Outcome	Duration of Follow-up	References
14	M 45 years	–	–	–	–	Stahlberg et al., 2004
15	M 18 years	Hyperactivity, impulsivity, insomnia, dyslexia, aggression, thrill-seeking behavior, self-harm, depression, delusions, cannabis use	methylphenidate XL 54 mg, amisulpride 800 mg	Full remission	18 months	Sambhi & Lepping, 2009
16	M 23 years	History of sexual and emotional abuse, hyperactivity, impulsivity, insomnia, concentration deficits	methylphenidate XL 36 mg, amisulpride 400 mg	Remission	–	Sambhi & Lepping, 2009
17	F 27 years	History of physical and emotional abuse, concentration deficits, limited attention span, insomnia, impulsivity, motoric restlessness, aggression, auditory hallucinations, delusions, alcohol use, cannabis use, amphetamine use, cocaine use, ecstasy use	methylphenidate 90 mg, olanzapine, fluoxetine	Remission	–	Mason, 2010
18	M 26 years	Concentration deficits, disorganization, impulsivity, irritability, aggression, auditory hallucinations, persecutory delusions, delusions of thought insertion	methylphenidate 72 mg, clozapine, amisulpride, sodium valproate			Mason, 2010

19	M 31 years	Motoric restlessness, concentration deficits, depressive mood, psychotrauma, paranoid delusions, cannabis use, amphetamine use, cocaine use	Long-acting methylphenidate 36 mg, olanzapine 15 mg	Remission	–	de Jong et al., 2010
20	F 31 years	Distractibility, impulsivity, motoric restlessness, concentration deficits, aggressive and depressive mood swings, suicide attempt, bodily hallucinations, cenaesthesias magical ideas, paranoid delusions, hyperreflectivity, ambivalence, catatonic stereotypes	–	–	–	Jandl et al., 2012
21	M 50 years	Distractibility, impulsivity, motoric restlessness, concentration deficits, aggression, formal thought disorder, delusions, tactile hallucinations, visual hallucinations, auditory hallucinations, alcohol use, amphetamine use	methylphenidate 220 mg, clozapine 50 mg	Full remission	8 years	Blom & Kooij, 2012; also described in present chapter

(*continued*)

Table 6.2. CONTINUED

Case Number	Sex and Age	Symptoms	Treatment	Outcome	Duration of Follow-up	References
22	M 42 years	Distractibility, impulsivity, motoric restlessness, concentration deficits, aggression, aggression, formal thought disorder, paranoid delusions, depression, apathy, social withdrawal, cannabis use, LSD use, amphetamine use, cocaine use	Long-acting methylphenidate 36 mg, aripiprazole 15 mg	Remission	6 months	Blom & Kooij, 2012
23	F 44 years	Distractibility, motoric restlessness, agitation, insomnia, formal thought disorder, mood swings, impulsivity, restlessness, disorganization, paranoid delusions, auditory hallucinations, cocaine use, methylphenidate abuse	methylphenidate 60 mg, quetiapine 400 mg	Remission	3 years	Blom et al., present chapter

Note: "Full remission" indicates remission without any reported relapse; "remission" indicates initial remission, followed by subsequent relapse.

THEORIES OF ETIOLOGY

On the basis of the supposed therapeutic actions of antipsychotics and psycho-stimulants, it has been speculated that schizophrenia spectrum disorders are caused by an excess of dopamine, and AD(H)D by a lack of dopamine. As a consequence, the two groups of disorders long have been considered conceptual opposites with very different prescribed treatments. Any theory designed to explain the etiology of ADD psychosis must come to terms with this conceptual problem.

Recent epidemiological and genetic studies, however, indicated that such a strict dichotomy may be ill-founded. Based on a prospective cohort study of 208 youths diagnosed with ADHD, the relative risk for these patients to develop schizophrenia later in life, as compared with a non-ADHD sample, was found to be 4.3 (Dalsgaard, Mortensen, Frydenberg, Maibing, Nordentoft, & Thomsen, 2014). Whether this elevated risk is due to a shared genetic vulnerability is as yet unknown, but with a heritability estimate of 80% for schizophrenia (Sullivan, Kendler, & Neale, 2003) and of 60%–80% for ADHD (Froehlich, Anixt, Loe, Chirdkiatgumchai, Kuan, & Gilman, 2011), the possibility of a shared genetic vulnerability is not unrealistic. As indicated by various studies, sometimes single nucleotide polymorphisms (SNPs) and copy number variants (CNVs) are associated with AD(H)D-like as well as schizophrenia-like symptoms, and, in at least some cases, a final common pathway would seem to exist for both groups of symptoms at the level of molecular biology (Hamshere et al., 2013; Niklasson, Rasmussen, Oskarsdóttir, & Gillberg, 2009; Mitchell & Porteous, 2010).

The possibility of a shared neurobiological substrate also is indicated by the work of Hasan et al. (2013), who found similar dysfucntional hemispheric patterns of cortical inhibition and facilitation in a group of 25 first-episode psychotic patients, 28 ADHD patients, and 41 healthy controls with the aid of transcranial magnetic stimulation (TMS). The impairments that both groups of patients share with each other include inattention, deficits of executive functioning, a reduced capacity for emotional processing, impulsivity, low frustration tolerance, and impairments in social functioning (Opler et al., 1991; Levy et al., 2015). Pathophysiologically, these symptoms would seem to hint at a shared mechanism of frontal lobe dysfunction.

Given that both groups of patients are also known for elevated risks of substance abuse, it has also been suggested that this factor might constitute the link between psychosis and AD(H)D. As indicated by a survey among 7,403 adults in the United Kingdom, however, the link between ADHD symptoms and psychosis would seem to involve dysphoric mood rather than the use of amphetamines, cocaine, or cannabis (Marwaha et al., 2015). As the authors concluded, "Our analyses contradict the traditional clinical view that the main explanation for people with ADHD symptoms developing psychosis is illicit drugs." As regards the role of psychostimulants, Dalsgaard et al. (2014) found that the chance for AD(H)D patients to develop schizophrenia later in life did not correlate with the duration of treatment with these substances, and, therefore, consider it unlikely that ADD psychosis is an iatrogenic condition caused by the prolonged use of stimulants.

In conclusion, the etiology of ADD psychosis is as yet unknown, although various studies point in the direction of a shared neurobiological substrate for psychotic and AD(H)D-like symptoms that may well be based on a shared genetic vulnerability. The role of epigenetic factors in such cases is currently the subject of further study (Pallanti et al., 2015).

ASSESSMENT OPTIONS

So far, no available assessment tools are specifically tailored to assess the symptoms of ADD psychosis. Based on the literature and our clinical experience, we recommend careful diagnosis of psychotic *and* AD(H)D symptoms with the aid of structured diagnostic interviews. For psychosis, various diagnostic tools are available, such as the *Comprehensive Assessment of Symptoms and History* (CASH) (Andreasen, Flaum, & Arndt, 1992) and the *Structured Clinical Interview for DSM-IV Axis I Disorders, Clinician Version* (SCID-CV) (First, Spitzer, Gibbon, & Williams, 1996). For the diagnosis of AD(H)D symptoms, we recommend the *Diagnostic Interview for ADHD in Adults* (DIVA 2.0) (Kooij & Francken, 2013).

DIFFERENTIAL DIAGNOSIS

The differential diagnosis of ADD psychosis obviously includes schizophrenia spectrum disorder, ADD, and ADHD, but also schizoaffective disorder, bipolar disorder, borderline personality disorder, and various types of substance abuse disorder. We recommend that clinicians attempting to diagnose ADD psychosis not only concentrate on clinical symptoms and medical history, but also on the patients' reported responses to stimulants such as cocaine, amphetamines, and methylphenidate (which may be used orally or nasally). When substances such as these appear to have a soothing, calming effect, accompanied by an increased attention span and a decrease in both impulsivity and formal thought disorders (rather than the usual effects of elevated or expansive mood, restlessness, irritability, and paranoia), the patient may be using them in an attempt at self-medication. Thus, they may benefit from proper stimulant treatment.

TREATMENT OPTIONS

As suggested by Bellak and his group, the treatment of ADD psychosis—after careful diagnosis—involves the equally careful prescription of antipsychotics *and* psychostimulants. Psychotic patients should first be stabilized with the aid of antipsychotics (Levy et al., 2015). Dosages of stimulants should subsequently be titrated stepwise, starting from low dosages of (preferably long-acting) methylphenidate or dexamphetamine, up to levels of optimal effect and acceptable side effects (Blom & Kooij, 2012). Meanwhile, strict monitoring should take place, preferably in a specialized clinical setting. This monitoring should focus on detecting any early signs of psychosis, substance abuse, and general side effects of both psychostimulants and antipsychotics. In addition, it is advisable to provide psychoeducation in order to promote proper use of the prescribed medication as well as abstinence from illicit substances.

As our first case vignette and overview of published cases indicate, some patients do indeed benefit from a combination of antipsychotics and psychostimulants. Nonetheless, some caution is required because of the risk of psychostimulant abuse (Wilens 2004; 2008). After all, the fear of inducing hallucinations and other psychotic symptoms due to the ability of stimulants to promote excess levels of dopamine is not without precedent (Cherland & Fitzpatrick, 1999; Curran, Byrappa, & McBride 2004). Therefore, in view of the dopamine hypothesis of schizophrenia, it seems crucial to prevent such a dysregulation of dopamine levels (Berman, Kuczenski, McCracken, & London, 2009).

On the other hand, amphetamine psychosis is a relatively rare side effect in healthy individuals, occurring almost exclusively in association with extremely high (or quickly increasing) dosages of amphetamines (Bulut et al., 2013; Curran et al., 2004; Berman et al., 2009). Moreover, various studies indicate that psychotic individuals using psychostimulants as an augmentation to classic antipsychotics may experience an improvement in their cognitive functioning (e.g., their concept formation, spatial working memory, language production, and Stroop task performance) without experiencing any increase of their psychotic symptoms (Goldberg, Bigelow, & Weinberger, 1991; Barch & Carter, 2005; Lindenmayer, Nasrallah, Pucci, James, & Citrome, 2013). A possible explanation for these benevolent effects in psychotic individuals may be that psychosis is associated primarily with excess levels of presynaptic dopamine in the mesolimbic pathways, whereas psychostimulants tend to affect the dopaminergic frontostriatal information processing system (Huber, Kirchler, Niederhofer, & Gruber, 2007; Blom & Kooij, 2012). An alternative hypothesis suggests that (low doses of) psychostimulants increase the tonic transmission of dopamine while simultaneously decreasing its phasic transmission, thus inducing a calming and attention-enhancing effect without evoking any psychotic symptoms (Opler et al., 2001; Lindenmayer et al., 2013).

As regards psychotherapeutic treatment options, ADHD-focused cognitive-behavioral therapy (CBT) may be an option, too. So far no studies have been published on CBT for this specific patient group, but in clinical practice this type of treatment has been shown to be useful for the treatment of AD(H)D, as well as for the prevention of transitions to psychosis in high-risk AD(H)D groups (Safren et al., 2011o; van der Gaag et al., 2012). For adults with AD(H)D who are already treated with medication, CBT can add a favorable effect to treatment as usual (Emilsson et al., 2011).

RECOMMENDATIONS FOR FUTURE WORK

Thirty years after its initial conception, Bellak's concept of ADD psychosis recently has re-emerged as a diagnostic concept worthy of scientific investigation, which, in designated and well-assessed cases, may imply the careful application of relatively novel treatment approaches. As a diagnostic category in its own right, it still lacks sufficient support from large-scale systematic studies, but recent advances in neurobiological and epidemiological research indicate the presence of a significant overlap between the group of psychotic disorders and AD(H)D at symptomatic, genetic, and pathophysiological levels. Now that the search for biological markers of psychiatric disorders is firmly on the agenda of international research consortia, it is not inconceivable that the traditional boundaries between specific disorders such as schizophrenia, ADD, and ADHD will become blurred and that, over time, our categorical diagnostic systems perhaps will be replaced by dimensional ones (van Os & Kapur, 2009; Blom & van Praag, 2011). Whether the ADD psychosis concept deserves a place in either type of system is as yet uncertain, but one of its undeniable virtues is that it increases awareness of the existence of individuals who experience psychotic symptoms as well as symptoms of AD(H)D. To establish the proportion of individuals in that area of categorical overlap, systematic clinical research is needed, preferably in combination with genetic and epidemiological research.

In addition, systematic pharmacoclinical research is needed to further chart the risks and benefits of combined treatments (i.e., antipsychotics and psychostimulants) in designated cases. As indicated above, the use of illicit substances may be one of the reasons for psychotic relapses in reported cases of ADD psychosis. Another reason may be that the self-administration of short-acting psychostimulants is a demanding task, partly due to the necessity for using them at regular and frequent intervals, and partly due to the rebound phenomena that they may cause whenever a dose is missed. Therefore, future studies might benefit from the use of long-acting psychostimulants (or nonstimulants such as bupropion) to minimize rebound symptoms, or, alternatively, the use of dextrorotatory stimulants (such as dexmethylphenidate) to minimize both the dosage and the severity of side effects. Another advantage of these long-acting types of medication is that they offer fewer opportunities for abuse.

REFERENCES

American Psychiatric Association. (2013). *Diagnostic and statistical manual of mental disorders. Fifth edition.* Washington, DC: American Psychiatric Association.

Andreasen, N.C., Flaum, M., & Arndt, S. (1992). The Comprehensive Assessment of Symptoms and History (CASH). An instrument for assessing diagnosis and pathology. *Archives of General Psychiatry, 49*, 615–623.

Barch, D.M., & Carter, C.S. (2005). Amphetamine improves cognitive function in medicated individuals with schizophrenia and in healthy volunteers. *Schizophrenia Research, 77*, 43–58.

Bellak, L. (1948). *Dementia praecox.* New York, NY: Grune & Stratton.

Bellak, L. (1976). A possible subgroup of the schizophrenic syndrome and implications for treatment. *American Journal of Psychotherapy, 30*, 194–205.

Bellak, L. (1977). Psychiatric states in adults with minimal brain dysfunction. *Psychiatric Annals, 7*, 575–589.

Bellak, L. (1979). An idiosyncratic overview. In L. Bellak (Ed.), *Disorders of the schizophrenic syndrome* (pp. 3–22). New York, NY: Basic Books.

Bellak, L. (1985). ADD psychosis as a separate entity. *Schizophrenia Bulletin, 11*, 523–527.

Bellak, L., & Charles, E. (1979). Schizophrenic syndrome related to minimal brain dysfunction: A possible neurologic subgroup. *Schizophrenia Bulletin, 5*, 480–489.

Bellak, L., Kay, S., & Opler, L. (1987). Attention deficit disorder psychosis as a diagnostic category. *Psychiatric Developments, 3*, 239–263.

Bellak, L., & Opler, L.A. (1994). Conceptualizing ADHD. *Journal of Clinical Psychiatry, 55*, 312–313.

Benjumea Pino, P., & Mojarro Práxedes, D. (1996). Psicosis tipo Bellak, ¿un subgrupo de esquizofrenia? *Annales de Psiquiatria, 12*, 375–388.

Berman, S.M., Kuczenski, R., McCracken, J.T., & London, E.D. (2009). Potential adverse effects of amphetamine treatment on brain and behavior: A review. *Molecular Psychiatry, 4*, 123–142.

Blom, J.D., & Kooij, J.J.S. (2012). De ADD-psychose: Behandeling met antipsychotica én methylfenidaat? *Tijdschrift voor Psychiatrie, 54*, 89–93.

Blom, J.D., & van Praag, H.M. (2011). Schizophrenia: It's broken and it can't be fixed. A conceptual analysis at the centenary of Bleuler's Dementia praecox oder Gruppe der Schizophrenien. *Israel Journal of Psychiatry and Related Sciences, 48*, 240–248.

Bulut, G.C., Kaynar, S.Y., & Sabuncuoglu, O. (2013). Stimulant-related psychosis in ADHD treatment: An update for past 10 years. *Current Psychopharmacology, 2*, 218–221.

Cherland, E., & Fitzpatrick, R. (1999). Psychotic side effects of psychostimulants: A 5-year review. *Canadian Journal of Psychiatry, 44*, 811–813.

Curran, C., Byrappa, N., & McBride, A. (2004). Stimulant psychosis: Systematic review. *British Journal of Psychiatry, 185*, 196–204.

Dalsgaard, S., Mortensen, P.B., Frydenberg, M., Maibing, C.M., Nordentoft, M., & Thomsen, P.H. (2014). Association between Attention-Deficit Hyperactivity Disorder in childhood and schizophrenia later in adulthood. *European Psychiatry, 29*, 259–263.

De Jong, M.H., Eussen, M.L.J.M., & van Gool, A.R. (2010). Antipsychotica en stimulantia: Een zinvolle combinatie? *Tijdschrift voor Psychiatrie, 52*, 57–61.

Emilsson, B., Gudjonsson, G., Sigurdsson, J. F., Baldursson, G., Einarsson, E., Olafsdottir, H., & Young, S. (2011). Cognitive behaviour treatment in medication-treated adults with ADHD and persistent symptoms: A randomized controlled trial. *BMC Psychiatry, 11*, 116.

Fayyad, J., de Graaf, R., Kessler, R., Alonso, J., Angermeyer, M., Demyttenaere, K., . . . Jin, R. (2007). Cross-national prevalence and correlates of adult attention-deficit hyperactivity disorder. *British Journal of Psychiatry, 190*, 402–409.

First, M.B., Spitzer, R.L., Gibbon, M., & Williams, J.B.W. (1996). *Structured clinical interview for DSM-IV Axis I disorders, clinician version (SCID-CV)*. Washington, DC: American Psychiatric Press.

Froehlich, T.E., Anixt, J.S., Loe, I.M., Chirdkiatgumchai, V., Kuan, L., & Gilman, R.C. (2011). Update on environmental risk factors for attention-deficit/hyperactivity disorder. *Current Psychiatry Reports, 13*, 333–344.

Goldberg, T.E., Bigelow, L.B., & Weinberger, D.R. (1991). Cognitive and behavioral effects of coadministration of dextroamphetamine and haloperidol in schizophrenia. *American Journal of Psychiatry, 148*, 78–84.

Hamshere, M.L., Stergiakouli, E., Langley, K., Martin, J., Holmans, P., Kent, L., ...
  Craddock, N. (2013). Shared polygenic contribution between childhood attention-
  deficit hyperactivity disorder and adult schizophrenia. *British Journal of Psychiatry*,
  203, 107–111.

Hasan, A., Schneider, M., Schneider-Axmann, T., Ruge, D., Retz, W., Rösler, M., ...
  Wobrock, T. (2013). A similar but distinctive pattern of impaired cortical excitability
  in first-episode schizophrenia and ADHD. *Neuropsychobiology*, *67*, 74–83.

Huber, M., Kirchler, E., Niederhofer, H., & Gruber, L. (2007). Neuropsychiatrie des
  Methylphenidat bei der Aufmerksamkeits-Defizit/Hyperaktivitäts-Störung (ADHS).
  Fortschritte der Neurologie und Psychiatrie, *75*, 275–284.

Huey, L.Y., Zetin, M., Janowsky, D.S., & Judd, L.L. (1978). Adult minimal brain dysfunction and schizophrenia: A case report. *American Journal of Psychiatry*, *135*,
  1563–1565.

Jandl, M., Steyer, J., & Kaschka, W.P. (2012). Adolescent attention deficit hyperactivity
  disorder and susceptibility to psychosis in adulthood: A review of the literature and a
  phenomenological case report. *Early Intervention in Psychiatry*, *6*, 11–20.

Kay, S.R., & Bellak, L. (1986). Attention deficit disorder psychosis: Psychometric distinction from schizophrenia. *Perceptual and Motor Skills*, *62*, 510.

Kay, S.R., Fiszbein, A., & Opler, L.A. (1987). The positive and negative syndrome scale
  (PANSS) for schizophrenia. *Schizophrenia Bulletin*, *13*, 261–276.

Kooij, J.J.S., & Francken, M.H. (2013). Diagnostic Interview for ADHD in Adults (DIVA
  2.0). In J.J.S. Kooij (Ed.), *Adult ADHD. Diagnostic assessment and treatment*(3rd ed.)
  (pp. 97–99). New York, NY: Springer. Available online in 17 languages via www.diva-
  center.eu.

Levy, E., Traicu, A., Iyer, S., Malla, A., & Joober, R. (2015). Psychotic disorders comorbid
  with attention-deficit hyperactivity disorder: An important knowledge gap. *Canadian
  Journal of Psychiatry*, *60*(3 Suppl 2), S48–S52.

Lieberman, J.A., Kane, J.M., & Alvir, J. (1987). Provocative tests with psychostimulant
  drugs in schizophrenia. *Psychopharmacology*, *91*, 415–433.

Lindenmayer, J.-P., Nasrallah, H., Pucci, M., James, S., & Citrome L. (2013). A systematic review of psychostimulant treatment of negative symptoms of schizophrenia: Challenges and therapeutic opportunities. *Schizophrenia Research*, *147*, 241–252.

Marwaha, S., Thompson, A., Bebbington, P., Singh, P., Freeman, D., Winsper, C., &
  Boome, M.R. (2015). Adult attention deficit hyperactivity symptoms and psycho-
  sis: Epidemiological evidence from a population survey in England. *Psychiatry
  Research*. doi: 10.1016/j.psychres.2015.07.075.

Mason, P. (2010). ADHD, schizophrenia and methylphenidate. *ADHD in Practice*,
  2, 8–10.

Mitchell, K.J., & Porteous, D.J. (2010). Rethinking the genetic architecture of schizophrenia. *Psychological Medicine*, *41*, 19–32.

Niklasson, L., Rasmussen, P., Oskarsdóttir, S., & Gillberg, C. (2009). Autism, ADHD,
  mental retardation and behaviour problems in 100 individuals with 22q11 deletion
  syndrome. *Research in Developmental Disabilities*, *30*, 763–773.

Opler, L.A., Frank, D.M., & Ramirez, P.M. (2001). Psychostimulants in the treatment of
  adults with psychosis and attention deficit disorder. *Annals of the New York Academy
  of Sciences*, *931*, 297–301.

Pallanti, S., & Salerno, L. (2015). Raising attention to attention deficit hyperactivity disorder in schizophrenia. *World Journal of Psychiatry*, *5*, 47–55.

Perälä, J., Suvisaari, J., Saarni, S.I., Kuoppasalmi, K., Isometsä, E., Pirkola, S., ... Lönnqvist, J. (2007). Lifetime prevalence of psychotic and bipolar I disorders in a general population. *Archives of General Psychiatry, 64,* 19–28.

Peralta, V., de Jalón, E.G., Campos, M.S., Zandio, M., Sanches-Torres, A., & Cuesta, M.J. (2010). The meaning of childhood attention-deficit hyperactivity symptoms in patients with a first-episode of schizophrenia-spectrum psychosis. *Schizophrenia Research, 126,* 28–35.

Pine, D.S., Klein, R.G., Lindy, D.C., & Marshall, R.D. (1993). Attention-deficit hyperactivity disorder and comorbid psychosis: A review and two clinical presentations. *Journal of Clinical Psychiatry, 54,* 140–145.

Regier, D.A., Kuhl, E.A., & Kupfer, D.J. (2013). The DSM-5: Classification and criteria changes. *World Psychiatry, 12,* 92–98.

Safren, S.A., Sprich, S., Mimiaga, M.J., Surman, C., Knouse, L., Groves, M., & Otto, M.W. (2010). Cognitive behavioral therapy vs relaxation with educational support for medication-treated adults with ADHD and persistent symptoms: A randomized controlled trial. *Journal of the American Medical Association, 304,* 875–880.

Sambhi, R.S., & Lepping, P. (2009). Adult ADHD and psychosis: A review of the literature and two cases. *Clinical Neuropsychiatry, 6,* 174–178.

Stahlberg, O., Soderstrom, H., Rastam, M., & Gillberg, C. (2004). Bipolar disorder, schizophrenia, and other psychotic disorders in adults with childhood onset AD/HD and/or autism spectrum disorders. *Journal of Neural Transmission, 111,* 891–902.

Sullivan, P.F., Kendler, K.S., & Neale, M.C. (2003). Schizophrenia as a complex trait: Evidence from a meta-analysis of twin studies. *Archives of General Psychiatry, 60,* 1187–1192.

Van der Gaag, M., Nieman, D.H., Rietdijk, J., Dragt, S., Ising, H.K., Klaassen, R.M., ... Linszen, D.H. (2012). Cognitive behavioral therapy for subjects at ultrahigh risk for developing psychosis: A randomized controlled clinical trial. *Schizophrenia Bulletin, 38,* 1180–1188.

Van Os, J., & Kapur, S. (2009). Schizophrenia. *Lancet, 374,* 635–645.

Vergouwen, T., & Gorissen, M. (2001). Een verantwoord experiment: Behandeling met methylfenidaat bij een psychotische patiënte. *Psychopraxis, 3,* 161–164.

Ward, M.F., Wender, P.H., & Reimherr, F.W. (1993). The Wender Utah Rating Scale: An aid in the retrospective diagnosis of childhood attention deficit hyperactivity disorder. *American Journal of Psychiatry, 150,* 885–890.

Wilens, T.E. (2004). Attention-deficit/hyperactivity disorder and the substance use disorders: The nature of the relationship, subtypes at risk, and treatment issues. *Psychiatric Clinics of North America, 27,* 283–301.

Wilens, T.E. (2008). Effects of methylphenidate on the catecholaminergic system in attention-deficit/hyperactivity disorder. *Journal of Clinical Psychopharmacology, 28*(3 Suppl 2), S46–S53.

World Health Organization (1993). International Classification of Diseases and Related Health Problems 10th revision. Geneva: World Health Organization.

7

Cotard's Syndrome

HANS DEBRUYNE ∎

VIGNETTE

A 46-year-old woman with rapid cycling bipolar disorder was admitted to the hospital. She presented in a depressive episode with psychotic features. Nihilistic delusions were also present. Specifically, she had the constant experience of having no identity or "self" and the sense of being only a body without any content. In addition, she was convinced that her brain had vanished, that her intestines had disappeared, and that her whole body was translucent. She refused to take a bath or shower because she was afraid she was soluble and might disappear down the drain. She had experienced several admissions to various hospitals due to depressive or manic episodes since the age of 29 years. In previous depressive episodes, she never reported Cotard's syndrome symptoms. When the depression and Cotard's syndrome resolved, she switched to a hypomanic state (Debruyne et al, 2009).

HISTORICAL AND CULTURAL CONTEXT

Cotard's syndrome is named for Jules Cotard (1840–1889), a French neurologist who first described this condition in 1880. He presented the following case report of a 43-year-old female. "Mlle X, affirms she has no brain, no nerves, no chest, no stomach, no intestines; there's only skin and bones of a decomposing body ... She has no soul, God does not exist, neither the devil. She's nothing more than a decomposing body, and has no need to eat for living, she cannot die a natural death, she exists eternally if she's not burned, the fire will be the only solution for her" (translation from Cotard, 1880).

He formulated the syndrome that would later bear his name as a new type of depression characterized by the following symptoms: anxious melancholia, ideas of damnation or rejection, insensitivity to pain, delusions of nonexistence concerning one's own body, and delusions of immortality. He categorized this under *lypémanie,* a kind of psychotic depression described by Esquirol (Debruyne et al., 2011). In 1882, Cotard introduced *délire des négations* ("delusion of negation") as new terminology for the syndrome. Séglas introduced the eponym "Cotard's syndrome" in 1887 in his book, *Le Délire de Négation.* A few years later, Régis (1893) linked the syndrome to other psychiatric disorders.

Tissot (1921) extracted two components from Cotard's syndrome: an affective component associated with anxiety and a cognitive component associated with the presence of a delusion. Loudet and Martinez (1933) tried to clarify the heterogeneity by defining different subtypes. They first described a nongeneralized *délire de négation* associated with paralysis, alcoholic psychosis, or dementia. They described the "real" Cotard's syndrome, however, as being only found in anxious melancholia and chronic hypochondria.

In 1968, Saavedra described 10 cases of Cotard's syndrome and classified them into three types: depressive, mixed, and schizophrenic. He drew a distinction between "genuine" Cotard's syndrome, occurring during depressive states, and what he described as a pseudonihilistic or pseudo–Cotard syndrome. He also termed the latter *coenesthetic schizophrenia.*

Berrios and Luque (1995) made the first evidence-based classification of Cotard's syndrome. They conducted a retrospective factor analysis of 100 cases in the literature and identified three types of Cotard's syndrome. The first is a form of psychotic depression in which anxiety, melancholia, delusions of guilt, and auditory hallucinations are the more prominent features. Second, they described Cotard's syndrome type I, which is associated with hypochondriac and nihilistic delusions and the absence of a depressive episode. The third is Cotard's syndrome type II, in which anxiety, depression, auditory hallucinations, delusions of immortality, nihilistic delusions, and suicidal behavior are characteristic features.

ROLE IN CURRENT DIAGNOSTIC SYSTEMS

In our current classification systems, *the Diagnostic and Statistical Manual of Mental Disorders* (DSM-5) (American Psychiatric Association, 2013) and the *International Classification of Diseases* (ICD-10) (World Health Organization, 2015), Cotard's syndrome is not defined as a separate entity. In DSM-5, nihilistic delusions (but not Cotard's syndrome) are mentioned in the description of delusions in the *Schizophrenia Spectrum and other Psychotic Disorders* section, as well as examples of mood-congruent psychotic features in one of the *Depressive Disorder specifiers.* A search for "Cotard syndrome" in the online ICD-10 (World Health Organization, 2015) directs the reader to delusional disorder. However, Cotard's syndrome is not mentioned in the description. Cotard's syndrome is currently diagnosed as a phenomenological syndrome within different underlying disorders (Debruyne & Audenaert 2009; 2012). I would advocate this current evolution and not recommend that Cotard's syndrome be a separate diagnostic entity in the existing classification systems. The etiology is broad, both psychiatric and somatic. Cotard's syndrome is more likely a possible symptomatic result of several underlying disorders, rather than a separate disorder as such. The specificity and severity of the symptomatology, however, can make the recognition of Cotard's syndrome clinically important.

SYMPTOMATOLOGY

Nihilistic delusions concerning the individual's body are the central features of Cotard's syndrome. In his first publication, Cotard pointed out six characteristic symptoms: anxious melancholia; ideas of damnation or possession; suicidal behavior and self-harm; analgesia; hypochondriac ideas of nonexistence or destruction of organs, the whole body, the soul, God, etc.; and ideas of immortality (Debruyne, 2009).

In an analysis of 100 cases, the most prominent symptoms were: depressive mood (89%), nihilistic delusions concerning one's own existence (69%), anxiety (65%), delusions of guilt (63%), delusions of immortality (55%), and hypochondriac delusions (58%) (Berrios & Luque, 1995).

The duration of the syndrome can vary from weeks to years, depending on the underlying disorder (Hansen & Bolwig, 1998). A classical description of the course of Cotard's syndrome is given by Enoch and Trethowan (1991):

In its early stages Cotard's syndrome is characterized by a vague feeling of anxiety, with a varying time-span from weeks to years. This anxious state gradually augments and can result in nihilistic delusions, where a denial of life or denial of body parts is the prominent features. The patient loses sense of reality. Despite the delusion of being dead, these patients show an increased tendency to automutilation or suicidal behaviour. Additional symptoms may include analgesia and mutism. The core symptoms always reflect a preoccupation with guilt, despair and death. Delusions can be accompanied by a délire d'énormité, a delusion of massive increase of body measures. This has been described as the manic Cotard's syndrome. As the syndrome often occurs in association with other psychotic states, symptoms of these specific disorders are likely to be present. As an example, nihilistic delusions grafted on a depressive illness are often associated by other characteristics of a depressive episode such as weight loss and sleeping difficulties and the syndrome associated with organic disease is often associated with other symptoms such as disorientation or neurological signs.

In 1999, Yamada made a proposal for the stages of development in Cotard's syndrome. Based on a case report, he defined three stages: germination stage, blooming stage, and chronic stage. The *germination stage* is characterized by significant hypochondria, cenesthopathy, and a depressed mood. A diagnosis of Cotard's syndrome cannot yet be made at this stage. In the *blooming stage*, the characteristic features of Cotard's syndrome (nihilistic delusions, delusions of immortality together with anxiety and negativism) are seen. The last, the *chronic* stage, is differentiated into two manifestations: one with persistent emotional disturbances (depressive type) and a second where depressive symptoms are less prominent (paranoid type). Evidence for this hypothesis is limited and only supported by two case reports (Yamada, 1999; Duggal, 2002). A recently published case report rejected this hypothesis (Nejad, Anari, & Pouya, 2013). In my opinion, it is important to take the heterogeneity of Cotard's syndrome into account. Depending upon underlying conditions, the evolution and manifestations of the symptoms can differ. For this reason a more general theory on the evolution or staging of Cotard's syndrome phenomenology is difficult to defend. Some common pathways may be found in etiologic (mostly neuropsychologic) pathways. On the phenomenological level, prudence is needed when attempting to generalize from specific cases to theories. For several patients, the staging theory certainly can be applied, but for others, perhaps not.

PREVALENCE RATE AND ASSOCIATED FEATURES

Good epidemiologic data about Cotard's syndrome are not yet available, but the available research will be presented below. There are a few prevalence studies available, though each study had only a very limited number of patients (Debruyne, 2012).

A prevalence study conducted in a selected psychogeriatric population in Hong Kong found Cotard's syndrome in two out of 349 patients. A higher prevalence rate of 3.2% was reached when only severely depressed elderly were included (Chiu, 1995). In a Mexican sample of primary psychiatric patients screened over a two-year period, 0.62% (n = 3) patients had Cotard's syndrome. Using the same methodology, a rate of 0.11% (n = 1) was found in a sample of neurological patients with mental disturbances (Ramirez-Bermudez et al., 2010). In an Austrian data set of 346 schizophrenia patients, 0.87% (n = 3) could be diagnosed with Cotard's syndrome (Stompe et al., 2013).

The likelihood of developing Cotard's delusion appears to increase with age (Edelstyn, 2006). A mean age of 56 years was found in a review of 100 cases (Berrios et al, 1995), and more recently, a mean age of 47.7 years was found when aggregating 138 case reports (Consoli et al., 2007). Women seem to be more vulnerable (Enoch & Trethowan, 1991). Caution should be exercised when interpreting these results, however, because a publication bias is likely in effect (i.e., special and interesting cases with scientific value are more likely to be published). Further, the syndrome is found across various ethnic groups (Edelstyn, 2006). Diagnosis of Cotard's syndrome in people under 25 years old has been thought to be associated with bipolar disorder (Consoli, 2007).

Cotard's syndrome currently is conceptualized as the phenomenological presentation of an underlying disorder (Debruyne, 2012). Several psychiatric and somatic diseases have been associated with the syndrome. Unipolar and bipolar depressions are the most common associated psychiatric disorders, but psychotic disorder also is frequently reported (Debruyne, 2012). Some reports describe the co-occurrence of Cotard's syndrome with other rare psychiatric syndromes (e.g., hydrophobia, lycanthropy, and *folie à deux* as in Debruyne, 2009). Examples of Cotard's coexistence with other rare delusions have been published. These include Capgras (a delusion wherein familiar persons are replaced by identical imposters) and the Fregoli delusion (a delusion wherein different people are, in fact, a single person who changes appearance or is in disguise—(see Chapter 5) (Enoch, 1991; Butler, 2000; Yalin et al., 2008; Joseph, 1986; Wolf & McKenzie, 1994; Shiraishi et al., 2004; Wright et al., 1993).

A recent review (Debruyne, 2012) cited numerous organic conditions associated with Cotard's: dementia, major depressive episode in mild cognitive impairment, depression in frontotemporal atrophy, semantic dementia, severe mental retardation, typhoid fever, tuberculosis infection, HIV, cerebral infarction, superior sagittal sinus thrombosis, brain tumors, temporal lobe epilepsy, limbic epileptic insults, postictal depression, cerebral arteriovenous malformation with and without epilepsy, migraine, Laurence-Moon-Bardet-Biedl syndrome, multiple sclerosis, Parkinson's disease, brain injury, noninfectious complication of heart transplantation, consequence of adverse drug reaction to acyclovir and valacyclovir and herpetic or nonherpetic encephalitis. Recently, reports of associations with right subdural hemorrhage (Perez et al., 2014), insular cortex atrophy in dementia (Chatterjee & Mitra, 2015), and postsurgical depression (Sharma & Biswas, 2012) were published.

THEORIES OF ETIOLOGY

Starting with a traditional view, depersonalization phenomena were reported to be an essential step in the development of Cotard's syndrome according to Séglas (1887). Alheid elaborated depersonalization in a Cotard's syndrome context using German terminology: "*Leib*" (body for me) and "*Körper*" (body as such). Depersonalization may occur when "*Körper*" prevails over "*Leib*," and when the body is less associated with the self ("*Leib*"). In depersonalization, however, patients feel as though they are dead (indifference of affect) while in Cotard's syndrome patients are convinced that they are dead (lack of feeling) (Saavedra, 1968; Enoch, 1991). Recently, a case report with a direct association of depersonalization and the development of Cotard's syndrome was published (Nejad et al., 2013).

Some scholars believe that personality characteristics have an essential role in the development of Cotard's syndrome (Cotard, 1882; Enoch, 1991). With regard to premorbid personality characteristics, it has been proposed that patients with a more internal attributional style (which often co-occurs with depression) are more vulnerable to developing the syndrome. Patients with a more external attributional style (which is more co-occurring with paranoia) are also more prone to develop Capgras syndrome (Gerrans, 2000). This hypothesis that Cotard's patients have a more internal attribution style was empirically tested in at least one case (McKay & Cipolotti, 2007). A significantly higher score on two attribution bias indices (internalizing bias index, internalizing bias for negative events) calculated on the *Internal, Personal, and Situational Attributions Questionnaire* was found in this one patient with Cotard's syndrome compared with control subjects. Several authors, however, reported the co-occurrence of Cotard's syndrome and Capgras syndrome (Enoch, 1991; Butler, 2000; Yalin, 2008; Joseph, 1986; Wolff, 1994; Shiraishi, 2004; Wright, 1993). Vinkers (2008) suggested that a combination of attribution styles occur in these patients, such that these patients are both depressed and paranoid or such that they suffer from delusions about self-identity and about the identity of others. Unfortunately, evidence-based proof for this hypothesis is lacking.

The neuropsychological origin of Cotard's delusion is thought to be related to a dysfunction of an information processing subsystem where face and body recognition is associated with a changed affective component (or changed feeling of familiarity). When this affective component is lacking, the patients may experience a feeling of de-realization and depersonalization (Young & Leafhead, 1996). The same hypothesis has been supported in other misidentification syndromes, especially Capgras (Ellis et al., 1997; Hirstein & Ramachandran, 1997; Breen et al., 2002). Interestingly, in studies using facial recognition tasks (using skin conductance as an outcome measure) a differential autonomic response to familiar faces compared to unknown faces was absent in patients with Capgras syndrome (Ellis, 1997; Hirstein, 1997). Another patient with atypical Capgras delusion showed impaired interpretation of facial expressions. This led the patient to mistake differences in expression for differences in identity (Breen, 2002). For Cotard's syndrome, the hypothesis of a lack of differential autonomic response to anything is suggested. This absence of affect of familiarity to anything could lead to the delusion of being dead, whereas in Capgras delusion there is only lack of familiarity to known faces, leading to the delusion of familiar persons being replaced by identical impostors. In this hypothesis, Cotard patients have a more pronounced and generalized loss of familiarity than Capgras patients (Coltheart, 2007a; 2012). For Cotard's syndrome, however, empirical evidence is very limited. In one patient with Cotard's syndrome due to right hemispheric infarction, the role for an affective component was indeed supported (Nishio & Mori, 2012).

The absence of a feeling of familiarity, along with a particular attribution style, cannot completely explain the pathophysiology of delusional misidentification syndromes. Patients with brain damage of the ventromedial region of the frontal cortex also demonstrate the aforementioned lack of differential autonomic responsivity to familiar faces in spite of the absence of delusions. The same is seen in patients suffering from pure autonomic failure (a neurodegenerative disease, with gradually worsening autonomic disturbances without other neurologic signs). In the absence of delusions, these patients also show a lack of differential autonomic responsivity to anything (Breen, 2002; Coltheart 2007a;Coltheart et al. 2007b; 2012; Davies, 2001). As patients with depersonalization disorders, they may report feeling as though they were dead, but this is quite different from the existential negation found in typical Cotard's patients (Young, 2013).

The idea of a changed affective component has been incorporated into most neuropsychological models, but the role for each differs. Several of these models will be described next.

One-Stage Model

In this model, the difference between normal and delusional subjects hinges upon perceptual (or other) malfunctions, which produce anomalous experience, and this anomalous experience gives subjects compelling evidence for their delusional beliefs (Breen, 2002). Formation of the delusional belief is, therefore, a rational process (Coltheart, 2010). Given that the lack of a feeling of familiarity, along with attributional style, cannot completely explain the pathophysiology of delusional misidentification syndromes, a two-stage model was a logical sequela.

Two-Stage Model

There are known disorders other than Cotard's syndrome wherein patients undergo an anomalous perceptual experience, but do not develop a delusional disorder (e.g., pure autonomic failure or depersonalization). Therefore, this perceptual or other type of malfunction is not sufficient for a delusional disorder to develop, and there must be at least a second factor involved. This second factor is presumably responsible for the failure to reject the characteristic Cotard's hypothesis (e.g., "I'm dead") as an explanation for the lack of feeling of familiarity to anything despite the presence of (often overwhelming) evidence against it (Breen, 2002; Coltheart, 2007a). In this two-factor explanation, an anomalous experience arises at the first stage, and some form of *cognitive* disruption manifests at the second stage (Young, 2011). The importance of the right dorsolateral prefrontal cortex (RDLPFC) for the hypothesis of this second factor was demonstrated with functional magnetic resonance imaging (fMRI) (Corlett et al., 2004; Fletcher et al., 2001; Turner, 2004). It also has been observed that right frontal damage commonly occurs in cases of delusional misidentification (including Cotard's syndrome, as in Edelstyn, 2006; McKay, 2007).

Expressive Theory

The delusional subject is not really expressing beliefs at all, given that a proposition so clearly falsifiable by other facts available to the subject (and hence disqualified by the proper application of procedural rationality) cannot be sincerely believed. Delusional subjects use what we might call the *language of beliefs* to express the bizarre and disorienting nature of the experience. Patients who know that their delusion would not be judged true by others applying normal standards cannot really be expressing a belief. This means that their pragmatic competence is intact. Experiencing beliefs "as if," with an impaired ability to use their intact pragmatic competence, leads to the delusion (Gerrans, 2001). Support for this theory is rather limited.

Change in Existential Orientation

In this model, the explanation for delusions of misidentification is grounded in changes to the patient's particular *existential feeling*; that is, the particular ways we have of experiencing ourselves in the world and with other people, which shape all of our thoughts and characteristic activity. This has to be *felt* in some sense (e.g., feeling dead/alive, feeling lost, things feeling right), as proposed by Ratcliffe (Young, 2011; Ratcliffe, 2008; 2012). Here, the delusional content is simply an expression of a more general alteration in existential feeling. Impairments in reasoning are thought to be embedded in a background of existential feeling, rather than manifesting after an anomalous experience (Young, 2011). This contrasts with other more "spectatorial models" (i.e., the patient as a spectator of an anomalous experience, wherein perceptions and experiences are constructed as a kind of input system through which perceptual contents are presented (Young, 2011).

Interactionist Model

An interactionist model was also proposed which provided a more bidirectional account with a greater emphasis on the patient's underlying phenomenal experience. The classic top-down process explanations of one- and two-stage models are thus integrated. Adherents of this model believe that the interaction of top-down and bottom-up processes better explains the maintenance of the delusional belief. In the bottom-up process, once a belief is formed, it will affect how the subject interprets subsequent observational data, thereby becoming predisposed to see what is expected. It also places a greater emphasis on the patient's underlying phenomenal experience in accounting for the specificity of the delusional content (Young, 2010; 2011).

For one Cotard's patient there were empirical data supporting this bottom-up process: neuropsychologic research with an emotional Stroop paradigm demonstrated an attentional bias for words related to death. The role of attentional biases was thought to reinforce and maintain the delusional beliefs by constantly focusing the patient's attention onto any relevant information (Turner, 2004).

Interestingly, most neuroimaging data show no gross structural changes in the brain in patients with Cotard's syndrome (Edelstyn, 2006). It also has been observed, however, that right frontal damage has commonly occurred in some cases of delusional misidentification (including Cotard's syndrome). Left lesions also have been described. Using molecular neuroimaging modalities, not all studies show right-sided hypofunctionality (Edelstyn, 2006; Swamy et al., 2007). There appears to be a correlation between prefrontal dysfunction and nihilistic beliefs in neurological patients (Edelstyn, 2006).

ASSESSMENT OPTIONS

There are limited publications on technical assessments of Cotard's, and the results appear to be conflicting. Several structural abnormalities have been reported (Debruyne, 2009; Swamy, 2007), but in most cases no gross structural changes on structural brain imaging are evident (Swamy, 2007). For the most part, there are no electroencephalogram abnormalities revealed in Cotard's syndrome, although nonspecific abnormalities and abnormalities suggestive of the underlying organic condition have occasionally been mentioned (Swamy, 2007). Functional brain imaging techniques (mostly Single Photon Emission Computed Tomography [SPECT]) showed several abnormalities, but normal cerebral perfusion also has been reported (e.g., Debruyne, 2009).

Only a few reports mentioned detailed neuropsychological examination. Most research was performed using face recognition tasks. It was suggested that a general impairment of all aspects of face processing could be attributed to loss of knowledge of familiar people. Interestingly, a normal recognition of emotional facial expressions is typically observed in Cotard's (Swamy, 2007).

As mentioned previously, damage to an affective component of the face recognition system was proposed as an etiological component (Gerrans, 2000; Young, 1996). Despite the normal regional brain perfusion, severe neuropsychological right-hemisphere abnormalities were discovered in one case of Cotard's syndrome (Debruyne, 2009).

Acquiring a precise history is essential when assessing Cotard's syndrome. Because Cotard's syndrome is part of an underlying disorder, several potential etiologies have to be taken into account. Next to psychiatric assessment, physical and technical investigations should be mandatory to rule out certain somatic etiologies. At present, there are no specific tests, questionnaires, clinical interviews, or well-established examinations for Cotard's syndrome. Because Cotard's syndrome is a phenomenological state of an underlying disorder, one could argue whether having such tests available has a clinical value.

DIFFERENTIAL DIAGNOSIS

Cotard's syndrome is a phenomenological diagnosis. Because the phenomenology forms part of an underlying disorder, differential diagnosis for different etiologies has to be made. Nihilistic delusions within depressive episodes with psychotic features (uni- and bipolar) are the most common, but Cotard's syndrome regularly is reported in psychotic disorders as well. It may be prudent to consider bipolar disorder in patients under the age of 25 years (Consoli, 2007). Several somatic disorders also can cause this syndrome, if only in rare cases. Thus, prudence in diagnostics is important, especially in patients without a previous history of depression or psychosis.

TREATMENT OPTIONS

Treatment initially should follow current treatment guidelines for the primary DSM-5 (American Psychiatric Association, 2013) or IDC-10 (World Health Organization, 2015) diagnosis in which Cotard's syndrome is manifesting. Several case reports detailing treatment of Cotard's syndrome have been published, but no randomized trials have yet been conducted. The most frequently reported treatment strategy appears to be electroconvulsive therapy (ECT) (Debruyne, 2012). In depressive disorder with psychotic features, ECT (often in combination with pharmacotherapy) seems to be the most empirically supported strategy (Debruyne, 2012).

Successful pharmacotherapeutic approaches also have been published. This primarily has consisted of antidepressants, antipsychotics, or a combination of both classes (Debruyne, 2012). Within published reports, the prescribed pharmaceuticals were heterogeneous, and no differences between agents can be determined at this time. A publication bias, favoring case reports with successful treatment, could also be a confound in the literature. As noted above, following international treatment guidelines for the underlying disorder is recommended.

Special measures may be needed due to the risk for suicide (Enoch, 1991). A heightened suicide risk for Cotard's, based on expert opinion, has been discussed in several reports. However, no statistical data are yet available to bear this out. The frequent association of a severe depressive episode with psychotic features is likely an important contributing factor. Following a case report of Cotard's syndrome in a schizophrenic patient, Huber and Agorastos (2012) suggested a thorough risk assessment for violent behavior. It is important to note that other reports do not mention violent risk. In my opinion, the risk for violent behavior in Cotard's syndrome is not higher than for any other psychiatric condition.

RECOMMENDATIONS FOR FUTURE WORK

Cotard's syndrome is a phenomenological diagnosis that does not fit neatly into our current classification system. In my work and review of the literature, Cotard's syndrome can be a phenomenological expression of several disorders, as well as somatic (mostly neurologic) and psychiatric disorders. The phenomenological similarity between these cases suggests a common psychopathologic pathway in which delusions are formed. Research on syndromes where isolated delusions are manifested, such as Cotard's syndrome, could provide additional knowledge about pathophysiologic/neuropsychologic mechanisms in these and other disorders with delusional symptoms. For this reason, future study of the phenomenology of Cotard's may help the field gain a better understanding of brain functioning and pathophysiology.

REFERENCES

American Psychiatric Association, (2013). *Diagnostic and statistical manual of mental disorders. Fifth edition (DSM-5)*. Washington, DC: American Psychiatric Publishing.

Berrios, G., & Luque, R. (1995). Cotard's syndrome: analysis of 100 cases. *Acta Psychiatrica Scandinavica, 91*(3), 185–188. doi:10.1111/j.1600-0447.1995.tb09764.x

Breen, N., Caine, D., & Coltheart, M. (2002). The role of affect and reasoning in a patient with a delusion of misidentification. *Cognitive Neuropsychiatry, 7*(2), 113–137. doi:10.1080/13546800143000203

Butler, P. (2000). Diurnal variation in Cotard's syndrome (copresent with Capgras delusion) following traumatic brain injury. *The Australian and New Zealand Journal of Psychiatry, 34*(4), 684–687. doi:10.1080/j.1440-1614.2000.00758.x

Chatterjee, S., & Mitra, S. (2015). "I do not exist"—Cotard syndrome in insular cortex atrophy. *Biological Psychiatry, 77*(11), e52–e53. doi:10.1016/j.biopsych.2014.11.005

Chiu, H. (1995). Cotard's syndrome in psychogeriatric patients in Hong Kong. *General Hospital Psychiatry, 17*(1), 54–55. doi:10.1016/0163-8343(94)00066-m

Coltheart, M. (2007a). The 33rd Sir Frederick Bartlett Lecture Cognitive neuropsychiatry and delusional belief. *The Quarterly Journal of Experimental Psychology, 60*(8), 1041–1062. doi:10.1080/17470210701338071

Coltheart, M., Langdon, R., & McKay, R. (2007b). Schizophrenia and monothematic delusions. *Schizophrenia Bulletin, 33*(3), 642–647. doi:10.1093/schbul/sbm017

Coltheart, M. (2010). The neuropsychology of delusions. *Annals of the New York Academy of Sciences, 1191*(1), 16–26. doi:10.1111/j.1749-6632.2010.05496.x

Consoli, A., Soultanian, C., Tanguy, M., Laurent, C., Perisse, D., Luque, R. Cohen, D., Berrios, G.E. (2007). Cotard's syndrome in adolescents and young adults is associated with an increased risk of bipolar disorder. *Bipolar Disorders, 9*(6), 665–668. doi:10.1111/j.1399-5618.2007.00420.x

Corlett, P., Aitken, M., Dickinson, A., Shanks, D., Honey, G., Honey, R., Fletcher, P.C., Robbins, T.W., Bullmore, E.T. (2004). Prediction error during retrospective revaluation of causal associations in humans: fMRI evidence in favor of an associative model of learning. *Neuron, 44*(5), 877–888. doi:10.1016/s0896-6273(04)00756-1

Cotard, J. (1880). Du délire hypocondriaque dans une forme grave de la mélancholie anxieuse. *Annales Médico-Psychologique, 4*, 168–174.

Cotard, J. (1882). Du délire des négations. *Archives De Neurologie, 4*, 282–295.

Davies, M., Coltheart, M., Langdon, R., & Breen, N. (2001). Monothematic delusions: Towards a two-factor account. *Philosophy, Psychiatry, & Psychology, 8*(2), 133–158. doi:10.1353/ppp.2001.0007

Debruyne, H., Portzky, M., Van den Eynde, F., & Audenaert, K. (2009). Cotard's syndrome: A review. *Current Psychiatry Reports, 11*(3), 197–202. doi:10.1007/s11920-009-0031-z

Debruyne, H., Portzky, M., Peremans, K., & Audenaert, K. (2011). Cotard's syndrome. *Mind & Brain, 2*(1), 67–72.

Debruyne, H., & Audenaert, K. (2012). Towards understanding Cotard's syndrome: an overview. *Neuropsychiatry, 2*(6), 481–486. doi:10.2217/npy.12.67

Duggal, H. (2002). Biological basis and staging of Cotard's syndrome. *European Psychiatry, 17*(2), 108–109. doi:10.1016/s0924-9338(02)00637-5

Edelstyn, N., & Oyebode, F. (2006). A review of the phenomenology and cognitive neuropsychological origins of the Cotard delusion. *Neurology Psychiatry and Brain Research, 13,* 9–14.

Ellis, H., Young, A., Quayle, A., & De Pauw, K. (1997). Reduced autonomic responses to faces in Capgras delusion. *Proceedings of the Royal Society B: Biological Sciences, 264*(1384), 1085–1092. doi:10.1098/rspb.1997.0150

Hansen, E.H., Bolwig, T.G. (1998). Cotard syndrome: An important manifestation of melancholia. *Nordic Journal of Psychiatry, 52*(6), 459–464. doi:10.1080/08039489850139238

Enoch, M., & Trethowan, W. (1991). *Uncommon psychiatric syndromes.* Oxford: Butterworth-Heinemann.

Fletcher, P., Anderson, J., Shanks, D., Honey, R., Carpenter, T., & Donovan, T. (2001). Responses of human frontal cortex to surprising events are predicted by formal associative learning theory. *Nature Neuroscience, 4*(10), 1043–1048. doi:10.1038/nn733

Gerrans, P. (2000). Refining the explanation of Cotard's delusion. *Mind and Language, 15*(1), 111–122. doi:10.1111/1468-0017.00125

Gerrans, P. (2001). Delusions as performance failures. *Cognitive Neuropsychiatry, 6*(3), 161–173. doi:10.1080/1354680004200016

Hirstein, W., & Ramachandran, V. (1997). Capgras syndrome: a novel probe for understanding the neural representation of the identity and familiarity of persons. *Proceedings of the Royal Society B: Biological Sciences, 264*(1380), 437–444. doi:10.1098/rspb.1997.0062

Huber, C., & Agorastos, A. (2012). We are all zombies anyway: aggression in Cotard's syndrome. *JNP: The Journal of Neuropsychiatry and Clinical Neurosciences, 24*(3), E21–E21. doi:10.1176/appi.neuropsych.11070155

Joseph, A. (1986). Cotard's syndrome in a patient with coexistent Capgras' syndrome, syndrome of subjective doubles, and palinopsia. *Journal of Clinical Psychiatry, 47,* 605–606.

Loudet, O., & Martinez, D. (1933). Sobre la psicogénesis y el valor pronóstico del síndrome de Cotard. *Archives Argent Neurologie, 1,* 1–12.

McKay, R., & Cipolotti, L. (2007). Attributional style in a case of Cotard delusion. *Consciousness and Cognition, 16*(2), 349–359. doi:10.1016/j.concog.2006.06.001

Nejad, A., Anari, A., & Pouya, F. (2013). Effect of cultural themes on forming Cotard's syndrome: reporting a case of Cotard's syndrome with depersonalization and out of body experience symptoms. *Iranian Journal of Psychiatry and Behavioral Sciences, 72*(2), 91–93.

Nishio, Y., & Mori, E. (2012). Delusions of death in a patient with right hemisphere infarction. *Cognitive and Behavioral Neurology, 25*(4), 216–223. doi:10.1097/wnn.0b013e31827504c7

Perez, D., Fuchs, B., & Epstein, J. (2014). A case of Cotard syndrome in a woman with a right subdural hemorrhage. *JNP: Journal of Neuropsychiatry and Clinical Neuroscience, 26*(1), E29–E30. doi:10.1176/appi.neuropsych.13020021

Ramirez-Bermudez, J., Aguilar-Venegas, L., Crail-Melendez, D., Espinola-Nadurille, M., Nente, F., & Mendez, M. (2010). Cotard syndrome in neurological and psychiatric patients. *Journal of Neuropsychiatry, 22*(4), 409–416. doi:10.1176/appi.neuropsych.22.4.409

Ratcliffe, M. (2008). *Feelings of being.* Oxford: Oxford University Press.

Ratcliffe M. (2012). The phenomenology of existential being. In J. Fingerhut & S. Marienberg (Eds.), *Feelings of being alive* (pp. 23–54). Berlin: Walter de Gruyter GmbH & Co.

Régis, E. (1883). Notre historique et clinique sur le délire de negations. *Gazette Médical De Paris, 2,* 61–64.

Saavedra, V. (1968). El syndrome de Cotard. Consideraciones psico- pathologicas y nosograficas. *Revista De Neuro-Psiquiatria, 11,* 175–211.

Séglas, J. (1887). *Mélancholie* anxieuse avec délire des négations. *Progrès Médical, 46,* 414–417.

Sharma, V., & Biswas, D. (2012). Cotard's syndrome in post-surgical patients. *JNP: Journal of Neuropsychiatry and Clinical Neuroscience, 24*(4), E42–E43. doi:10.1176/appi. neuropsych.11110329

Shiraishi, H., Ito, M., Hayashi, H., & Otani, K. (2004). Sulpiride treatment of Cotard's syndrome in schizophrenia. *Progress in Neuro-Psychopharmacology and Biological Psychiatry, 28*(3), 607–609. doi:10.1016/j.pnpbp.2004.01.011

Stompe, T., & Schanda, H. (2013). Das Cotard-Syndrom bei schizophrenen Erkrankungen. *Neuropsychiatrie, 27*(1), 38–46. doi:10.1007/s40211-012-0046-2

Swamy, N., Sanju, G., & Mathew Jaimon, M. (2007). An overview of the neurological correlates of Cotard syndrome. *European Journal of Psychiatry, 21*(2). doi:10.4321/ s0213-61632007000200002

Tissot, F. (1921). Délire des negations terminé par guérison. Considérations sur l'hypochondrie et la mélancholie. *Annales Médico-Psychologique, 79,* 321–328.

Turner, D. (2004). The role of the lateral frontal cortex in causal associative learning: exploring preventative and super-learning. *Cerebral Cortex, 14*(8), 872–880. doi:10.1093/cercor/bhh046

Vinkers D. (2008). Reactie op "Het syndroom van Cotard. Een overzicht." *Tijdschrift voor Psychiatrie, 50*(6), 391–392.

Wolff, G., & McKenzie, K. (1994). Capgras, Fregoli and Cotard's syndromes and Koro in folie Ã deux. *British Journal of Psychiatry, 165*(6), 842.

World Health Organization. (2015). *ICD-10 Version:2015.* Retrieved July 7. 2015 from http://apps.who.int/classifications/icd10/browse/2015/en

Wright, S., Young, A., & Hellawell, D. (1993). Sequential Cotard and Capgras delusions. *British Journal of Clinical Psychology, 32*(3), 345–349. doi:10.1111/j.2044-8260.1993. tb01065.x

Yalin, S., Varol Tas, F., & Güvenir, T. (2008). The coexistence of Capgras, Fregoli and Cotard's syndromes in an adolescent case. *Archives of Neuropsychiatry, 45,* 149–151.

Yarnada, K., Katsuragi, S., & Fujii, I. (1999). A case study of Cotard's syndrome: stages and diagnosis. *Acta Psychiatrica Scandinavica, 100*(5), 396–398. doi:10.1111/j.1600-0447.1999.tb10884.x

Young, A., & Leafhead, K. (1996). Betwixt life and death: case studies of Cotard delusion. In P. Halligan & J. Marshall (Eds.), *Method in madness: case studies in cognitive neuropsychiatry* (1st ed., pp. 147–171). Hove: Taylor & Francis.

Young, G. (2010). *Delusional misidentification.* New York: Nova Science.

Young, G. (2011). Beliefs, experiences and misplaced being: an interactionist account of delusional misidentification. *Phenomenology and the Cognitive Sciences, 10*(2), 195–215. doi:10.1007/s11097-010-9168-9

Young, G. (2013). *Philosophical psychopathology, philosophy without thought experiments.* Basingstoke: Palgrave Macmillan.

Sexual Disorders/ Disorders of Desire

8

Persistent Genital Arousal Disorder

DAVID GOLDMEIER AND SHALINI ANDREWS ■

VIGNETTE

Clara is a 60-year-old semiretired solicitor who has been happily married for 30 years. A year ago she started going to fitness classes, which included 10 minutes of "spinning" and five minutes of "squats." Looking back to that time, she recalls that she was rather surprised that she had become vaginally orgasmic then, whereas in the past she could not achieve this in spite of being clitorally orgasmic. About nine months ago she developed an irritating sensation around the clitoris that seemed to arise spontaneously and persisted for hours. At about the same time she was treated on three occasions for "cystitis" by her general practitioner (GP).

Six months ago the genital sensations changed to what Clara now describes as "being turned on" in the genital area. This happened every day and came unbidden. In other words, it was not associated with situations that usually switched on sexual desire for her (e.g., watching romantic films or talking to good-looking men). The sensation had a painful quality at times. By this time she had become panicky about the whole process and decided to see if masturbation/orgasm could help. This, however, seemed only to relieve the symptoms for approximately five minutes.

At this stage, she reconsulted her GP, who referred her to a gynecologist. This doctor could find nothing physically wrong with Clara, and suggested that stress might be the underlying issue.

Clara came to see the author DG a few weeks ago. She told us that she had had a good childhood with very supportive parents who had a positive attitude toward sexual matters. Her first sexual experience occurred at university when she was 17 years old. This was with one of the academic staff who at the time was 40 years of age. She recalled that the experience was overwhelming for her and that she really did not understand her emotions at that time or the painful sex that seemed to persist throughout their six-month relationship. He ended the relationship. She later met her husband, who was then a 21-year-old. Their physical relationship was slow, enjoyable, and romantic.

Over the years Clara has suffered two periods of depression. She also described a perfectionistic personality.

Clara takes no medication and is otherwise currently well. She drinks six units of alcohol per day.

She was examined genitally and was found to have hyperesthesia in the distribution of the dorsal clitoral nerve. She appeared tense and weepily told us she found life unbearable because of the constant arousal. Clara said, "I think something is terribly wrong with my genitals," "I think it will be with me always," "I am worried I may orgasm in public" (she never has), and that "it will take over my mind and my life."

Pelvic and lumbosacral magnetic resonance imaging (MRI) scans were reported as normal.

We explained to Clara that she had persistent genital arousal disorder (PGAD) largely because of a pudendal/dorsal clitoral neuralgia, but exacerbated by her affective state. It may have been initiated by pelvic trauma at the gym, and perpetuated by past negative associations with unwanted and inappropriate genital arousal.

She was taught mindfulness, which helped her accept the unbidden genital feelings. Cognitive therapy helped her by challenging her catastrophic associations with PGAD, such as worries about a progressive disease of the genitals and fear of orgasms in public. She was put onto duloxetine 30 milligrams a day. She also saw a pelvic floor physiotherapist who found tense musculature around the pelvic floor in the path of the pudendal nerve. We discussed her high alcohol intake as a possible aggravating factor of her symptoms and contributing factor to neuropathy of the pudendal nerve. She decided to decrease alcohol consumption.

Two months later Clara's symptoms had decreased in severity from 9/10 to 2/10. On many days she has no symptoms at all. On days she does, the symptoms last for one to two hours at most. Intercourse with her husband is still enjoyable.

HISTORICAL AND CULTURAL CONTEXT

The earliest historical reference to PGAD is probably found in the early descriptions of satyriasis and nymphomania. The second-century Greek physician Soranus, in his four-volume treatise on gynecology, described satyriasis in women as "intense itching of the genitals together with pain, so that they continually bring their hands to this region . . . they develop an irresistible desire for sexual intercourse and a certain alienation of mind (because of the sympathetic relation of the meninges with the uterus) which throws aside all sense of shame" (Temkin, 1956, p. 148). The Scottish physician Dr. William Cullen was the first to medically utilize the term nymphomania in his 1769 taxonomy of nervous diseases, *Synopsis Methodicae*. He mentioned it as a common female disorder but did not give any further descriptions. In 1771 the European doctor Bienville published *"De La Nymphomanie Ou Traité De La Fureur Utérine,"* wherein he used the terms metromania and nymphomania interchangeably to describe an insatiable desire for sexual stimulation. He described the condition as a "fury of the womb," and attributed the pathology to "imagination" and excessive uterine nerves (Bouce, 1982). Since then, nymphomania in women has been variously described in medical literature as wanting or having too much coitus, too much sexual desire, or excessive masturbation. This has been complicated by a societal expectation of sexual passivity in women with the result that behaviors such as wearing lewd clothes, flirting, and committing adultery were added as symptoms of the condition (Groneman, 1994). The diagnoses of satyriasis, nymphomania, and metromania do not exist in current medical literature. Although some of the descriptions are now considered "normal sexual behavior," others may represent a diagnosis of PGAD or sexual compulsivity. It is difficult to know how many of these women with "an insatiable desire for sexual stimulation" or wanting "excessive masturbation" suffered from the unbidden sexual arousal of PGAD.

The understanding of female sexuality vastly increased with Kinsey's work normalizing female sexual desire and clitoral orgasm as well as Masters and Johnson's descriptions of the sexual response cycle (Kinsey, 1953; Angel, 2010). There are several case reports in the 1980s and 1990s of drug-induced clitoral engorgement and clitoral priapism and unwanted orgasms induced by an epileptic focus. Some of these may have been presentations of PGAD (Modell, 1989; Blin, Schwertschlag, & Serratrice, 1991; Levenson, 1995; Berk & Acton, 1997; Brodie-Meijer, Diemont, & Buijs, 1999). At the turn of this century, Leiblum and Nathan (2001) described five cases of women with persistent physiological arousal in the absence of conscious feelings of sexual desire. This was the first description in medical and sexuality literatures of this condition, which was named "persistent sexual arousal syndrome." Goldmeier and Leiblum (2006) later renamed it "persistent genital arousal disorder" to reflect more accurately the presence of genital arousal as opposed to sexual arousal.

ROLE IN CURRENT DIAGNOSTIC SYSTEMS

Persistent genital arousal was provisionally suggested to be included in female sexual dysfunction at the second edition of the *International Consultation on Sexual Medicine* (ICSM) in July 2003 (Basson et al., 2004). The third edition of the ICSM in 2009 included "Persistent Genital Arousal Dysfunction" in its list of sexual dysfunction in women. The ICSM, hosted by the *International Organisation of Sexual Medicine Professionals, International Society of Sexual Medicine* bring together international experts to produce guidelines based on consensus.

PGAD is not, however, included in the *Diagnostic and Statistical Manual of Mental Disorders*, DSM-5 (American Psychiatric Association, 2013) or the International Classification of Diseases, ICD-10 (World Health Organization, 1992). This is perhaps not surprising, given that it is a relatively newer recognized condition that demands further research to elucidate its place in a scientific classification.

SYMPTOMATOLOGY

The following criteria are descriptive features of PGAD (Goldmeier, Mears, Hiller, & Crowley, 2009):

1. Symptoms that are characteristic of sexual arousal (genital fullness/ swelling and sensitivity with or without nipple fullness/swelling) that persists for an extended period of time (hours or days) and do not subside completely on their own.
2. Symptoms of physiological arousal that do not resolve with ordinary orgasmic experience and may require multiple orgasms over hours or days to remit.
3. Symptoms of arousal are usually experienced as unrelated to any subjective sense of sexual excitement or desire.
4. Symptoms are experienced as unbidden, intrusive, and unwanted.
5. The symptoms cause the woman at least a moderate degree of distress.
6. The persistent sexual arousal may be triggered not only by a sexual activity but also by seemingly nonsexual stimuli or by no apparent stimulus at all.

The initial diagnostic criteria for persistent sexual arousal disorder (Basson et al., 2003) included the first five of these six symptoms prior to the recognition that sexual arousal was not the only trigger. These sometimes continue to be referred to in literature as the five criteria for PGAD. In an anonymous online survey by Leiblum, Seehuus, and Brown (2007) of 206 women who met the five criteria, the most common sites of genital arousal and symptoms experienced were clitoral tingling (86%), vaginal congestion (80%), vaginal wetness (77%), vaginal contractions (71%), vaginal tingling (71%), clitoral pain (20%), and vaginal pain (17%). The most common nongenital arousal site was the nipple (37%). In this study, 48% of participants experienced continuous symptoms.

A smaller and more in-depth study by Waldinger and Schweitzer (2009) of 18 Dutch women with PGAD who experienced continuous symptoms reported the most common sites of arousal were the clitoris (78%), vagina (55%), labia (28%), or a combination of all three (44%). The pubic bone and groin were other reported sites. Genital contractions and a feeling of imminent orgasm or persistently being on the verge of orgasm without completion (i.e., the pleasurable feeling of orgasm) were commonly reported. The triggers for exacerbation of symptoms were tension, being frightened, anger, anxiety, annoyance, stress, and alcohol, particularly red wine. Women also experienced fatigue and severe loss of energy.

Another study (Leiblum, Brown, Wan, & Rawlinson, 2005) reported exacerbation of symptoms by both touch and visual stimulation that led to arousal. In this study, masturbation and intercourse both exacerbated and relieved symptoms. Other relieving factors were orgasm, distraction, intercourse, exercise, and the application of cold compresses.

PREVALENCE RATE AND ASSOCIATED FEATURES

There are no population-based estimates of the prevalence of PGAD. A survey of 96 women attending a sexual-health clinic found one who fulfilled all five criteria (Garvey, West, Latch, Leiblum, & Goldmeier, 2009). Although there is not much published data and many professionals are unaware of this condition, many experts working within the field of sexual medicine have encountered it in their working practice and consider it to be less rare than initially thought (Goldstein, 2013).

The median age in the two large published studies was 38 years and 55 years respectively (Leiblum et al., 2007; Waldinger & Schweitzer, 2009). In their study of 23 women with PGAD, Waldinger, Venema, Van Gils, & Schweitzer (2009) found a strong association with restless leg syndrome, overactive bladder, and urethral hypersensitivity. They termed this clinical cluster "Restless Genital Syndrome" (ReGS). In their subsequent literature review, Facelle, Sadeghi-Nejad, and Goldmeier (2013) identified several psychological and biological associations including anxiety, depression, obsessive compulsive disorder, previous sexual assault, pudendal neuralgia, Tarlov's cysts, pelvic varices, medication, clitoral priapism, central nervous system lesions and epileptic foci, and dietary products. These associations will be discussed further in the next section on etiology.

THEORIES OF ETIOLOGY

The association of PGAD with several conditions has helped to postulate the probable cause and mechanisms of this intriguing condition. These associated conditions are as follows:

Atypical Pudendal Nerve Neuropathy

Sensory neuropathy of the pudendal nerve, particularly the dorsal clitoral nerve is thought to be the etiology of the condition, especially in women with ReGS. The pudendal nerve originates in the second to fourth sacral level of the spinal cord. In the upper half of the pudendal (or Alcock's) canal it branches into the inferior rectal nerve. The inferior rectal nerve provides motor innervation to the levator ani muscle and sensory innervation to the perianal skin and labia. At the end of the pudendal canal it branches into the perineal nerve and dorsal nerve of the clitoris. The perineal nerve divides into the labial branch and two branches toward the bulbocavernosus and the striated urethral sphincter. The dorsal nerve of the clitoris is thought to be a purely sensory nerve supplying the clitoris.

Waldinger et al. (2009) conducted a detailed study of 23 women that included in-depth interviews, routine and hormonal investigations, electroencephalo-graphs, and magnetic resonance imaging (MRI) of brain and pelvis included sensory testing of the skin of the genital area with a cotton swab (genital tactile mapping test or GTM test). All women demonstrated orgasmic or preorgasmic sensation along various points within the sensory areas of the pudendal and dorsal clitoral nerve, and investigators were able to map mechanical "trigger points" based on hypersensitivity to static pressure. Five of the eight women who received local anesthetic injections at these trigger points reported resolution of symptoms for the duration of anesthesia. This theory of hyperesthesia was supported by the reports of symptom exacerbation with tight clothes and prolonged sitting by women with PGAD. The authors further assumed that the neuropathy is a small fiber neuropathy, which may explain the sensations of paresthesia, dysesthesia, allodynia (triggering of pain sensation by a usually painless stimulus such as contact with clothing), association with restless leg syndrome, and the waves of extreme fatigue during the day. All women in this study had pelvic varices raising the possibility of the varices causing neuropathy. Thorne and Stuckey (2008) reported a case of pelvic congestion syndrome presenting with PGAD, where symptoms improved by 70% when the ovarian vein was occluded to relieve variceal dilatation in the vaginal wall. Although it is possible that the primary etiology in this case was vascular, vascular dilatation causing peripheral neuropathy is also a plausible explanation. The case of a woman with PGAD, thought to be secondary to cardiac defects and elevated atrial natriuretic peptide, is now being followed up by the author DG (Bell et al., 2007). She later was diagnosed with Ehlers-Danlos syndrome and developed severe peripheral and autonomic neuropathy, with the PGAD related to neuropathy.

Other case reports support this theory of pudendal neuropathy. Rosenbaum (2010) reported the case of a 27-year-old pregnant woman with PGAD and multiple trigger points in the hypertonic obturator internus muscle. Soft tissue mobilization massage by the author led to immediate and complete resolution of symptoms. It is postulated that the massage relieved the pelvic floor hypertonicity that caused compression of the pudendal nerve in the Alcock's canal. A woman with PGAD that did not resolve with clitoridectomy reported temporary but complete resolution of symptoms with local anesthetic injections at two trigger points (Waldinger, Venema, Van Gils, Schutter, & Schweitzer, 2010). The same group also reported successful treatment with transcutaneous electrical nerve stimulation (TENS) in the pudendal dermatome in two women with PGAD (Waldinger, De Lint, Venema, Van Gils, & Schweitzer, 2010). Other treatment modalities for neuropathy such as duloxetine, pregabalin, and botulinum injections have been used successfully in treating PGAD (Philippsohn & Kruger, 2012; Nazik, Api, Aytan, & Narin, 2014).

Psychological

A psychological model was proposed by Leiblum and Chivers (2007) whereby preexisting anxiety is exacerbated by symptoms of genital arousal, causing increased sympathetic tone and further augmenting the genital arousal. This causes a cognitive narrowing that more sharply focuses attention on the perceived arousal symptoms and contributes to the vicious cycle. This theory was based upon work done by Leiblum et al. (2007), which showed a high rate of psychological pathology such as panic attacks (31.6%) and depression (57.9%) in women with PGAD who accessed their online survey. The anxiety and depression predated symptoms of PGAD. A large number (53%) of women in these surveys also reported childhood sexual abuse but only 16.7% thought that symptoms could be attributed to the abuse. In contrast to these findings, a Dutch study of 18 women found that none reported preexisting anxiety, only one had depression, and the rate of childhood sexual abuse (17%) was lower than that of the general population (Waldinger & Schweitzer, 2009).

In the authors' clinical experience, many patients with PGAD appear to have either a primarily psychological etiology or a pudendal neuropathy. Those with a psychological etiology often report past sexual abuse. In these cases, normal genital arousal appears to cause distress, leads to anxiety, and eventuates in the development of PGAD. They do not have hyperesthesia and respond to treatments aimed at addressing anxiety and restoring healthier cognition around arousal.

A recent online survey of 43 women with PGAD showed that women reporting PGAD symptoms presented significantly more dysfunctional sexual beliefs (e.g., sexual conservatism, sexual desire as a sin), as well as more negative thoughts (e.g., thoughts of sexual abuse and of lack of partner's affection) and dysfunctional affective states (more negative and less positive affect) during sexual activity than non-PGAD women (Carvalho, Veríssimo, & Nobre, 2013). It is difficult to know whether the psychological state is a cause or consequence of PGAD in these women, but nonetheless, addressing dysfunctional beliefs and negative cognitions is important in managing patients with PGAD.

Other Potential Causes

Certain pharmaceutical medications are associated with the development of PGAD, both on initiation and withdrawal. Several authors have noted associations between both selective serotonin reuptake inhibitors (SSRI) and serotonin norepinephrine reuptake inhibitors (SNRI) and PGAD, upon both initiation and withdrawal of these drugs (Leiblum & Goldmeier, 2008). The proposed mechanisms include increased atrial natriuretic peptide and vasodilatation following antidepressant withdrawal, as well as return to baseline awareness of genital sensation, which was previously suppressed by medication. Some of the well-recognized symptoms found in SSRI withdrawal include numbness, paresthesia, and electric shock-like sensations (Haddad, Lejoyeux, & Young), which is similar to sensations recognized by women with PGAD. Drug induced clitoral priapism is another probable mechanism of spontaneous genital arousal in these cases. As mentioned previously, there are several case reports of clitoral priapism prior to the formal recognition of PGAD, and the drugs implicated include citalopram, nefazodone, bupropion, and bromocriptine.

Central nervous system pathology including epilepsy, space-occupying lesions, and vascular insufficiency are associated with PGAD. There are several case reports of localized seizure activity in the brain causing genital symptoms. Anzellotti et al. (2010) reported the case of a woman with PGAD, which was characterized by genital spasms followed by genital pain. EEG showed bilateral frontocentrotemporal epileptic activity with a specific focus in left posterior insular gyrus on magnetoencephalography; symptoms resolved when treated with topiramate. Sexual aura, defined as erotic feelings accompanied by sexual arousal and orgasm have been described in women and men with temporal lobe epilepsy (Aull-Watschinger, Pataraia, & Baumgartner, 2008). Goldstein and Johnson (2006) reported four cases of central nervous system pathology (arteriovenous malformation and stroke) causing PGAD.

There are two case reports of women with bipolar disorder and PGAD who were successfully treated with elecroconvulsive therapy (Korda, Pfaus, Kellner, & Goldstein, 2009; Yero, McKinney, Petrides, Goldstein, & Kellner, 2006). The authors suggested that, at least in these cases, PGAD was related to a lack of central nervous system control of sexual arousal. Electroconvulsive therapy resulted in lowering of the hyperstimulated central dopamine release and also led to an increase in sexual inhibition by stimulating serotonin activity.

A study of 12 women with PGAD using pelvic MRI showed a 66.7% prevalence of Tarlov cysts (Komisaruk and Lee, 2012). These are cysts of the sacral nerve root sheath (viz., usually in the S2-S3 region) present in 1.2%–9% of the population. They are predominantly asymptomatic but are reported to cause back pain, coccyx pain, low radicular pain, bowel/bladder dysfunction, leg weakness, paresthesia, and genital pain. Further studies are needed to explain the high prevalence of these cysts in women with PGAD. There is a case report of PGAD following drainage of a presacral abscess, suggesting that neurological pathology at this site may cause PGAD symptoms (Spoelstra, Waldinger, Nijhuis, & Weijmar, 2012).

There is one case report of PGAD following massive ingestion of soy products, which resolved with dietary modification; the authors postulate the hyperestrogenic state caused by soy phytoestrogen as the likely etiology (Amsterdam, Abu-Rustum, Carter, & Krychman, 2005).

ASSESSMENT OPTIONS

Because PGAD is a complex condition with an uncertain etiology, the patient will benefit from assessment by a multidisciplinary team (e.g., a physician, psychologist, and pelvic floor physical therapist).

The initial interview is important for both the treating professional and the patient. The professional needs to understand the problem, especially in light of the fact that the patient may have felt rejected or not listened to by previous healthcare workers. The history-taking should include a full description of the PGAD symptoms, the site, quality and duration, aggravating and relieving factors, whether genital arousal is preceded by desire, and whether there is concomitant pain. The degree of distress should be assessed. A full psychological history should be taken including history of anxiety, depression, obsessive-compulsive behavior, and sexual abuse. A psychosexual history is important to assess sexual functioning and relationship issues. The drug history should include current and previous use of psychotropic medication such as SSRI/SNRI and trazodone. A medical history must be taken and attention paid to symptoms relating to syndrome clusters (restless leg syndrome, overactive bladder), neurological (paresthesia, dysesthesia, autonomic dysfunction, epilepsy, temporal lobe events), and vascular pathology (leg varices).

All patients with suspected PGAD should be offered a genital examination. The patient may experience orgasm during the course of the examination and must be reassured that this is not unusual in women with PGAD. The examination is important to identify clitoral, vulvar, or labial hyperesthesia, engorgement, or visible varices. Bimanual palpation is necessary to assess pelvic floor tone and identify pelvic masses.

Further investigations may be necessary depending on history and examination findings. These investigations may include hematological and biochemical tests and assessment of hormone profile, as well as imaging such as pelvic Doppler ultrasound, pelvic MRI and spinal MRI, and CT/MRI brain scan. An electroencephalogram (EEG) may be needed if the history suggests an epileptic focus.

DIFFERENTIAL DIAGNOSIS

PGAD needs to be differentiated from hypersexuality. Hypersexuality has been defined as persistent and recurrent intensive sexual fantasies, urges, and behaviors that are difficult to control and pose harm to the individual's mental or physical well-being (Kafka, 2010; Goldmeier & Petrak, 2011). One of the features of hypersexuality is compulsive masturbation. However, unlike with PGAD, masturbation is prompted by sexual desire and not by unbidden genital arousal or dysesthesia.

PGAD also should be differentiated from the spectrum of normal sexuality, wherein women report spontaneous genital arousal but are not distressed by these sensations. Leiblum et al. (2007) in their online survey of 388 women who reported features of PGAD, found that there is a cohort of women who regularly, if intermittently, experience unprovoked and persistent genital arousal and find it mildly pleasurable. Their genital arousal differs from that of women who meet all five criteria for a diagnosis of PGAD. Moreover some women with persistent genital arousal can be distressed by their condition some of the time but may actually welcome it at other times.

The understanding of "normality" in women is complicated by two important aspects of the female sexual response cycle. First, it is well known that sexual desire and arousal are overlapping concepts in women, both in the way they are perceived and experienced. Unlike the male sexual response cycle, female arousal does not necessarily follow desire, and desire may, in fact, be triggered by arousal.

Secondly, a lack of correlation between subjective feelings of genital arousal and objective measures (e.g., vaginal lubrication and swelling) has been noted in women (Bancroft & Graham, 2011). Hence, it can be difficult for patient and therapist to know when unbidden arousal is unwanted.

TREATMENT OPTIONS

There are no published treatment trials for PGAD, although potentially effective solutions may be found in the case report literature. When an underlying cause is found (e.g., excess soy intake or large ovarian veins) treatment of the cause may lead to resolution of PGAD symptoms. For the majority of women with PGAD, however, the aim of treatment is to help the patient manage and cope with symptoms, given that there is as of yet no clearly definitive "cure." A biopsychosocial approach to treatment is likely to be successful given the complex nature of this condition. This would include psychological, medical, and physical therapy, as well as addressing sexual and relationship issues.

Psychological Therapy

Cognitive behavior therapy (CBT) has been found to be potentially beneficial in treating PGAD. Leiblum and Chivers (2007) conceptualized that a patient's moral judgment of genital sensations (e.g., "it is wrong to feel aroused") leads to anxiety. This anxiety, in turn, increases focus on genital symptoms and catastrophizing of symptoms. Carvalho et al. (2013) confirmed this in their study and recommended a CBT-based approach to therapy that targeted maladaptive cognitions and reduced the cognitive dissonance between core sexual beliefs and bodily signs of genital arousal. Mindfulness-based CBT for PGAD is known to decrease anxiety, depression, and feelings of pain, as well as to alter brain structure, function, and immune responses (Goldmeier & Mears, 2010). The practice of mindfulness requires the patient to focus on the present (e.g., one's breath) while being aware of distracting thoughts and feelings. Awareness of the distracting thoughts can help the patient move them to the periphery, instead of remaining entangled in them in ways that are not useful, thereby decreasing stress and anxiety. Thus patients with PGAD can develop a better awareness of their genital sensation without allowing catastrophic thoughts such as, "Will this ever stop?" "I cannot deal with this," and "When will I have to masturbate again?" to come to the fore. Patients are taught to focus on the PGAD sensations for 10– 20 minutes while mindfully observing the mind's reaction. This leads to greater acceptance of the symptoms and increases the patient's ability to cope. Such acceptance has been shown to be helpful in other painful conditions (Vowles, McCracken, & O'Brien, 2011).

Psychological therapies are also likely important in treating anxiety, depression, obsessive-compulsive disorder, and the trauma of previous sexual assault. These are all conditions that may coexist in patients with PGAD and may complicate the diagnostic picture.

Physiotherapy

Pelvic physiotherapy may be a useful adjunct to treatment as illustrated by the case report wherein the obturator internus muscle was successfully manipulated to relieve probable nerve entrapment (Rosenbaum, 2010). Physiotherapists also can identify trigger points and help patients use this knowledge to apply treatment such as TENS (transcutaneous electric nerve stimulation).

Pharmacological Therapy

There are no pharmacotherapeutic trials reported in patients with PGAD. There are anecdotal reports of symptom improvement with various medications. Clonazepam ameliorated symptoms in 11 of 18 women with PGAD and ReGS, and those that were refractory to clonazepam responded to oxazepam or tramadol (Waldinger et al., 2009). Drugs used to treat peripheral neuropathy, such as duloxetine and pregabalin, have been used successfully (Philippsohn & Kruger, 2012). Amitriptyline or nortriptyline, antidepressants, and SSRIs have been found to be useful, especially in patients with psychiatric comorbidity (Facelle et al., 2013). There are isolated case reports of success with varenicline tartrate (a smoking cessation agent and partial nicotine receptor agonist) and risperidone, an antipsychotic with antidopaminergic activity (Korda, Pfaus, & Goldstein, 2009; Wylie, Levin, Hallam-Jones, & Goddard, 2006). Antiepileptic agents such as topiramate and carbamazepine have been used in cases with an epileptic focus (Anzellotti et al., 2010; Reading & Will, 1997). These medications may be prescribed in patients along with psychotherapy in order to manage symptoms. The choice of mediation will depend on whether the symptoms are predominantly related to ReGS, neuropathy, or psychological comorbidity.

Managing Sexual Functioning

PGAD affects sexual functioning in women in different ways. Genital touching or sexual arousal can exacerbate symptoms (Leiblum et al., 2005), and anticipatory anxiety about impending symptoms can disrupt sexual activity. Leiblum and Seehuus (2009) found, using the *Female Sexual Function Index* (FSFI) questionnaire, that women with PGAD had a sexual function intermediate between controls and those with female sexual arousal disorder (FSAD) for all categories except desire; and pain ratings similar to the FSAD group. The management of PGAD must include addressing sexual functioning. Women with intermittent PGAD may be encouraged to have sex between exacerbations. Nongenital stimulation may be more pleasurable for some.

RECOMMENDATIONS FOR FUTURE WORK

PGAD is a newly recognized condition of uncertain etiology with limited data on successful treatment. A biopsychosocial model of evaluation that includes a detailed history, psychological assessment, and comprehensive examination and investigation will enable an increased understanding of etiology. Clinical trials to identify the best treatment option are clearly needed. Although the majority of PGAD cases have been identified in women, there are three case reports in men—two with ReGS and one with isolated PGAD (Waldinger, Venema, van Gils, de Lint, & Schweitzer, 2011; Stevenson & Köhler, 2015). There is no data on prevalence in men and little is known about whether PGAD in men shares a common etiology with PGAD in women; future research needs to address this.

REFERENCES

American Psychiatric Association. (2013). *Diagnostic and statistical manual of mental disorders (DSM-5)*. Washington, DC: American Psychiatric Publishing.

Amsterdam, A., Abu-Rustum, N., Carter, J., & Krychman, M. (2005). Persistent sexual arousal syndrome associated with increased soy intake. *The Journal of Sexual Medicine, 2*(3), 338–340.

Angel, K. (2010). The history of "female sexual dysfunction" as a mental disorder in the 20th century. *Current Opinion in Psychiatry, 23*(6), 536.

Anzellotti, F., Franciotti, R., Bonanni, L., Tamburro, G., Perrucci, M.G., Thomas, A., ... Onofrj, M. (2010). Persistent genital arousal disorder associated with functional hyperconnectivity of an epileptic focus. *Neuroscience, 167*(1), 88–96.

Aull-Watschinger, S., Pataraia, E., & Baumgartner, C. (2008). Sexual auras: predominance of epileptic activity within the mesial temporal lobe. *Epilepsy & Behavior, 12*(1), 124–127.

Bancroft, J., & Graham, C.A. (2011). The varied nature of women's sexuality: Unresolved issues and a theoretical approach. *Hormones and Behavior, 59*(5), 717–729.

Basson, R., Leiblum, S., Brotto, L., Derogatis, L., Fourcroy, J., Fugl-Meyer, K., ... Schultz, W.W. (2003). Definitions of women's sexual dysfunction reconsidered: advocating expansion and revision. *Journal of Psychosomatic Obstetrics & Gynecology, 24*(4), 221–229.

Basson, R., Leiblum, S., Brotto, L., Derogatis, L., Fourcroy, J., Fugl-Meyer, K., ... Schultz, W.W. (2004). Revised definitions of women's sexual dysfunction. *The Journal of Sexual Medicine, 1*(1), 40–48.

Bell, C., Richardson, D., Goldmeier, D., Crowley, T., Kocsis, A., & Hill, S. (2007). Persistent sexual arousal in a woman with associated cardiac defects and raised atrial natriuretic peptide. *International Journal of STD & AIDS, 18*(2), 130–131.

Berk, M., & Acton, M. (1997). Citalopram-associated clitoral priapism: a case series. *International Clinical Psychopharmacology, 12*(2), 121.

Blin, O., Schwertschlag, U.S., & Serratrice, G. (1991). Painful clitoral tumescence during bromocriptine therapy. *Lancet, 337* (8751), 1231–1232.

Boucé, P.G. (Ed.). (1982). Sexuality in eighteenth-century Britain. Manchester, UK: Manchester University Press.

Brodie-Meijer, C.C., Diemont, W.L., & Buijs, P.J. (1999). Nefazodone-induced clitoral priapism. *International Clinical Psychopharmacology, 14*(4), 257–258.

Carvalho, J., Veríssimo, A., & Nobre, P.J. (2013). Cognitive and emotional determinants characterizing women with persistent genital arousal disorder. *The Journal of Sexual Medicine, 10*(6), 1549–1558.

Facelle, T.M., Sadeghi-Nejad, H., & Goldmeier, D. (2013). Persistent genital arousal disorder: characterization, etiology, and management. *The Journal of Sexual Medicine, 10*(2), 439–450.

Garvey, L.J., West, C., Latch, N., Leiblum, S., & Goldmeier, D. (2009). Report of spontaneous and persistent genital arousal in women attending a sexual health clinic. *International Journal of STD & AIDS, 20*(8), 519–521.

Goldmeier, D., & Leiblum, S.R. (2006). Persistent genital arousal in women—a new syndrome entity. *International Journal of STD & AIDS, 17*(4), 215–216.

Goldmeier, D., Mears, A., Hiller, J., & Crowley, T. (2009). Persistent genital arousal disorder: a review of the literature and recommendations for management. *International Journal of STD & AIDS, 20*(6), 373–377.

Goldmeier, D., & Mears, A.J. (2010). Meditation: A review of its use in western medicine and, in particular, its role in the management of sexual dysfunction. *Current Psychiatry Reviews, 6*(1), 11–14.

Goldmeier, D., & Petrak, J. (2011). How to recognise sexual addiction in the sexual health clinic setting? *Sexually Transmitted Infections, 87*(5), 370–371.

Goldstein, I., De, E.J.B., & Johnson, J. (2006). *Persistent sexual arousal syndrome and clitoral priapism. Women's sexual function and dysfunction: Study, diagnosis and treatment.* London: Taylor and Francis, 674–685.

Goldstein, I. (2013). Persistent genital arousal disorder—Update on the monster sexual dysfunction. *The Journal of Sexual Medicine, 10*(10), 2357–2358.

Groneman, C. (1994). Nymphomania: the historical construction of female sexuality. *Signs, 19*(2), 337–367.

Haddad, P., Lejoyeux, M., & Young, A. (1998). Antidepressant discontinuation reactions. *BMJ, 316*(7138), 1105–1106.

Kafka, M.P. (2010). Hypersexual disorder: A proposed diagnosis for DSM-V. *Archives of Sexual Behavior, 39*(2), 377–400.

Kinsey, A.C. (Ed.). (1953). *Sexual behavior in the human female.* Bloomington, Indiana, Indiana University Press.

Komisaruk, B.R., & Lee, H.J. (2012). Prevalence of sacral spinal (Tarlov) cysts in persistent genital arousal disorder. *The Journal of Sexual Medicine, 9*(8), 2047–2056.

Korda, J.B., Pfaus, J.G., & Goldstein, I. (2009). Persistent genital arousal disorder: A case report in a woman with lifelong PGAD where serendipitous administration of varenicline tartrate resulted in symptomatic improvement. *The Journal of Sexual Medicine, 6*(5), 1479–1486.

Korda, J.B., Pfaus, J.G., Kellner, C.H., & Goldstein, I. (2009). Persistent genital arousal disorder (PGAD): Case report of long-term symptomatic management with electroconvulsive therapy. *The Journal of Sexual Medicine, 6*(10), 2901–2909.

Leiblum, S.R. & Nathan, S. (2001). Persistent sexual arousal syndrome: A newly discovered pattern of female sexuality. *Journal of Sex & Marital Therapy, 27*(4), 365–380.

Leiblum, S., Brown, C., Wan, J., & Rawlinson, L. (2005). Persistent sexual arousal syndrome: a descriptive study. *The Journal of Sexual Medicine, 2*(3), 331–337.

Leiblum, S., Seehuus, M., & Brown, C. (2007). Persistent genital arousal: Disordered or normative aspect of female sexual response? *The Journal of Sexual Medicine, 4*(3), 680–689.

Leiblum, S.R., & Chivers, M.L. (2007). Normal and persistent genital arousal in women: new perspectives. *Journal of Sex & Marital Therapy, 33*(4), 357–373.

Leiblum, S.R., & Goldmeier, D. (2008). Persistent genital arousal disorder in women: case reports of association with anti-depressant usage and withdrawal. *Journal of Sex & Marital Therapy, 34*(2), 150–159.

Leiblum, S.R., & Seehuus, M. (2009). FSFI scores of women with persistent genital arousal disorder compared with published scores of women with female sexual arousal disorder and healthy controls. *The Journal of Sexual Medicine, 6*(2), 469–473.

Levenson, J.L. (1995). Priapism associated with bupropion treatment. *The American Journal of Psychiatry, 52*(5), 813–813.

Modell, J.G. (1989). Repeated observations of yawning, clitoral engorgement, and orgasm associated with fluoxetine administration. *Journal of Clinical Psychopharmacology, 9*(1), 63.

Nazik, H., Api, M., Aytan, H., & Narin, R. (2014). A new medical treatment with botulinum toxin in persistent genital arousal disorder: Successful treatment of two cases. *Journal of Sex & Marital Therapy, 40*(3), 170–174.

Philippsohn, S., & Kruger, T.H. (2012). Persistent genital arousal disorder: successful treatment with duloxetine and pregabalin in two cases. *The Journal of Sexual Medicine, 9*(1), 213–217.

Reading, P.J., & Will, R.G. (1997). Unwelcome orgasms. *Lancet, 350*(9093), 1746.

Rosenbaum, T.Y. (2010). Physical therapy treatment of persistent genital arousal disorder during pregnancy: A case report. *The Journal of Sexual Medicine, 7*(3), 1306–1310.

Spoelstra, S.K., Waldinger, M., Nijhuis, E.R., & Weijmar, S.W. (2012). [A woman with restless genital syndrome: a difficult-to-treat condition]. *Nederlands tijdschrift voor geneeskunde, 157*(16).

Stevenson, B.J., & Köhler, T.S. (2015). First reported case of isolated persistent genital arousal disorder in a male. *Case Reports in Urology, 2015.*

Temkin, O. (Ed.). (1956). *Soranus' gynecology* (Vol. 3). Baltimore: JHU Press.

Thorne, C., & Stuckey, B. (2008). Pelvic congestion syndrome presenting as persistent genital arousal: A case report. *The Journal of Sexual Medicine, 5*(2), 504–508.

Vowles, K.E., McCracken, L.M., & O'Brien, J.Z. (2011). Acceptance and values-based action in chronic pain: a three-year follow-up analysis of treatment effectiveness and process. *Behaviour Research and Therapy, 49*(11), 748–755.

Waldinger, M.D., & Schweitzer, D.H. (2009). Persistent genital arousal disorder in 18 Dutch women: Part II—A syndrome clustered with restless legs and overactive bladder. *The Journal of Sexual Medicine, 6*(2), 482–497.

Waldinger, M.D., Venema, P.L., Van Gils, A.P., & Schweitzer, D.H. (2009). New insights into restless genital syndrome: Static mechanical hyperesthesia and neuropathy of the nervus dorsalis clitoridis. *The Journal of Sexual Medicine, 6*(10), 2778–2787.

Waldinger, M.D., Venema, P.L., Van Gils, A.P., Schutter, E.M., & Schweitzer, D.H. (2010). Restless genital syndrome before and after clitoridectomy for spontaneous orgasms: A case report. *The Journal of Sexual Medicine, 7*(2pt2), 1029–1034.

Waldinger, M.D., De Lint, G.J., Venema, P.L., Van Gils, A.P., & Schweitzer, D.H. (2010). Successful transcutaneous electrical nerve stimulation in two women with restless genital syndrome: The role of Aδ- and C-nerve fibers. *The Journal of Sexual Medicine*, 7(3), 1190–1199.

Waldinger, M.D., Venema, P.L., van Gils, A.P., de Lint, G.J., & Schweitzer, D.H. (2011). Stronger evidence for small fiber sensory neuropathy in restless genital syndrome: two case reports in males. *The Journal of Sexual Medicine*, 8(1), 325–330.

World Health Organization. (1992). *The ICD-10 classification of mental and behavioural disorders: clinical descriptions and diagnostic guidelines*. Geneva: World Health Organization.

Wylie, K., Levin, R., Hallam-Jones, R., & Goddard, A. (2006). Sleep exacerbation of persistent sexual arousal syndrome in a postmenopausal woman. *The Journal of Sexual Medicine*, 3(2), 296–302.

Yero, S.A., McKinney, T., Petrides, G., Goldstein, I., & Kellner, C.H. (2006). Successful use of electroconvulsive therapy in 2 cases of persistent sexual arousal syndrome and bipolar disorder. *The Journal of ECT*, 22(4), 274–275.

9

Necrophilia

SARA G. WEST AND PHILLIP J. RESNICK ■

VIGNETTE

Through a literature review, small studies, and brief synopses of the lives of several necrophiles, we will attempt to convey some understanding of the what, who, and why of necrophilia. We will begin with an in-depth case study of one necrophile in an effort to demonstrate many of the points made later in the chapter. The following information was obtained from a sanity report dated February 25, 1986 (Resnick):

Mr. P was born in the Dominican Republic and reported that he was adopted by a quiet mother and a father whom he described as loud, quick tempered, and physically abusive. He endorsed cruelty to animals as a youth, noting that he cut off the legs of frogs and placed firecrackers in their mouths. He smoked marijuana and used LSD and Mescaline regularly as well as experimented with other substances. He expressed ideas about Satan and the Antichrist (which did not rise to the level of delusional or psychotic beliefs).

When asked about his sexual history, Mr. P stated that, at the age of four years, he was sexually abused (forced to both give and receive oral sex) by an adult man. Between the ages of 12 and 14, he engaged in sexual activities with two boys his age. He coerced them into having oral and anal sex and also had one of the boys defecate on his genitals then lay on it. Between the ages of 16 and 20, he engaged in a variety of sexual activities with a girlfriend his own age, noting that he was only able to have anal sex on a few occasions because it was painful for her. Between the ages of 18 and 21, he had sex with prostitutes, who, among other sexual acts, had anal intercourse and urinated on his face upon his request. He also stated that he was excited by women's lingerie and would steal dirty underwear from the hampers in friends' homes. Starting at the age of 18, he reported that he enjoyed "unusual" pornographic material, including sex involving bondage and male transvestites. He said that he masturbated four to five times per day.

Mr. P also engaged in sex with animals. At the age of 18 or 19, he performed fellatio on and was the recipient of anal sex with the family dog, a German Shepherd. He took Polaroid pictures of this on occasion as well. He then purchased a female Great Dane. Once he discovered that he was unable to have vaginal or anal sex with the dog, he killed the dog and then attempted to have sex with the dog again. He also killed a cat for sexual reasons but decided it was "too ugly" for sex. Around this time, Mr. P worked as a hospital orderly and would steal urine and fecal samples to enhance his sexual pleasure. He would drink the urine and eat the feces while masturbating. He also inserted the pilfered feces into his own anus.

Mr. P first developed fantasies about sex with a dead body after killing the Great Dane, and these fantasies became more clearly defined and intensified over time. He thought about drowning a woman, taking her into the crawl space under his house, undressing her and mutilating her body. More specifically this included, "Eating her feces, drinking urine, anal sex, biting her ear . . . licking eyeballs, opening the abdomen . . ." It occurred to him that he could either abduct a body from the morgue or kill someone, but he expressed concern that he would get caught. He did have sex (vaginal and anal) with the recently deceased in the morgue of the hospital in which he worked. While he had a partial erection and was able to ejaculate, he noted that he was anxious about being caught while engaging in these activities.

On September 15, 1985, Mr. P (age 25) was home alone when an eight-year-old neighbor girl came over to see his girlfriend's pet tarantula. He took her into the bathroom, turned on the water in the bathtub and attempted to drown her. He then took her to the crawl space and struck her in the head many times with a brick, which was the cause of her demise. Mr. P described the experience as "horrible." He then covered her body with a piece of plastic and cleaned up the house. The victim's five-year-old brother, the police (on two separate occasions), and Mr. P's girlfriend all came to the house following the incident that evening. The following day (after his girlfriend had gone to work), Mr. P returned to the crawl space. Using Vaseline as a lubricant, Mr. P inserted his penis in the victim's anus and his finger in her vagina. He was only able to maintain a partial erection but was able to ejaculate. The police returned for a third time later that afternoon, discovered the body and arrested Mr. P.

Upon psychiatric evaluation (in 1986 using DSM-III), Mr. P was diagnosed with Atypical Paraphilia with interest in coprophilia (feces), urophilia (urine), zoophilia (animals), and necrophilia (corpses) as well as Schizotypal Personality Disorder and Cannabis Abuse. He was ineligible to use the insanity defense because he was opined to not suffer from a mental illness that impacted his knowledge of wrongfulness or ability to refrain from his actions. He was convicted for his crimes and is currently still incarcerated in Ohio.

HISTORICAL AND CULTURAL CONTEXT

Reading the above case undoubtedly generates strong reactions, and Finbow (2014, p. 14) succinctly captures the dichotomous nature of these feelings: "Haunters of graveyards and morgues, the necrophile embodies our worst fears and our most base desires." This simultaneous repulsion and curiosity concerning necrophilia is often reflected in the culture of a society. Countless stories about vampires throughout history sexualize the so-called undead by focusing on the vampires' ability to bite and suck blood from the exposed necks of their victims. Even seemingly innocuous and romantic children's fairy tales, such as *Sleeping Beauty* and *Snow White*, make those women, who appear dead, the object of men's desire. Shakespeare employed the same technique in *Romeo and Juliet* (Rosman & Resnick, 1989). The Marquis de Sade made frequent mention of necrophilia in his writings (Aggrawal, 2011). A 1987 West German horror film, *Nekromantik*, has been banned in a number of countries due to its controversial subject matter, including a scene during which the main character presents his wife with a corpse that they then involve in their sexual escapades (Mullin, 2014). Common, and seemingly benign, societal practices also may reflect elements of necrophilia. Browne (1875) described a "healthy necrophilism" in the "mementoes cherished in every household of those who passed away" (pp. 551–560), which could certainly extend to retaining the ashes of lovers who have died. Halloween is another societally sanctioned homage in which people, through the use of costumes, are encouraged to be both gruesome and sexually appealing. Even college campuses may be the home of activities on the continuum with necrophilia, more specifically, intoxicated coeds engaging in sexual activities with those rendered unconscious by deceptive or voluntary substance use.

Throughout recorded history, there has been both a recognition and a fear of necrophilia. Circa 440 B.C., Herodotus (1988, p. 167) recorded the ancient Egyptians' attempts to prevent necrophilia, noting, "The wives of distinguished men ... they do not give for embalmment right away ... Only when they have been dead three or four days do they hand them over to the embalmers. This is done to prevent the embalmers from copulating with these women" (Herodotus, 1988, p. 167). Another group accused of necrophilia were the sailors charged with transporting bodies across oceans for last funeral rights. Long periods at sea, loneliness, and few witnesses may have been responsible for encouraging this behavior (Aggrawal, 2009). Below are summaries of the lives of a variety of infamous necrophiles, whose sensational and horrific stories certainly captivated the attention of the popular press and the public.

Sergeant Francois Bertrand—Vampire of Montparnasse (1824–1878)

As a youth in 19th-century France, Bertrand attended the theological seminary of Langres and later joined the army. Growing up, he mutilated the bodies of dead animals (horses, dogs, and cats); more specifically, he disemboweled them and masturbated over their entrails. He then engaged in the same activity after killing live animals. In 1847, while in a graveyard, he unearthed his first corpse, mutilated the body with a shovel and then a knife. This led to an orgasm. He continued to disinter women, and, when unable to do so completely, he would remove a piece of their clothing and masturbate with or over it. The following year, he exhumed the body of a teenage girl and, for the first time, fondled and had sexual intercourse with the remains, which he later eviscerated. In the process of breaking into graveyards, shots were fired at Bertrand on several occasions. He was ultimately arrested after presenting to the hospital to seek treatment for a gunshot wound and confessed to his surgeon. Because necrophilia was not a crime, Bertrand was convicted of vampirism and sentenced to one year in jail (Finbow, 2014, pp. 53–62).

Carl Tanzler (1877–1952)

Tanzler was born in Germany, was married in 1920, and immigrated to the United States in 1926. In 1930, while working at a hospital in Florida, Tanzler met Maria Milagro de Hoyos, whom he treated for tuberculosis. He fell in love with her and showered her with gifts. When she succumbed to the illness in 1931, he paid for her funeral services, including a mausoleum that he visited almost daily. In 1933, Tanzler removed her remains from the cemetery and transported them to his home. He attempted, through a variety of mechanisms, to preserve the body and slept with it his bed. In 1940, Hoyos's sister, after hearing rumors about Tanzler sleeping with Hoyos's corpse, confronted him and subsequently discovered the body in his home. Tanzler was charged with "wantonly and maliciously destroying a grave and removing a body without authorization." Some reports indicated that a paper tube was inserted in Hoyos' vagina to allow for posthumous sexual intercourse. After discovery, Hoyos's body was returned to an undisclosed grave, but Tanzler reportedly created a life-size effigy of her, with which he lived until his death (Harrison, 2009).

Jerome "Jerry" Brudos (1939–2006)

As a child, Brudos found a pair of high-heeled shoes while playing at the local junkyard. He returned home with them and was chastized severely by his mother when she discovered him wearing them. He began stealing shoes, then later women's underwear. At the age of 17 he, at knifepoint, forced a woman to strip, took photographs of her naked body, and beat her. Following this, he was court-ordered to the Oregon state psychiatric facility for nine months where he was diagnosed with "borderline schizophrenia." He enlisted briefly in the military but was discharged for "delusional tendencies." He later became an electrician.

In 1961, Brudos married a 17-year-old woman and had two children. He took pictures of his wife while she was naked doing household tasks and wearing high-heeled shoes. In 1968, Brudos killed his first victim by beating her with a piece of wood then strangling her. Following her death, he stripped her and dressed her in his lingerie. He cut off her left foot, placed it in a stiletto heeled shoe and stored it in the freezer. He subsequently took photos of it and masturbated over the foot until it began to decompose, at which point he disposed of it. After again dressing up and photographing the body of his next victim, he had vaginal and anal intercourse with the corpse. Prior to disposing of the body, he cut off one of the breasts. He did much the same with his third victim. With the fourth victim, he raped her while strangling her to death. He also had sex with the body postmortem. A few days after her death, he connected electrical wires to the body and used electricity to make the corpse move. In 1969, Brudos was caught after the police set a trap for him. He pleaded guilty to murder, was sentenced to life in prison, and died there in 2006 from liver cancer (Finbow, 2014, pp.142–150).

Dennis Nilsen (1945)

Nilsen was raised in Scotland and served 11 years in the military. He later worked as a police officer then a civil servant in London. He killed a minimum of 12 victims between 1978 and 1983. Nilsen lured his male victims back to his apartment by offering them shelter and food. He then strangled his victims (using ligatures, neckties, headphone cords, or his bare hands) while they ate a meal that he had prepared for them. He then drowned them in buckets, sinks, and baths. Once dead, he washed and dressed the victims, placed them in his bed, masturbated over them, and even placed them in chairs to greet him when he returned home. He also took pictures using a Polaroid camera. Nilsen would store the corpses, often under the floorboards, for a few weeks and took them out for sex or companionship. He then dismembered his victims, which was followed by boiling them, burning them, or cutting the bodies into small pieces to flush them down the toilet. After other tenants complained of drainage issues in the building, a drain cleaning company was called and found what they believed to be chicken in the pipes. The police were notified and questioned Nilsen, who showed them body parts he had stored in a wardrobe. In 1983, Nilsen was sentenced to life for six murders and two attempted murders. While in prison, Nilsen asked to receive *Vulcan*, a hardcore gay pornographic magazine. Nilsen also penned a 400-page unpublished autobiography, which he titled, *The History of a Drowning Boy* (Finbow, 2014, pp. 129–142; Masters, 1985).

Theodore "Ted" Bundy (1946–1989)

Unbeknownst to him, Bundy was raised by his grandparents (who said that they were his parents) and his mother (who said that she was his sister); his father was absent. He was a straight-A student but was teased and bullied in school. On a ski trip, he fell in love with a woman, who ultimately rejected him because she felt that he lacked ambition. Bundy became more goal-oriented, worked on political campaigns, applied to law school and was accepted. He rekindled his romance with his former girlfriend only to reject her when she began to express interest in him.

In the beginning of his decades-long crime spree, Bundy was known to lure woman into seclusion by feigning injury (wearing a plaster cast on his arm), requesting assistance, and then rendering his victims unconscious. His early victims shared a number of commonalities: they were thin, Caucasian, had long hair parted in the middle, and wore pants, features which were reminiscent of his ex-girlfriend. After killing his victims, Bundy would later return to visit the bodies, have sex with the corpses, and beautify them by applying makeup and washing their hair. He would continue to do so until the decomposition disgusted him. He also kept trophies, including taking photographs of the victims and even decapitating them. Once his crimes were discovered, Bundy was arrested. He managed to escape from jail on two different occasions. While on the run, he stole clothing and food to avoid capture. He fled from Colorado to Florida and continued his killing spree. He was ultimately captured, tried, convicted, and executed. Shortly after his conviction in 1979, Bundy granted a series of interviews to offer up the lurid details of his crimes, and once his execution date was set in 1988, he confessed to other murders, some of which were unknown to the authorities (Finbow, 2014, pp. 101–127; Rule, 2000).

Karen Greenlee (1957)

1n 1979, Greenlee was a 22-year-old mortuary attendant. In lieu of delivering the body of a 33-year-old man to the cemetery, she drove to the next county and had sex with the corpse. She then wrote a letter detailing her necrophilic acts with an estimated 20 to 40 men and overdosed on medication. The police found her, took her to a hospital, and then arrested her. She was charged with illegally driving a hearse and interfering with a burial (necrophilia was not illegal in California). She was sentenced to 11 days in jail, fined $255, and placed on two years of probation. The deceased man's mother also sued her. She asked for $1 million but settled for $117,000 in general and punitive damages.

Five years later, Greenlee granted an interview. When asked, she stated that necrophilia was "something I've been attracted to all my life." She added that she used to hold funeral services for her pets after they died and would walk around mortuaries whenever she had the opportunity as a youth. She worked in several nursing homes and broke into others. She often attended the funeral services of those with whom she had had sex. Greenlee stated that she had grown more comfortable with her sexuality, noting, "When I wrote that letter, I was still listening to society. Everyone said necrophilia was wrong, so I must be doing something wrong. But the more people tried to convince me I was crazy, the more sure of my desires I became" ("Badass Digest," n.d.; "The Unrepentant Necrophile," n.d.).

Jeffrey Dahmer (1960–1994)

Dahmer grew up in Ohio, served two years in the military, and then worked in a chocolate factory in Milwaukee. He was 18 years old when he killed his first victim, a 19-year-old hitchhiker whom he picked up and took home. The two drank and had sex. When the man attempted to leave, Dahmer killed him, had sex with the body, dismembered him, and ultimately buried him alongside dead animals that he had dissected years before. Later, much like Nilsen described earlier, Dahmer met his victims in bars and offered money, food, or shelter to lure his homosexual victims back to his apartment. He incapacitated his victims, injecting boiling water or acid through holes in their skulls to create "zombies." He had a predilection for hard core pornography and photographed his victims both alive and dead in a variety of pornographic poses. He kept the bodies for weeks, dismembering them, and storing various body parts throughout his apartment. He also ate pieces of at least one victim. Between 1978 and 1991, Dahmer killed 17 men. Once captured, Dahmer provided a 160-page confession. In 1992, he was sentenced to life in prison, and in 1994, he was beaten to death by a fellow inmate (Finbow, 2014, pp. 128–141).

The vast majority of people view the act of necrophilia as fundamentally immoral, but it was only recently that legal systems began to criminalize this conduct. As noted earlier, in 19th-century France, there was no specific law prohibiting necrophilia, so Sergeant Bertrand was convicted of "vampirism." In the 1940s, Tanzler was convicted of "wantonly and maliciously destroying a grave and removing a body without authorization." And Greenlee was convicted of illegally driving a hearse and interfering with a burial. More recently, the Philippines handled this issue differently. In 2009 and 2010, the sexually abused corpses of five females were discovered laid out on their graves. The Philippine government proposed Senate Bill 1038, making necrophilia a crime punishable by death. The bill noted, "... this vicious bestiality is notoriously offensive and revolting to the feelings of the living even as it grossly desecrates the dead" (Senate of the Philippines, n.d.). In the United States, necrophilia is illegal in the large majority of states (Aggrawal, 2011).

ROLE IN CURRENT DIAGNOSTIC SYSTEMS

Necrophilia is not a standalone diagnostic category in either the *Diagnostic and Statistical Manual of Mental Disorders, Fifth Edition* (DSM-5) or the *International Classification of Disease, Tenth Edition* (ICD-10). The DSM-5, however, does specifically mention necrophilia in its definition of *Other Specified Paraphilic Disorders*, which are noted to be disorders characterized by "recurrent and intense sexual arousal involving telephone scatologia (obscene phone calls), necrophilia (corpses), zoophilia (animals), coprophilia (feces), klismaphilia (enemas) or urophilia (urine) that has been present for at least six months and causes marked distress or impairment in social, occupational or other important areas of functioning" (American Psychiatric Association, 2013, p. 705). According to the ICD-10, necrophilia is specifically mentioned under Other Paraphilias, a subcategory of Paraphilias, which also includes fetishism, transvestic fetishism, exhibitionism, voyeurism, pedophilia, and sadomasochism (Centers for Medicaid and Medicare Services, n.d.).

SYMPTOMATOLOGY

The core features of necrophilia are erotic fantasies about and/or sexual contact with the dead. Given that it is natural to attempt to further define and classify what we struggle to understand, a variety of authors have done so with necrophilia in recent times. In 1866, von Krafft-Ebbing (1965) divided necrophiles into two categories: passive (used corpses for sexual purposes) and active (killed for the purpose of having sex with the dead). In 1910, Erich Wulffen added a third category, necrophagy (consumption of the dead's flesh), which appears to be synonymous with cannibalism. In 1931, Ernest Jones further defined passive necrophilia, describing two subcategories: sex with the corpse of a loved one versus sex with an unknown dead body.

In 1989, Rosman and Resnick based their own classification system on 122 cases of necrophilic acts and/or fantasies from around the world. They described three subcategories of genuine necrophila: necrophilic homicide, "regular" necrophilia, and necrophilic fantasy. In necrophilic homicide, the perpetrator commits murder to obtain a corpse. Regular necrophiles obtain sexual pleasure from the previously deceased. With necrophilic fantasies, the necrophile simply fantasizes about corpses but does not carry out any necrophilic acts. Additionally, they defined a fourth category, the pseudonecrophile, defined as an individual with a transient attraction to corpses but who prefers contact with living sexual partners. They further define this term through the case example of a man who accidentally shot and killed his wife, became sexually aroused while hiding her body, and had anal sex with the corpse. Of note, other authors have used the term pseudonecrophilia to refer to those who have sex with an individual pretending to be dead (Shaffer & Penn, 2006) or just masturbate to fantasies about sex with a corpse (in lieu of actual physical contact with the dead) (Lazarus, 1968; Rauch, 1947; Segal, 1953). The latter would be consistent with Rosman and Resnick's necrophilic fantasy category.

In 2009, Aggrawal created the most extensive system for classifying necrophilia. He described 10 categories: (1) *Role Players*—those who are aroused by sex with a living person pretending to be dead; (2) *Romantic Necrophiles*—bereaved individuals who preserve their loved one's body (or body parts) and continue to relate to them sexually as they did during the life of the deceased (often transient in nature); (3) *Necrophilic Fantasizers*—those who only fantasize about sexual intercourse with the dead; (4) *Tactile Necrophiles*—people who need to touch a corpse in an erotic manner in order to achieve orgasm; (5) *Fetishistic Necrophiles*—those who remove a part of a previously dead body and use it for sexual pleasure; (6) *Necromutilomaniacs*—people who derive sexual pleasure from mutilating a corpse while simultaneously masturbating; (7) *Opportunistic Necrophiles*—those who are generally content having sex with the living but would have sex with a corpse if the opportunity arose (i.e., Rosman & Resnick's definition of pseudonecrophilia); (8) *Regular Necrophiles*—individuals who derive pleasure from having sexual intercourse with the dead (and prefer them to the living); (9) *Homicidal Necrophiles*—people who resort to killing in order to obtain a body with which to have sex; and (10) *Exclusive Necrophiles*—those who will only have sex with the dead.

PREVALENCE RATE AND ASSOCIATED FEATURES

Necrophilia is a rare disorder, and given the stigma associated with it, its true prevalence may never be known (Stein, Schlesinger, & Pinizzotto, 2009). The conclusions drawn about the subject are significantly limited by the dearth of systematic empirical literature addressing the topic. Although only a handful of cases are discussed above, and the results of any analyses may be confounded by the high profile nature of these cases, there are a few commonalities among them worth noting. Growing up, necrophiles tend to be raised by inadequate (e.g., abusive, neglectful) parents. Brudos had a harsh, domineering mother. Bundy's mother and grandparents lied about their identity, while his father was absent. Some of these necrophiles (Bertrand, Brudos, and Dahmer) engaged in antisocial or sexually dysfunctional behavior as youths. Both Bertrand and Dahmer had sexual contact with dead animals prior to engaging in sexual activities with corpses. Perhaps this behavior served as a rehearsal for contact with humans, where the consequences could be much more significant. Other paraphilias, such as Zoophilia (Bertrand), Transvestic Disorder and Fetishistic Disorder (Brudos), were comorbid in a few of the cases. Also, prior to their necrophilic acts, several (Bertrand, Brudos, Nilsen, and Dahmer) served in the military, and others (Brudos and Bundy) committed acts of theft, which led to incarceration. Of note, Greenlee stole the body with which she had sex.

During the acts, some collected trophies or items that represented the victims. Brudos, Nilsen, Bundy, and Dahmer retained body parts, while Bertrand removed pieces of clothing from the deceased. Brudos, Nilsen, Bundy, and Dahmer also photographed their victims. Following the necrophilic act, Bertrand, Brudos, Nilsen, Bundy, and Dahmer mutilated or dismembered their victims. At some point after their arrest, Nilsen, Bundy, Greenlee, and Dahmer also provided detailed descriptions of their actions.

In general, these necrophiles demonstrate some features consistent with Antisocial Personality Disorder, which is described as "a pervasive pattern of disregard for and violation of the rights of others," and includes, more specifically, a failure to conform to social norms with respect to lawful behavior and a lack of remorse (American Psychiatric Association, 2013, p. 659).

The literature demonstrates some common trends as well. The vast majority of necrophiles are men (especially those who commit homicide) (Rosman & Resnick, 1989). Necrophiles commonly are employed as gravediggers or mortuary attendants, giving them much freer access to the deceased. This does raise the question: Do people become necrophiles because of loneliness coupled with easy access to corpses? Or, do necrophiles seek out jobs in which access to bodies is guaranteed (Aggrawal, 2009)? Though they often are viewed as such by the public, Rosman and Resnick (1989) noted that necrophiles are typically not intellectually disabled or psychotic. They also noted that necrophiles may use drugs or alcohol to decrease inhibition and promote their commission of, what would be to most, such a distasteful act.

THEORIES OF ETIOLOGY

Given the paucity of empirical work with this population, we are left to hypothesize about the reasons for their behavior. Rosman and Resnick (1989, p. 161) concluded that the overarching motive for necrophilia is "a profound lack of self-esteem." They suggested that the necrophile may be fearful of rejection and wish to totally possess a partner incapable of resisting or rejecting him; or, the necrophile may fear the dead and, through reaction formation, develop an attraction to them. Other motives include reuniting with a romantic partner or loneliness. Stein, Schlesigner, and Pinizzotto (2009) noted that necrophilia associated with homicide may require different explanations, including a means of further degrading the victim (DeRiver, 1958; Masters, 1963) or calling greater attention to their disdain for society (Hazelwood & Douglas, 1980).

ASSESSMENT OPTIONS

Given the shameful and illicit nature of the behavior, necrophiles do not often seek help on their own. As described in multiple instances earlier, necrophiles frequently come to light in the context of legal charges. From that point, they likely disclose the details of their histories and behavior for the purposes of completing a police report, a sanity evaluation, or participation in a court hearing. There do not appear to be any clinical measures (e.g., questionnaires or structured interviews) to assess for the presence and features associated with necrophilia.

DIFFERENTIAL DIAGNOSIS

Society accepts a continuum of behavior as "normal" sexual functioning, and one could argue necrophilia sits at the extreme end of what is tolerable, given that the victim has suffered no physical or emotional pain as a result of the necrophile's actions. Necrophilia also may be viewed as a form of Fetishism, which the DSM-5 defines as "recurrent and intense sexual arousal from either the use of non-living objects or a highly specific focus on non-genital body part(s), as manifested by fantasies, urges or behaviors." (American Psychiatric Association, 2013, pp. 700–702). In this interpretation, the corpse would serve as the fetishistic object. This is, however, a very literal interpretation of fetishism, and it appears the spirit of the definition refers to objects that were never living (e.g., shoes).

TREATMENT OPTIONS

In 1989, Rosman and Resnick stated, "No one has treated a sufficient number of necrophiles to determine effective treatment on a scientific basis," and since that time, little has changed. These authors do suggest that, in an effort to treat necrophilia, one should address comorbid psychopathology, encourage healthy sexual and social relationships, and consider antiandrogen therapy in males with heightened sex drives. Given that necrophilia has been characterized as a paraphilia, it stands to reason that therapeutic interventions, such as cognitive behavioral therapy, that are used to treat these other dysfunctional sexual behaviors would be appropriate for the treatment of necrophilia (Lazarus, 1968). One specific technique that may be of some utility involves the pairing of normal sexual fantasy with orgasm and the deviant fantasy (in this case, sex with the dead) with the refractory period following orgasm in order to uncouple the deviant fantasy from sexual arousal.

RECOMMENDATIONS FOR FUTURE WORK

Sex and death in combination lead to both disgust and fascination, thus the practice of necrophilia has been documented since ancient times. Classification systems highlight the differences among necrophiles, but in reviewing the available literature and the aforementioned cases, there are some potential commonalities evident as well. Some of these may include inadequate parenting, contact with dead animals as a youth, previous theft charges, the acquisition of trophies, mutilation of corpses, and confessions in great detail. Given the comorbid nature of paraphilias, perhaps it may also be worthwhile to screen for the presence of . necrophilia when evaluating individuals who present with other deviant sexual behavior. This may provide some sense of the prevalence of the disorder. Future research with a larger number of subjects is required to further define these associations.

REFERENCES

Aggrawal, A. (2009). A new classification of necrophilia. *Journal of Forensic and Legal Medicine, 16,* 316–320.

Aggrawal, A. (2011). *Necrophilia: Forensic and medico-legal aspects.* Boca Raton, FL: CRC Press.

Badass Digest. (n.d.). Retrieved on April 20, 2015 from http://badassdigest.com/2013/10/31/ghoul-of-your-dreams-proud-necrophiliac-karen-greenlee/

Brown, W.A.F. (1875). Necrophilism. *Journal of Mental Science, 20,* 551–560.

Centers for Medicaid and Medicare Services. (n.d.). Retrieved on June 23, 2015 from https://www.cms.gov/Medicare/Coding/ICD10/downloads/6_I10tab2010.pdf

DeRiver, J.P. (1958). *Crime and the sexual psychopath.* Springfield, IL: Thomas.

Finbow, S. (2014). *Grave desire: A cultural history of necrophilia.* Winchester, UK: Zero Books.

Harrison, B. (2009). *Undying love: the true story of a passion that defied death.* Key West, FL: The Ketch & Yawl Press.

Hazelwood, R.R., & Douglas, J.E. (1980). The lust murder. *FBI Law Enforcement Bulletin, 49*, 3.

Herodotus. (1988). *The history* (D. Grene, Trans.). Chicago: University of Chicago.

Jones, E. (1931). *On the nightmare.* New York: Liverright.

Lazarus, A.A. (1968). A case of pseudonecrophilia treated with behavioral therapy. *Journal of Clinical Psychology, 24(1),* 113–115.

Masters, B. (1985). *Killing for company: the case of Dennis Nilsen.* New York: Random House.

Masters, R.E.L. (1963). *Perverse crimes in history: Evolving concepts of sadism, lust-murder and necrophilia—from ancient to modern times.* New York: Julian Press.

Merriam-Webster. (n.d.). Retrieved on April 18, 2015 from http://www.merriamwebster.com/dictionary/necrophilia

Mullin, F. (2014, September 4). Cult film shocker "Nekromantik" to get UK release after BBFC grants 18 certificate. *The Guardian.* Retrieved from http://www.theguardian.com/film/filmblog/2014/sep/04/nekromantik-film-uk-release-horror-censorship

Rauch, H.J. (1947). Uber nekrophile. *Archiv fur Psychiatrie und Nervenkrankheiten, 179*, 54.

Resnick, P.J. (February 25, 1986). Insanity Report. 1–20.

Rosman, J., & Resnick, P.J. (1989). Sexual attraction to corpses: A psychiatric review of necrophilia. *Bulletin of the American Academy of Psychiatry and the Law, 17(2),* 153–163.

Rule, A. (2000). *The stranger beside me.* New York: WW Norton & Company.

Segal, H. (1953). A necrophilic fantasy. *International Journal of Psychoanalysis, 34,* 98–101.

Senate of the Philippines. (n.d.). Retrieved on April 18, 2015 from http://www.senate.gov.ph/lis/bill_res.aspx?congress=14&q=SBN-1038

Shaffer, L., & Penn, J. (2006). A comprehensive paraphilia classification system. In E.W. Hicky (Ed.), *Sex crimes and paraphilia* (1st ed.) (p. 87). New Jersey: Pearson Prentice Hall.

Stein, M., Schlesinger, L., & Pinizzotto, A. (2009). Necrophilia and sexual homicide. *Journal of Forensic Sciences, 55(2),* 443.

The Unrepentant Necrophile. (n.d.). Retrieved on April 20, 2015 from http://www.nokilli.com/sacto/karen-greenlee.htm

von Krafft-Ebbing, R. (1965). *Psychopathia sexualis.* New York: G.P. Putnam's Sons.

Wulffen, E. (1910). *Enzyklopaedie der modernen kriminalistik.* Berlin: Langenscheidt.

10

Frotteurism

RICHARD McANULTY ■

VIGNETTE

Charles was 45 years old when he was referred for psychiatric consultation by his parole officer following his second arrest for rubbing up against a woman in the subway. According to Charles, he had a "good" sexual relationship with his wife of 15 years when he began to touch women in the subway approximately 10 years ago. A typical episode would begin with his decision to go into the subway to rub against a woman, usually in her twenties. He would select the woman as he walked into the subway station, move in behind her, and wait for the train to arrive at the station. He would be wearing plastic wrap around his penis so as not to stain his pants after ejaculating while rubbing up against his victim. As riders moved on to the train, he would follow the woman he had selected. When the doors closed, he would begin to push his penis up against her buttocks, fantasizing that they were having intercourse in a normal, noncoercive manner. In about half of the episodes, he would ejaculate and then go on to work. If he failed to ejaculate, he would either give up for that day or change trains and select another victim. According to Charles, he felt guilty immediately after each episode but would soon find himself ruminating about it and anticipating the next encounter. He estimated that he had done this about twice a week for the last 10 years and thus had probably rubbed up against approximately a thousand women. During the interview, Charles expressed extreme guilt about his behavior and often cried when talking about fears that his wife or employer would find out about his second arrest. However, he apparently had never thought about how his victims felt regarding what he did to them. His personal history did not indicate any obvious mental problems other than being rather socially inept and unassertive, especially with women (Spitzer et al., 2002).

HISTORICAL/CULTURAL CONTEXT

The earliest published reports of individuals rubbing against unsuspecting women for sexual purposes were reported by European psychiatrists at the turn of the 19th century. Both Magnan (1890) and von Krafft-Ebing (1906) described cases of men who were arrested for such acts. In each case, these behaviors were described as having a compulsive quality in an oversexed man. Such aberrations were viewed as deviant and rare. Today, however, unwanted sexual "groping" or "grinding," as it is known in the popular press, is rather commonly reported on crowded public transportation in large metropolitan areas in several cultures, including the United States. It virtually always consists of a male rubbing up against or fondling an unsuspecting female stranger.

Individuals who engage in this behavior typically do so by positioning themselves next to a lone attractive female, taking advantage of the crowded situation to rub their genitals against the victim's buttocks or thighs or to fondle her crotch or breasts from behind. The physical contact generally occurs without face-to-face interaction or verbal exchanges (Lussier & Piche´, 2008).

"Forcible touching" is the most prevalent sex crime in the New York subway system (Ryley & Donohue, 2014). Between 2008 and 2013, 1,322 incidents of forcible touching were reported to law enforcement officials. These incidents typically occurred during morning rush hour on this, the busiest subway line in the nation. The actual number of incidents is likely much higher because most victims never report them to authorities due to the hassle of filing reports, embarrassment, doubt, or being resigned to it as part of the cost of daily commuting in crowded places. In one study of college students in New York City, nearly 25% of female students reported having been victims of unwanted touching or groping by a stranger (Clark, Jeglic, Calkins, & Tatar, 2014). Despite feeling violated and upset by the experience, only 5% of female student victims reported it to police (Clark et al., 2014). Forcible touching was reportedly such a serious phenomenon in the Tokyo subway system that authorities implemented some female-only cars (Beech & Harkins, 2012). The problem is so common that such terms as "subway groper" and "transit grinder" have emerged in recent years (Bayona, 2010). Previously considered nuisances, recent legislation in New York could make such acts subject to prosecution as felony class offenses (Conley, 2015). Frotteurism is also reported in other settings that are crowded and bustling with activity, such as nightclubs, dance halls, elevators, and other busy social venues.

ROLE IN CURRENT DIAGNOSTIC SYSTEMS

Unwanted touching or groping is officially known as frotteurism (from the French *frotter*, "to rub"). The actual act is sometimes referred to as frottage, a term also used for any form of consensual sexual rubbing. As a sexual disorder, frotteurism was first included as an atypical paraphilia (formerly referred to as *Sexual Deviations*) in the third edition of the *Diagnostic and Statistical Manual of Mental Disorders* (DSM, American Psychiatric Association [APA], 1980). Paraphilias entailed "unusual or bizarre imagery or acts" that were necessary for sexual arousal and that deviated from normal sexual patterns while also interfering with the capacity for reciprocal sexual activity (APA, 1980, p. 261). Frotteurism currently is classified as a full-fledged paraphilia, a group of conditions involving intense and persistent sexual interest other than normal interest in sexual activity with an appropriate and consenting sexual partner (APA, 2013). Paraphilic sexual interest may involve unusual sexual activities (e.g., spanking), unusual sexual targets (e.g., children), or some combination. Paraphilic *disorders* entail paraphilic *sexual interest* that is causing distress or impairment in functioning for the individual or posing a risk of harm to the individual or to others. In the *International Classification of Diseases* (ICD-10) (World Health Organization, 1993), frotteurism is classified as a disorder of sexual preference involving rubbing up against people for sexual stimulation in crowded public places.

Some researchers have distinguished between frotteurism, consisting only of rubbing one's genitals against an unsuspecting person, and toucherism, which involves fondling a stranger, usually from behind (Freund, Seto, & Kuban, 1997; McAnulty, Adams, & Dillon, 2001). The current DSM diagnostic system makes no such distinction, and the limited literature does not seem to support one. Frotteurism is considered one of the more common paraphilic sexual interests, along with voyeurism, exhibitionism, sexual masochism, sexual sadism, pedophilia, fetishism, and transvestic fetishism (APA, 2013).

Unfortunately, there is very little empirical research on the phenomenon of frotteurism. For example, in an earlier version of the official diagnostic system (DSM-IV-TR; APA, 2000), it was stated that the person engaging in frotteuristic acts usually fantasized about having an "exclusive, caring relationship" with the victim (p. 270). This descriptor was dropped in DSM-5, however, probably because of the lack of any supporting data (Lussier & Piche´, 2008; McConaghy, 1993).

SYMPTOMATOLOGY

In DSM-5, frotteuristic disorder involves recurrent and persistent sexual arousal from touching or rubbing against a nonconsenting person. The arousal is evident in the individual's sexual fantasies, urges, or behaviors. The official diagnosis requires that the person has either acted upon these sexual urges or that they cause significant distress or impairment in social, occupational, or other important areas of functioning (APA, 2013). A person with such urges who experiences no distress over them (e.g., guilt or shame), and is not impaired by them in some way, and who has not acted upon these impulses, could be described as having frotteuristic sexual interest, but *not* the full-blown disorder.

The diagnosis implies that it represents a problematic pattern, rather than an isolated incident. Therefore, a situation in which an eager male dancer rubs his groin against an unsuspecting stranger on the dance floor would not qualify unless it becomes a persistent pattern that is causing distress, impairment in functioning, or harm to self or others. In all likelihood, such an individual would prefer a more conventional sexual encounter with a consenting partner over opportunistic frottage (see Wakefield, 2011).

These diagnostic criteria are admittedly controversial. Blanchard (2011) complained that the diagnostic criteria for the paraphilias in the recent versions of

DSM were essentially developed without any field trials. Wakefield (2011) persuasively argued that the "most valid indicators of true paraphilic disorder," rather than just paraphilic sexual interest, are exclusiveness (preference for the paraphilic interest over normative sexual interest), fixation (necessary or required for sexual arousal), and compulsiveness (relatively irresistible). None of these are included in the current diagnostic criteria (APA, 2013). A pattern of deviant sexual arousal is considered "the core of the paraphilias" by several researchers (First, 2010, p. 1242) rather than actual behaviors. Such conceptual problems with DSM paraphilia criteria add to the difficulties in collecting useful information about these "disorders," including frotteurism.

PREVALENCE RATE AND ASSOCIATED FEATURES

According to DSM-5, "uninvited sexual touching or rubbing" may occur in 30% of the male population, making it a very common phenomenon. Twenty-five percent of the male college students in one survey admitted to having engaged in frotteuristic behavior (Templeman & Stinnett, 1991). Most of these males, however, probably did not have the problematic pattern, but rather engaged in opportunistic sexual contact. It is estimated that 10% to 14% of men in treatment for paraphilic disorders have frotteurism (APA, 2013). The frotteuristic urges reportedly develop in adolescence or early adulthood after a sexually arousing experience of surreptitiously touching an unsuspecting person. Although there are no longitudinal studies to verify this claim, it is estimated that sexual urges in general decline with advancing age, as do most paraphilic sexual interests (APA, 2013).

For some individuals, frotteurism has a compulsive quality. In a large study (N = 561) of nonincarcerated individuals with paraphilias, Abel et al. (1987) interviewed 62 self-proclaimed frotteurs. The mean number of reported victims was 901 (Median = 29.5). Frotteurs accounted for the second largest number of paraphilic acts (18.1%) in the sample, second only to exhibitionists. A frotteur may repeatedly board crowded subway cars during rush hour, affording access to multiple victims in a short period of time. He will rub against an unsuspecting victim until he climaxes or until she protests, taking advantage of regular stops to escape if needed. One individual in New York City, the so-called Subway Rat, was arrested 53 times for allegedly groping women on the subway. A 49-year-old man, he had reportedly engaged in frotteurism for 25 years, having started after witnessing another man do so unpunished (Long, 2008). Interestingly, he allegedly had an identical twin who was sentenced for the same offense (Sederstrom & Gendar, 2008).

Like other men with other paraphilias, frotteurs tend to rationalize their behavior. As one offender put it, "attractive women should expect to be groped on trains." "When there's this many attractive women in the city and on the subways, don't they know this will happen?" (Sederstrom & Gendar, 2008). Many men with frotteurism apparently insist that they never would harm a woman and are not violent, thereby downplaying the impact on their victims.

Comorbidity in DSM-5 includes other paraphilic disorders, particularly exhibitionism, voyeurism (APA, 2013), and hypersexuality. Freund and colleagues (1997) found that the majority (68%) of their sample of 144 men with frotteuristic disorder had other paraphilic interests, mostly exhibitionism and voyeurism, leading the authors to conclude that these are differing aspects of a common disturbance. From his literature review, Kafka (2010) concluded that hypersexuality, usually in the form of compulsive masturbation, commonly co-occurs with most paraphilic disorders. He estimated that 72% to 80% of individuals seeking treatment for paraphilias and related problems had histories of hypersexuality. Other comorbid disorders may include conduct disorder, antisocial personality disorder, mood disorders, anxiety disorders, and substance use disorders (APA, 2013).

Several writers have emphasized the nonconsensual and impersonal nature of the interaction between the frotteur and his victims (Lussier & Piche´, 2008). Money (1986) claimed that the impersonal nature of the sexual contact was essential to the individual's satisfaction. Langevin (1983) classified it as a form of sexual aggression on the basis of the lack of consent. For the frotteur, the contact with an unsuspecting stranger provides immediate sexual enjoyment with minimal investment of time or effort (Långström, 2010).

The literature on risk factors for frotteurism is sparse. In DSM-5, antisocial behavior and sexual preoccupation/hypersexuality are possible nonspecific risk factors for frotteurism (APA, 2013). From their review, Lussier and Piche´ (2008) concluded that lifelong antisocial behavior was characteristic of most offenders against women, including frotteurs. Traumatic brain injuries and other neurological impairments are possible risk factors for frotteurism and other anomalous sexual behavior (Cannas et al., 2006; Simpson, Blaszczynki, & Hodgkinson, 1999; Solla, Bortolato, Cannas, Mulas, & Marrosu, 2015), although it seems likely that these impairments are most related to pervasive disinhibition rather than to frotteurism per se. A history of sexual abuse might also be a risk factor for various inappropriate sexual behaviors, but not specifically for frotteuristic acts (Lussier & Piche´, 2008).

THEORIES OF ETIOLOGY

The courtship disorders model proposed by Freund and colleagues is based on the premise that normal human sexual interaction, or courtship, typically proceeds through four phases: (1) finding a potential partner; (2) making overtures to the partner; (3) making physical contact; and (4) engaging in sexual intercourse (Freund, 1990; Freund et al., 1997). According to the model, several of the paraphilias represent extreme distortions of one of these phases. Voyeurism is a distortion of the process of locating a prospective sexual partner. Exhibitionism represents a distorted approach to making a sexual overture to a sexual partner. Frotteurism is an aberration of the phase of making physical contact with a partner, and preferential rape is a distortion of the final phase because it involves omitting all of the previous phases. Although the courtship disorders model may be a useful heuristic for describing some of the deficits that characterize several of the impersonal paraphilias, it offers little insight into the developmental pathways to these disorders.

Lussier and Piche' (2008) reduced most theoretical models of frotteurism to the sex drive and social incompetence hypotheses. According to the sex drive hypothesis, frotteurs suffer from hypersexuality, or an usually high sex drive. Krafft-Ebing (1906) was the first to suggest that "frottage is a masturbatorial act of a hypersexual individual who is uncertain about his virility" (p. 525), thereby combining both hypotheses into its etiology. As previously noted, sexual preoccupation/hypersexuality is listed as a possible risk factor for frotteurism in DSM-5 (APA. 2013).

Kafka (2010) considers hypersexuality to be a defining feature of the majority of paraphilias. In a review, he noted that individuals with the highest number of paraphilias and other related problems also reported the greatest amount of time fantasizing and engaging in sexual activity (mean: 2–4 hours per day) and the highest number of orgasms (mean: 10 per week), mostly in the form of compulsive masturbation. Unfortunately, there have been no systematic studies of hypersexuality and frotteurism, so these conclusions are speculative, unless one assumes that paraphilias constitute a fairly homogeneous group with a common underlying pathology.

According to the social incompetence hypothesis, which is not incompatible with the sex drive hypothesis, several writers have speculated on presumed deficits that prevent frotteurs from forming meaningful consensual relationships. Krafft-Ebing (1906) alluded to heterosocial inadequacy. Others have proposed developmental disabilities (Fedoroff, 2003) and social anxiety (Brockman & Bluglass, 1996). Unfortunately, none of these hypotheses have been tested with a sample of men with frotteurism. Social incompetence hypotheses have been tested with individuals with other paraphilias, and there is evidence that some of them, but not all, suffer from social-skill deficits, emotional loneliness, and insecure attachment (see, for example, McAnulty, 2006; Marshall, 1989; Seto, 2004). Clearly, there is a need for empirical research on the etiology of frotteurism.

ASSESSMENT OPTIONS

As Banse and colleagues (2010) noted, "the assessment of enduring sexual preference is fraught with difficulties, mainly due to the problematic psychometric properties of the most commonly used measures" (p. 320). There is currently no standard assessment procedure for frotteurism. Krueger and Kaplan (2008) recommend a comprehensive diagnostic interview, with an emphasis on sexual history, following a review of available records (arrest record, victim statements, and criminal history). As with other self-report methods, the validity hinges on the individual's truthfulness and other factors (such as memory). Individuals charged with criminal behavior, especially sex offenses, are notoriously reluctant to self-disclose and, even when presented with incontrovertible evidence, they are prone to minimization and denial (Schneider & Wright, 2004; Seto, 2004). Denial can take many forms, ranging from denial of the offense itself or denial of a sexual motivation for it, to denial of any potential for future offending. Some clinicians advocate polygraph testing as a tool for evaluating alleged perpetrator's truthfulness (Konopasek, 2015). It is used in the majority of sex offender treatment programs (McGrath, Cumming, Burchard, Zeoli, & Ellerby, 2010). Its use is controversial, however, because of the mixed research findings on utility and validity (see Rosky, 2013).

Similar questions have been raised about the penile plethysmograph (also known as phallometry) with paraphilias. There is no standardized set of test materials (audiotaped descriptions or visual images of sexual acts), therefore, the psychometric properties cannot be evaluated (Murphy, Ranger, Stewart, Dwyer, & Fedoroff, 2015). Clinicians and researchers have consistently cautioned that the penile plethysmograph be used only for treatment purposes because of its limitations for diagnosis and assessment (Prentky, Gabriel, & Coward, 2010). Although the sensitivity and specificity of the procedure with pedophiles may be adequate, it has not proven useful with other paraphilias, including exhibitionism (Kalmus & Beech, 2005; Marshall, 2014).

Viewing time is another assessment methodology that has been used in a few studies with paraphilias. The *Abel Assessment of Sexual Interest* (AASI, Abel, Huffman, Warberg, & Holland, 1998) is a measure of viewing time based on the finding that, when shown photographs of targets of varying age and gender, viewers tend to inspect those that they find attractive for longer periods than less attractive targets. Studies have shown that viewing time can effectively discriminate child molesters from nonoffenders (Abel et al., 1998; Banse, Schmidt, & Clarbour, 2010). This methodology, however, has not been used with most other paraphilias, including frotteurism. Krueger and Kaplan (2008) anecdotally reported that they had not found it useful with this population.

There are currently no validated self-report measures for frotteuristic tendencies or acts. The *Multiphasic Sex Inventory-II* (MIS-II; Nichols & Molinder, 1984) is designed to evaluate the "sexual characteristics" of individuals who are alleged to have perpetrated a sexual offense of sexual misconduct. This 506-item true/false questionnaire includes validity scales, molester and rapist comparison scales, psychosexual scales (e.g., social sexual inadequacy, emotional neediness, cognitive distortions, and paraphilia scales (e.g., fetishism, masochism, obscene calling, bondage/ discipline), among others. There is no frotteurism scale per se, but the questionnaire does provide a sexual misconduct index. In their review, Kalmus and Beech (2005) concluded that there are no "published data to suggest that the MSI can actually differentiate sexual preference" (p. 207). It may be most useful in detecting denial rather than in assessing sexual interest. There are, however, simpler and less time-intensive methods for evaluating denial and deception (see Rogers, 2012).

DIFFERENTIAL DIAGNOSIS

According to DSM-5 (2013), frotteuristic disorder should be differentiated from conduct disorder, antisocial personality disorder, and substance use disorders. In the case of conduct disorder and antisocial personality disorder, the individual's history would involve a larger pattern of rule-breaking and norm violations beyond rubbing against or fondling unsuspecting women. For substance use disorders, particularly involving alcohol or stimulants, the individual might engage in frotteurism while intoxicated, but there should be no evidence of a pervasive pattern of sexual interest in frotteurism. Other conditions to consider for a differential diagnosis include a manic episode of bipolar disorder and a neurocognitive disorder (First, 2010). Essentially, any condition that involves lowered or impaired impulse control should be considered in cases of sexual misconduct.

Differential diagnosis is complicated by perpetrators' denial and the lack of sensitive and precise assessment tools. Perhaps the most effective indicator of frotteurism among individuals who deny such urges or acts would be a record of repeated allegations (i.e., two or more) of illicit grinding or groping in crowded places. The absence of such a record, of course, does not guarantee an accurate diagnosis because plea bargaining could result in a reduced and less telling charge (such as misdemeanor harassment). It would, therefore, be essential to review an individual's history of allegations and criminal charges critically. Finally, the possibility of risk for sexual aggression should be considered with any case of alleged frotteurism. In a study of convicted rapists, Freund and Seto (1998) found that almost 20% admitted to engaging in frotteuristic acts, again suggesting that the nonconsensual aspect of frotteurism requires additional study (Langevin, 1983).

TREATMENT OPTIONS

Aside from a few case studies, there are no treatment outcome studies for frotteurism (Beech & Harkins, 2012). Considering paraphilias as a group, the most common interventions have been pharmacological and cognitive behavioral therapies. As Krueger and Kaplan (2008) concluded, the literature on the effectiveness of treatment for paraphilias (usually meaning sex offenders) has produced mixed results. For example, one large treatment outcome study based on cognitive behavioral therapy found no significant benefits at six-year follow-up (Marques, Wiederanders, Day, Nelson, & van Ommeren, 2005). Meta-analyses, however, have revealed reductions in recidivism among treated sex offenders (Hanson et al., 2002). Beech and Harkins (2012) reported that the evidence for treatment effectiveness of paraphilias was "not strong" (p. 536), although there were not enough data to draw conclusions about the treatment of frotteurism specifically.

Garcia and Thibaut (2011) recommend considering antidepressant medications (i.e., selective serotonin reuptake inhibitors) in cases of mild paraphilias that have a compulsive quality. The use of hormonal treatments, such as antiandrogens, remains controversial. Although they have been shown in a few studies to lower sex drive, the side effects are potentially severe (e.g., hypertension, diabetes, testicular atrophy, and pulmonary embolism), and, therefore, compliance is problematic (Garcia & Thibaut, 2011).

Research on the treatment of paraphilias is limited by small sample sizes, brief follow-ups, lack of adequate controls, and diagnostic challenges (McManus, Hargreaves, Rainbow, & Alison, 2013). From their literature review, Kaplan and Krueger (2012) concluded that the evidence base for cognitive behavioral treatment of paraphilias is limited. A more optimistic appraisal was offered by Marshall and Marshall (2015) who reviewed treatment studies of various types of sex offenders. According to them, treatment often produces significant decreases in recidivism over long periods of follow-up. Effective treatment programs are those that target dynamic risk factors (e.g., loneliness, empathy deficits, and sexual preoccupation), use effective methods to modify risks, and deliver treatment in a compassionate fashion. Because none of the studies include a sample of frotteurs, no definitive conclusions can be generalized to this population.

RECOMMENDATIONS FOR FUTURE WORK

There is clearly a need for a substantial amount of research on all aspects of frotteuristic disorder. Such research could have important implications for classification, assessment, and treatment. As noted above, the field currently lacks well-validated and useful assessment instruments, and this will likely impede future research efforts. Wakefield (2011) has persuasively argued that the diagnostic criteria for any paraphilia should include the exclusiveness, fixation, and compulsiveness that characterize the deviant sexual interest. These proposed criteria might create more homogeneous categories, which would facilitate research on the common characteristics of bona fide paraphilias.

Several questions about frotteurism are particularly intriguing. Freund and colleagues proposed that frotteurism be placed under the rubric of "courtship disorders." Could frotteurism, along with exhibitionism and voyeurism, simply be different aspects of this broader syndrome? Some of the similarities, including the impersonal and nonconsensual nature of the sexual interest, are consistent with such a formulation. What is the developmental pathway to such sexual fantasies, urges, and behaviors? Freud (1905/1953) was one the first to observe that "perversions" were distortions, even approximations, of normative sexual behavior. Frotteurism as such may represent a distortion in the evolutionary male sexual strategy of seeking numerous sexual partners while minimizing investment and effort (Buss, 2011). Lussier and Piche' (2008) noted that it was the *context* in which the sexual behavior occurs, an interpersonal transgression against a stranger, rather than the sexual activity per se that renders frotteurism a paraphilia. Frotteuristic behavior is powerfully reinforced by immediate sexual gratification with little cost (unless apprehended) and investment, although at the expense of an unwilling stranger (Långström, 2010).

Although many men might find the prospect of a brief and impersonal encounter with an attractive stranger to be sexually arousing, the majority resist such opportunistic encounters. Other variables are probably implicated including hypersexuality and impulsivity. Individuals who have an abnormally high sex drive might find impersonal sexual encounters to be even more desirable than most men would, particularly if their elevated sex drive is combined with deficient inhibitions, perhaps due to intoxication, impulse control disorders, and other factors. Such individuals might be especially prone to acting on these urges if they lack adequate social skills for forming meaningful consensual relationships, struggle with chronic loneliness, or suffer from insecure attachment. Most of these hypotheses have received some empirical support, but there are many limitations to the existing research base. Conceptual problems with diagnoses, the absence of psychometrically sound assessment instruments, and the dearth of evidence for effective treatment have greatly hampered our understanding of this unusual and perplexing disorder.

REFERENCES

Abel, G.G., Becker, J.V., Mittelman, M., Cunningham-Rathner, J., Rouleau, J.L., & Murphy, W.D. (1987). Self-reported sex crimes of nonincarcerated paraphiliacs. *Journal of Interpersonal Violence, 2*, 3–25.

Abel, G.G., Huffman, J., Warberg, B., & Holland, C.L. (1998). Visual reaction time and plethysmography as measures of sexual interest in child molesters. *Sexual Abuse: A Journal of Research & Treatment, 10*, 81–95.

American Psychiatric Association. (1980). *Diagnostic and statistical manual of mental disorders (3rd ed.)*. Arlington, VA: American Psychiatric Association.

American Psychiatric Association. (2000). *Diagnostic and statistical manual of mental disorders (4th ed. text rev.)*. Arlington, VA: American Psychiatric Association.

American Psychiatric Association. (2013). *Diagnostic and statistical manual of mental disorders (5th ed.)*. Arlington, VA: American Psychiatric Association.

Banse, R., Schmidt, A.F., & Clarbour, J. (2010). Indirect measures of sexual interest in child molesters: A multi-method approach. *Criminal Justice and Behavior, 37*, 319–335.

Bayona, J. (2010, October 10). Crowded NYC subway not an excuse for groping. *Sandeep*. Retrieved from http://sandeep.journalism.cuny.edu/2010/10/15/crowded-nyc-subway-not-an-excuse/

Beech, A.R., & Harkins, L. (2012). DSM-IV paraphilia: Descriptions, demographics and treatment interventions. *Aggression and Violent Behavior, 17*, 527–539.

Blanchard, R. (2011). A brief history of field trials of the DSM diagnostic criteria for paraphilias. *Archives of Sexual Behavior, 40*, 861–862.

Brockman, B., & Bluglass, R.S. (1996). A general approach to sexual deviation. In I. Rosen (Ed.), *Sexual deviation* (3rd ed., pp. 1–42). New York: Oxford University Press.

Buss, D.A. (2011). *Evolutionary psychology: The new science of the mind* (4th ed.). Boston, MA: Pearson.

Cannas, A., Solla, P., Floris, G., Tacconi, P., Loi, D., Marcia, E., & Marrosu, M.G. (2006). Hypersexual behaviour, frotteurism and delusional jealousy in a young parkinsonian patient during dopaminergic therapy with pergolide: A rare case of iatrogenic paraphilia. *Progress in Neuro-Psychopharmacology and Biological Psychiatry, 30*, 1539–1541.

Clark, S. K., Jeglic, E. L., Calkins, C., & Tatar, J. R. (2014). More than a nuisance: The prevalence and consequences of frotteurism and exhibitionism. *Sexual Abuse: A Journal of Research and Treatment, 28* (1), 3–19.

Conley, K. (2015, May 20). Subway perverts to face felony charges under new bill. *New York Post.* Retrieved from http://nypost.com/2015/05/20/subway-grinders-to-face-felony-charges-under-new-bill/

First, M.B. (2010). DSM-5 proposals for paraphilias: Suggestions for reducing false positives related to use of behavioral manifestations. *Archives of Sexual Behavior, 39,* 1239–1244.

Fedoroff, J.P. (2003). The paraphilic world. In S.B. Levine, C.B. Risen, & S.E. Althof (Eds.), *Handbook of clinical sexuality for mental health professionals* (pp. 333–356). New York: Brunner-Routledge.

Freud, S. (1905/1953). Three essays on the theory of sexuality. In J.M. Strachey (Ed.) (1953), *The standard edition of the complete psychological works of Sigmund Freud, Volume VII (1901–1905): A case of hysteria, three essays on sexuality and other works* (pp. 123–245). London: The Hogarth Press.

Freund, K. (1990). Courtship disorders. In W.L. Marshall, D.R. Laws, & H.E. Barbaree (Eds.), *Handbook of sexual assault: Issues, theories, and treatment of the offender* (pp. 195–207). New York: Plenum.

Freund, K., & Seto, M.C. (1998). Preferential rape in the theory of courtship disorder. *Archives of Sexual Behavior, 27,* 433–443.

Freund, K., Seto, M.C., & Kuban, M. (1997). Frotteurism and the theory of courtship disorder. In D.R. Laws & W.T. O'Donohue (Eds.), *Sexual deviance: Theory, assessment, and treatment* (pp. 111–130). New York: Guilford.

Garcia, F. D., & Thibaut, F. (2011). Current concepts in the pharmacotherapy of paraphilias. *Drugs, 71 (6),* 771–790.

Hanson, R. K., Gordon, A., Harris, A. J. R., Marques, J. K., Murphy, W., Quinsey, V. L., & Seto, M. C. (2002). First report of the collaborative outcome data project on the effectiveness of psychological treatment for sex offenders. *Sexual Abuse: A Journal of Research and Treatment, 14 (2),* 169–194.

Kalmus, E., & Beech, A.R. (2005). Forensic assessment of sexual interest: A review. *Aggression and Violent Behavior, 10,* 193–217.

Kaplan, M.S., & Krueger, R.B. (2012). Cognitive-behavioral treatment of the paraphilias. *Israeli Journal of Psychiatry and Related Sciences, 49,* 291–296.

Konopasek, J.E. (2015). Expeditious disclosure of sexual history via polygraph testing: Treatment outcome and sex offense recidivism. *Journal of Offender Rehabilitation, 54,* 194–211.

Krafft-Ebing, R.v. (1906). *Psychopathia sexualis with especial reference to the antipathic sexual instinct: A medico-forensic study.* New York: Medical Art Agency.

Krueger, R.B., & Kaplan, M.S. (2008). Frotteurism: Assessment and treatment. In D.R. Laws & W.T. O'Donohue (Eds.), *Sexual deviance: Theory, assessment, and treatment* (2nd ed., pp.150–163). New York: Guildford Press.

Langevin, R. (1983). *Sexual strands: Understanding and treating sexual anomalies in men.* Hillsdale, NJ: Erlbaum.

Laws, D.R., & O'Donohue, W. T. (Eds.) (2013). *Sexual deviance: Theory, assessment, and treatment.* New York: Guilford.

Långström, N. (2010). The DSM Diagnostic criteria for exhibitionism, voyeurism, and frotteurism. *Archives of Sexual Behavior, 39,* 317–324.

Lussier, P., & Piche´, L. (2008). Frotteurism: Psychopathology and theory. In D.R. Laws & W.T. O'Donohue (Eds.), *Sexual deviance: Theory, assessment, and treatment* (2nd ed., pp.131–149). New York: Guildford Press.

Long, C. (2008, April 14). NYC subway groper could get life in prison. *USA Today*. Retrieved from http://usatoday30.usatoday.com/news/nation/2008-04-14-subway-groper_N.htm

Marques, J.K., Wiederanders, M., Day, D.M., Nelson, C., & Van Ommeren, A. (2005). Effects of a relapse prevention program on sexual recidivism: Final results from California's Sex Offender Treatment and Evaluation Project (SOTEP). *Sexual Abuse: A Journal of Research and Treatment, 17*, 79–107.

Marshall, W.L. (1989). Intimacy, loneliness and sexual offenders. *Behaviour Research and Therapy, 27*, 491–504.

Marshall, W.L. (2014). Phallometric assessments of sexual interests: An update. *Current Psychiatry Reports, 16*, 428–435.

Marshall, W.L., & Marshall, L.E. (2015). Psychological treatment of the paraphilias: A review and an appraisal of effectiveness. *Current Psychiatry Reports, 17*, 47–53.

McAnulty, R.D. (2006). Pedophilia. In R.D. McAnulty & M.M. Burnette (Eds.), *Sex and sexuality* (Vol. 3, pp. 81–95). Westport, CT: Praeger.

McAnulty, R.D., Adams, H.E., & Dillon, J. (2001). Sexual deviation: Paraphilias. In P.B. Sutker & H.E. Adams (Eds.), *Comprehensive handbook of psychopathology* (3rd ed., pp. 749–773). New York: Kuwer Academic/Plenum.

McConaghy, N. (1993). *Sexual behavior: Problems and management*. New York: Plenum.

McGrath, R.J., Cumming, G.F., Burchard, B.L., Zeoli, S., & Ellerby, L. (2010). *Current practices and emerging trends in sexual abuser management: The Safer Society 2009 North America Survey*. Brandon, VT: Safer Society Press.

McManus, M.A., Hargreaves, P., Rainbow, L., & Alison, L.J. (2013). Paraphilias: Definition, diagnosis and treatment. *F1000 Prime Reports, 5*. Retrieved from http://f1000.com/prime/reports/m/5/36

Money, J. (1986). *Lovemaps: Clinical concepts of sexual/erotic health and pathology, paraphilia, and gender transposition in childhood, adolescence, and maturity*. New York: Irvington.

Murphy, L., Ranger, R., Stewart, H., Dwyer, G., & Fedoroff, J.P. (2015). Assessment of problematic sexual interests with the penile plethysmograph: An overview of assessment laboratories. *Current Psychiatry Reports, 17*, 29–34.

Nichols, H.R., & Molinder, I. (1984). *Multiphasic Sex Inventory manual: A test to assess the psychosexual characteristics of the sexual offender*. Tacoma, WA: Author.

Prentky, R.A., Gabriel, A.M., & Coward, A.I. (2010). Sexual offenders. In J.C. Thomas & M. Hersen (Eds.), *Handbook of clinical psychology competencies* (pp. 1063–1094). New York: Springer.

Rogers, R. (Ed.) (2012). *Clinical assessment of malingering and deception* (3rd ed.). New York: Guilford Press.

Rosky, J.W. (2013). The (f)utility of post-conviction polygraph testing. *Sexual Abuse: A Journal of Research and Treatment, 25*, 259–281.

Ryley, S., & Donohue, P. (2014, June 23). Grand Central more like sex crimes central: Nearly half of all subway sex crimes reported along Lexington Avenue line in Manhattan. *New York Daily News*. Retrieved from http://www.nydailynews.com/new-york/nyc-crime/daily-news-analysis-reveals-perverted-subway-stations-article-1.1836952

Schneider, S.L., & Wright, R.C. (2004). Understanding denial in sexual offenders: A review of cognitive and motivational processes to avoid responsibility. *Trauma, Violence, & Abuse, 5*, 3–20.

Sederstrom, J., & Gendar, A. (2008, April 16). 6 train pervert's twin is also evil. *NY Daily News.* Retrieved from http://www.nydailynews.com/news/crime/6-train-pervert-twin-evil-article-1.283152

Seto, M.C. (2004). Pedophilia and sex offenses against children. *Annual Review of Sex Research, 14,* 321–361.

Simpson, G., Blaszczynki, A., & Hodgkinson, A. (1999). Sexual offending as a psychosocial sequela of traumatic brain injury. *Journal of Head Trauma Rehabilitation, 14*(6), 567–580.

Solla, P., Bortolato, M., Cannas, A., Mulas, C.S., & Marrosu, F. (2015). Paraphilias and paraphilic disorders in Parkinson's disease: A systematic review of the literature. *Movement Disorders, 30,* 604–613.

Spitzer, R.L., Gibbon, M., Skodol, A.E., Williams, J.B.W., & First, M.B. (Eds.) (2002). *DSM-IV-TR casebook: A learning companion to the diagnostic and statistical manual of mental disorders (4th ed. text rev.).* Arlington, VA: American Psychiatric Publishing.

Templeman, T.N., & Stinnet, R.D. (1991). Patterns of sexual arousal and history in a "normal" sample of young men. *Archives of Sexual Behavior, 20,* 137–150.

Wakefield, J.C. (2011). DSM-5 proposed diagnostic criteria for sexual paraphilias: Tensions between diagnostic validity and forensic utility. *International Journal of Law and Psychiatry, 34,* 195–209.

World Health Organization. (1993). Other disorders of sexual preference. *The ICD-10 classification of mental and behavioral disorders.* Retrieved from http://www.who.int/classifications/icd/en/bluebook.pdf

Zolondek, S.C., Abel, G.G., Northey, W.F., Jr., & Jordan, A. (2001). Self-reported behaviors of juvenile sexual offenders. *Journal of Interpersonal Violence, 16,* 73–85.

11

Autoerotic Asphyxia and Asphyxiophilia

STEPHEN HUCKER ■

VIGNETTE

Josh, a 17-year-old male student, reported that he began masturbating as early as age five or six years to thoughts of girls and young women. However, after the onset of puberty at age 12 he also became sexually interested in other boys. He stated that it was mainly the boys' necks that appealed to him, but only if they were "smooth, tender, and feminine-looking"; facial hair had no allure for him.

He also described how from age 15 he had engaged in self-hanging roughly once per week. During these sessions he would masturbate to fantasies of having sex with both males and females. He explained that one of his fantasies involved someone else strangling him and that he could become sexually aroused simply by thinking about this. He stated that it was essentially the feeling of choking that aroused him sexually. He denied any interest in cross-dressing, bondage, or any other paraphilias. He further indicated that he disliked pain of any kind.

Josh could not recall what first prompted him to attempt self-asphyxiation but believed that he had discovered it by accident. He would attach both ends of a rope to a hook on the wall above his bed, lie down and place his head in the loop. He was unable to fashion a knot to make a noose because of a birth injury, which will be described later. Usually he performed this self-hanging while clothed, and he masturbated over his clothes rather than take out his penis. Sometimes, however, he did this naked after he came out of the shower. As an alternative asphyxiating technique he would bury his face in a pillow while he masturbated.

He was ambivalent about these sexual behaviors, saying, "The more unusual, the more the turn on." And he relished his "secret life." At the same time, he was fearful he might inadvertently "blurt it out and explode the secret."

Josh was well aware of the risks involved in self-hanging because he had heard from other students about deaths resulting from this activity. On one occasion he blacked out while he was suspended but he recovered consciousness. This brush with death scared him and he stopped for a while but soon resumed. By the time of the assessment he asserted that he was in no danger because he placed the rope in such a way that he could "easily escape." He added, however, that he hoped to be able to curtail this behavior and at times had been able to reduce the frequency.

He also described feelings of depression and difficulties socializing with his peers such that he often experienced suicidal thoughts. These were woven into his sexual fantasies, however, and, as he put it, "There's a strange relation between sex and death through suicide."

Josh's birth was difficult and his umbilical cord was wrapped around his neck, causing some anoxic brain damage. His milestones were delayed and his motor development was noticeably late. He also walked awkwardly and had difficulties with fine motor control.

Psychological testing indicated a superior verbal IQ on the WAIS-R but with an average score on performance items, all consistent with his early history of cerebral damage. Other neuropsychological tests also pointed to this. There were problems with manual dexterity and response speed but his memory, attention, and concentration were all unimpaired.

After his assessment, Josh continued working with his referring psychiatrist, but he dropped from sight until the present writer discovered him among a group of auto-erotic fatalities that he was researching. Josh had died from self-hanging at 20 years of age.

HISTORICAL AND CULTURAL CONTEXT

Deliberate self-hanging, self-strangulation, or self-suffocation with the intent of inducing sexual arousal has been referred to by various names including sexual asphyxia (Brittain, 2004), auto-erotic asphyxia (Walsh, Stahl, Unger, Lilienstern, & Stephens, 1977), asphyxiophilia (Money, 1988), eroticized repetitive hangings (Resnik, 1972), hypoxyphilia, and Kotzwarraism, after the Czech musician who died during this activity (Dietz, 1983; Ober, 1984).

Early anthropologists reported that Inuit children and Yahgan Indians used self-hanging to arouse themselves (Resnik, 1972), and it also has been suggested that the practice was known to the Maya of ancient Mexico who recognized Ixtab, a goddess of the hanged (Hazelwood, Dietz, & Burgess, 1983). In the Middle Ages, it was apparently common to observe that those who were executed by hanging often had an erection or even ejaculated (Ober, 1984; Resnik, 1972). The Marquis de Sade also described the practice in his erotic novel, *Justine* (1791), in which he described the voluptuous sensations induced by hanging and choking. It is known from contemporary accounts in the late 19th century that there were brothels catering to men who wished to be strangled as a remedy for impotence (Bloch, 1938; Resnik, 1972). Also from around that time, we know of the erotic death of Franticek Kotzwarra, a noted musician, through the publication of a now rare pamphlet entitled *Modern Propensities: Or an Essay on the Art of Strangling* (Bloch, 1938; Hirschfeld, 1948; Wolfe, 1984). Based on the court proceedings against a young prostitute, this illicit account was created after the presiding judge ordered the official records of the trial to be destroyed. The girl was convicted of accidental manslaughter rather than murder and was released. She testified that Kotzwarra initially had requested that she cut his penis in two, but when she refused, he then asked her to hang him for five minutes, indicating that it would "raise his passions." He had her obtain a cord, which he placed around his neck, and suspended himself from the back of a door, then bent his knees so that he was suspended. This scenario is depicted in the pamphlet (see Figure 11.1). Previous

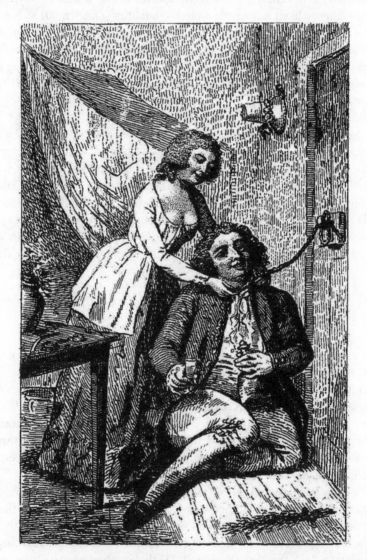

MODERN PROPENSITIES.

Figure 11.1 Kotzwarra and the Prostitute © The British Library Board. Frontpiece for late eighteenth century pamphlet entitled "Modern Propensities or An Essay on the Art of Strangulation." Courtesy of the British Library, where the only known original is retained. Reproduced by permission of the British Library.

scars, a bunch of twigs [for flagellation], and request for penile mutilation all suggest sexual masochism.

In the earliest known reference in the medical literature (Ryan, 1832) the author indicated his awareness that "examples are recorded of both sexes, who, to excite the venereal appetite, allowed themselves to be suspended for some time; and some of them lost their lives in not having been taken down before asphyxia occurred."

A contemporary forensic pathologist has suggested that some deaths in Europe from the early 19th century, which were reported at the time to be "atypical suicides," were more likely autoerotic asphyxial fatalities (Lunetta, 2013). It appears that the phenomenon was not described again until the beginning of the early 20th century, first in German (Seitz, 1913; Ziemke, 1925) and then in English (Auden, 1927) though again without the sexual nature of the fatality being recognized. Krafft-Ebing did not mention the phenomenon in his classic *Psychopathia Sexualis* (Krafft-Ebing, 1903), but it was later reported in the works of Stekel (1929), Ellis (1936), Bloch (1938), and Hirschfeld (1948).

Unusual suicides became correctly identified as autoerotic fatalities by investigators and pathologists only over time and typically with little or no appreciation that a sexological and psychiatric literature had been independently evolving (Dietz, 1983). Gradually, single case reports appeared, then small series, and then larger series of cases in the United States (Hazelwood, Dietz, & Burgess, 1983) and Canada (Hucker & Blanchard, 1992) were published, as well as reviews of cases over longer periods of time (e.g., Uva, 1995; Behrendt & Modvig, 1995; Breitmeier et al., 2003; Janssen et al., 2005; Shields et al., 2005; and Sauvageau & Racette, 2006).

ROLE IN CURRENT DIAGNOSTIC SYSTEMS

Sexual asphyxiation was mentioned for the first time in the *Diagnostic and Statistical Manual of Mental Disorders* of the American Psychiatric Association in the revision of its third edition (DSM-III-R, 1987) and has been included in subsequent editions, always as a subtype of Sexual Masochism. In DSM-IV-TR (American Psychiatric Association, 2000) the term "hypoxyphilia" was used and characterized as a "particularly dangerous form of Sexual Masochism that involves sexual arousal by oxygen deprivation obtained by means of chest compression, noose, ligature, plastic bag, mask or chemical" (p. 572).

In the current fifth edition, DSM-5 (American Psychiatric Association, 2013), the description is again subsumed under Sexual Masochism and uses the term "asphyxiophilia" as a specifier for cases where "an individual engages in the practice of achieving sexual arousal related to restriction of breathing." This change in terminology reflects the view (Hucker, 2011) that cerebral hypoxia is more likely the result, not the intention, of the behavior. Moreover, asphyxiophilic behavior did not appear to be sufficiently distinct from other types of masochistic behavior to justify a separate category or code with its own diagnostic criteria in DSM-5. Other research on sexual masochists clearly placed asphyxiophilia among other behaviors practiced by masochists (Alison, Santtila, Sandnabba, & Nordling, 2001; Rehor, 2015; Sandnabba, Santtila, Alison, & Nordling, 2002) and, therefore, reinforces this view.

Asphyxiophilia also is mentioned in *the International Classification of Mental and Behavioural Disorders* or ICD-10 (World Health Organization, 1992) though separately from the combined term "sadomasochism" and under the category of Other Disorders of Sexual Preference (Code F65.8), which includes a pattern of sexual preference and activity involving the "use of strangulation or anoxia for intensifying sexual excitement . . ." (p. 172).

SYMPTOMATOLOGY

Initially the only source of information about erotic asphyxiation and asphyxiophilia was from fatalities. These were the result of a failure of the strategy or device used by the individual with the intent of avoiding the fatal outcome. The findings from studies of these deaths have been very consistent and are summarized later in the chapter.

Among autoerotic fatalities, males far outnumber females and, indeed, the latter are more often initially considered to be suicides because of the absence of features such as unusual clothing, props, or other devices commonly seen with men (Byard, Hucker, & Hazelwood, 1990). In the present author's series of autoerotic deaths only one was female (S. Hucker & Blanchard, 1992).

Although there have been reports of aged individuals dying during autoerotic practices (Sauvageau & Geberth, 2009), most of the deceased are under 30 years of age. In our own series, the mean age was 26 years with the range 10 to 56 years. In nearly all the published series, self-hanging was the commonest method employed. Of our cases, 82% used this method, either alone or in combination with some other asphyxiating mechanism. Strangulation was used in only seven, suffocation in 13, and use of gases, solvents, etc. in only one (Hucker & Blanchard, 1992). Evidence of prior experience of autoerotic asphyxiation was indicated by the presence of permanently attached padding under the rope to make it more comfortable and to avoid burns (two of our cases had this feature). More commonly, however, the padding was temporary, and a towel or cloth may have been used (31 of our cases but one of our suicides also had done this). In other cases investigators may find multiple grooves on a beam used to support the rope or other evidence that the procedure had been repeated a number of times.

In addition to evidence of repetition, to distinguish an autoerotic fatality from a suicide the investigator must determine how the deceased would have tried to avoid such a mishap (Hazelwood et al., 1983). Sometimes a slip-knot mechanism is used to ensure a quick release of pressure on the neck and allow return of consciousness. In a few autoerotic fatalities the deceased may have used an elaborate asphyxiating device or apparatus that requires careful investigation to demonstrate how the person could have applied it and then disentangled themselves.

When investigators observe the body of an autoerotic asphyxia victim they are often struck by the clothing, or lack of it, on the body. In our series, the body was cross-dressed in about 30% of the cases, though a slightly higher figure has been reported in others. Nudity was found in 34% of our autoerotic asphyxia cases and nudity below the waist in six. None in our comparison group of asphyxial suicides was nude or cross-dressed.

Bondage is evident in many cases. By this it is meant that there were physical restraints on the body that were independent of the method of asphyxiation. Thus, the neck, head, ankles, thighs, chest or abdomen may have been bound, the genitals ligated, the hands bound or handcuffed and sometimes there will be a hood or blindfold. In our series 25% had such bindings.

Various fantasy aids, mirrors or cameras for self-photography, self-written fantasy material, items of leather, or other fetish objects are often found (34% of our cases). There may be signs of cigarette burns, clamps or clips applied to the body, self-flagellation, or other signs of masochism. Pornography also may be found at the scene, in front of the victim in many cases (22% of ours, for instance). Often this will depict bondage or other relevant themes.

Apart from the presence of obviously sex-related material or female clothing there may be evidence in males of penile erection or ejaculation (Rupp, 1980).

A suicide note would obviously point to an act of deliberate self-destruction, but some who have died due to autoerotic asphyxia have written ambiguous notes that often are interpreted initially as evidence of suicide (Hazelwood et al., 1983).

Our knowledge of what motivates those who asphyxiate themselves to achieve sexual arousal has until recently been dependent upon studying scenes such as those described above, supplemented by the rare descriptions of those who have survived and described the experience. In single-case reports of the latter the details are often meager, but reference to commonly associated paraphilias sometimes may be found. As with fatal cases, transvestitic and other types of fetishism often are mentioned, as well as more common features of sexual sadism, sexual masochism, and sometimes other rarer paraphilias.

There have also been descriptions of small samples of those who asphyxiate themselves for sexual purposes (Friedrich & Gerber, 1994; Litman & Swearingen, 1972; Lunsen, 1991). These studies, in contrast to individual case reports, often provide considerable detail about the fantasy lives of living asphyxiophiliacs. Typical masochistic fantasies such as being raped or beaten, humiliated, or forced into submission with obedience to a master, have been commonly reported. Others have described being in a dangerous situation as erotically exciting (Jenkins, 2000).

The present author has had the opportunity to interview 16 asphyxiophilic patients over 35 years of practice, and these interviews provided similar details to those just described. Clearly masochistic fantasies (being raped, physically abused, or humiliated) were reported by all the patients. Sadistic themes were reported by seven and being in a dangerous situation was reported by three patients. Three had autogynephilic fantasies (i.e., of themselves as a woman) (Blanchard, 1993). One man described being sexually aroused by thinking about choking and another by being "totally helpless." Indeed, for most of the patients, being choked, strangled, or suffocated was an especially potent stimulus for their sexual arousal.

The Internet has helped make available further information concerning autoerotic asphyxia and asphyxiophilia. This availability enables a phenomenon to be studied that would otherwise be beyond the reach of researchers (Kim & Bailey, 1997; Griffiths, 2012).

The present author conducted a study of living asphyxiophiliacs using a website set up specifically for this purpose. Over the course of a year, over 130 individuals responded by completing the online questionnaire. Upon reviewing all the responses, it was apparent that a small number were not, in fact, asphyxiophiliacs. As a result, 115 cases were left available for the study. In addition to their responses to the questions, some respondents submitted very detailed descriptions of their backgrounds, sexual interests, behaviors, and fantasies.

The sample comprised 91 men and 24 women. This large proportion of women contrasts strikingly with the aforementioned studies of fatalities in which very few were female. Fifty-four percent of the online sample were married or living common-law compared with 23% among our fatalities (Blanchard & Hucker, 1991) . Fifty-five percent were heterosexual, almost 7% homosexual, and 32% bisexual, with 5% unsure of their orientation. In most of the fatalities sexual orientation was not recorded.

More than half conducted their practice in the nude, 20% when cross-dressed, both figures being similar to those found in studies of fatalities, though fewer than in our earlier study. Seventy-three percent claimed that others knew about their practice whereas very few of the deceased's relatives or friends were aware of it. More than half knew that their activity was risky, and worried about it, but 27% were unconcerned, often believing that they had developed a "fail safe" method. Compared with the majority of fatal cases, only 47% of the living asphyxiophiliacs used self-hanging as their asphyxial method.

Seventy-four percent reported that they used bondage, either during asphyxiation or at other times; 44% affixed clips or clamps to sensitive areas such as nipples; 37% reported transvestic fetishism; 17% used electrical stimulation; 64% reported various other fetishes; and 35% used self-flagellation . Seventy-one percent regarded themselves as masochistic and 35% as sadistic, though a number endorsed both behaviors. Small numbers of less frequently encountered paraphilias also were reported. Once again, the overlap between transvestic and other fetishism, bondage, sadism, and masochism is consistent with the published literature on autoerotic fatalities.

Cases in which a partner has facilitated the act are known (Hazelwood, Deitz, & Burgess, 1982), and 13% of the present author's living asphyxiophiliacs reported this. There also have been cases in which the two participants jointly engaged in sexual asphyxiation (Roma, Pazzelli, Pompili, Girardi, & Ferracuti, 2013). Despite this and earlier, historical examples such as Kotzwarra, pathologists and investigators almost always emphasize the most common finding that the deceased died alone rather than with a partner (Sauvageau & Geberth, 2013).

Some studies of sexual masochism, both from clinical samples and consensual S & M partners in the community (Alison et al., 2001; Freund, Seto, & Kuban, 1995; Sandnabba et al., 2002), have found asphyxiophilia in about 15% of the subjects. In another very recent study of female masochists about two-thirds had engaged in "breath play, choking, strangling, hanging" (Rehor, 2015). All these strengthen the idea that asphyxiophilia belongs naturally among the wide variety of masochistic behaviors. There is no support for the notion that it represents a separate category.

PREVALENCE RATE AND ASSOCIATED FEATURES

Several estimates have been offered for the prevalence of erotic asphyxial fatalities though these may have been based on different methods of ascertainment. Forensic specialists in Denmark, Norway, and Sweden reported similar frequencies of 0.5–1.0 cases per million of the population per year (Innala & Ernulf, 1989). In Sweden, specifically, Flobecker et al. (1993) later estimated 0.1 per million per year. In Denmark, Behrendt and Modvig (1995) found an incidence of 0.5 deaths/million/year. In Germany, Breitmeier and colleagues (Breitmeier et al., 2003) report 0.49 cases per million inhabitants per year in the Hannover region. Byard and Winsog (2012) used national databases in Australia and Sweden. In Australia a rate of 0.3 deaths per million of the population was found, but Sweden reported only 0.14 deaths/million annually, leading the authors to conclude that "lethal sexual asphyxia is very uncommon in the Australian and Swedish populations." In Canada a low rate of 0.2 deaths/million/year is reported from the province of Quebec (Sauvageau, 2008). In another province, Ontario, data from our earlier published study (Hucker & Blanchard, 1992) allows a prevalence rate of 0.88 deaths/million/year to be calculated. The reasons for the disparity between these figures from various jurisdictions remain to be explored further.

THEORIES OF ETIOLOGY

Because asphyxiophiliacs rarely present to clinicians for evaluation or treatment, possible etiological factors have not been studied extensively. One researcher suggested, on the basis of his small series of living cases, that an experience of hypoxia in the developing years might be a predisposing factor (Friedrich & Gerber, 1994; Money, 1988). This was not confirmed, however, in the author's Internet study, in which 84% of respondents reported no history of asthma, lung disease, a cord around the neck at birth, etc. The possibility of childhood abuse also was canvassed, given that this has been suggested as a possible common factor of etiological significance among other masochists (Sandnabba et al., 2002), among whom 7.9% of men and 22.7% of women reported this experience

(Nordling, Sandnabba, & P., 2000). In comparison, 20% of the Internet sample endorsed this.

ASSESSMENT OPTIONS

There are no specific assessment procedures for asphyxiophilia. Moreover, those available for the assessment of sexual masochism more broadly are very limited. This is chiefly because paraphilias that have received the most attention are those encountered in the offender population. Masochists in the community are largely free of any criminal background (Moser & Levitt, 1987).

Various questionnaires that include items relating to sexual masochism are available. Those commonly used include the *Clarke Sex History Questionnaire for Males—Revised* (SHQ-R; Paitich & Langevin, 1977) and the *Multiphasic Sex Inventory-II* (MSI-II; Nichols and Molinder Assessments, Inc, 2000). The shorter *Wilson Sexual Fantasy Questionnaire* (Wilson, 1978) also includes masochistic items and the masochism subscales of other questionnaires also may be useful (O'Donohue, Letourneau, & Dowling, 1997). Kurt Freund worked with several of his own questionnaires, including one for masochism with references to asphyxiophilia. These are available through the personal website of one of his distinguished colleagues, Dr. Ray Blanchard (http://individual.utoronto.ca/ray_blanchard/index_files/EPES.html).

Phallometry, or penile plethysmography, has not been used to examine masochism except experimentally (Chivers, Roy, Grimbos, Cantor, & Seto, 2014).

DIFFERENTIAL DIAGNOSIS

From the psychiatric perspective asphyxiophilia, like most other paraphilias, has a tendency to cluster with other sexual anomalies (Abel, Becker, Cunningham-Rathner, Mittelman, & Rouleau, 1988; Bradford, Boulet, & Pawlak, 1992). The commonest reported include sexual sadism and sexual masochism (with which, as already noted, it is included) and fetishistic transvestism (Gosselin & Wilson, 1980; 1984).

Obviously, psychotic disorders may present with strange and unusual sexual feelings and behaviors, and some patients may engage in self-asphyxiation for nonsexual motives (Colón, Popkin, & Carlson, 1989). The gross distortions in reality-testing, however, will not be found in most individuals with asphyxiophilia.

More typically, asphyxiophilia may be associated with nonpsychotic psychiatric disorders. Anxiety and mood disturbances are commoner than would be expected among paraphiliacs in general (Kafka & Hennen, 2002). This often has been interpreted as a reaction to social embarrassment or worse, especially if the disorder is kept secret. This does not seem to be the case in most instances, but there does appear to be an association between mood disorders and paraphilias, which has been suggested to be a manifestation of a monoamine disturbance (Kafka, 2003).

TREATMENT OPTIONS FOR LIVING ASPHYXIOPHILIACS

Looking at sexual masochism in general, as opposed to asphyxiophilia specifically, the first treatments to be offered were psychoanalytic in nature. More often, however, the treatments have been behavioral, typically aversive methods such as the use of electric shocks or induction of nausea. These were based on the dubious premise that sexual preferences are conditioned and so likewise can be deconditioned. Some early studies that used such approaches did, however, yield positive results (Bancroft & Marks, 1968; Brownell, Hayes, & Barlow, 1977; Pinard & Lamontagne, 1976). It must be noted, however, that some questioned whether a painful or unpleasant experience such as electric shocks would be experienced as aversive or pleasurable. This issue was examined (Marks, Rachman, & Gelder, 1965) in a masochistic man who did experience the shocks as aversive and his longstanding masochistic urges and fantasies ceased after two treatments indicating that the approach was appropriate in such patients. However, short follow-up, lack of objective assessment measures, and confounding asphyxiophilia with other paraphilias such as sexual sadism, are problems with many of these studies.

Traditional behavioral techniques (Haydn-Smith, Marks, Buchaya, & Repper, 1987) have been largely supplanted by cognitive behavioral approaches (CBT). One case of a female asphyxiophiliac was treated with desensitization to her sexual fantasies as well as CBT and interpersonal process therapy (IPT). The treatment is reported as a success (Martz, 2003). Other reports (Thompson & Beail, 2002; Williams, Phillips, & Ahmed, 2000) have provided details of multidisciplinary approaches. Another reported art therapy, the course of which is described in detail (Innes, 1997). Treatment with a combination of psychodynamic psychotherapy, sex education, social skills training, aversive therapy, antiandrogens, and antidepressants was used in a patient who was sexually aroused by being burned or crushed. Apparently, antiandrogens and aversion therapy were at first successful, but he had relapsed when followed up not long afterward (Shiwach & Prosser, 1998).

Various medications have been used, as with other more common paraphilias, though none have emerged as a preferred treatment (Cesnik & Coleman, 1989; Faccini & Saide, 2012; Masand, 1993). Given the potentially lethal consequences of asphyxiophilia, the use of antiandrogens is worthy of serious consideration. One early case of the present author's was treated with medroxyprogesterone acetate (Provera). When this lost effect and the asphyxiation returned, the patient agreed to chemical castration (Lykins & Hucker, 2013). The one time the behavior returned was when his family doctor administered testosterone for other medical reasons. Asphyxiation returned within 48 hours after many years of absence.

It ceased when the testosterone was withdrawn. Currently, gonadotropin ago-nists are the preferred testosterone lowering agents (Assumpção, Garcia, Garcia, Bradford, & Thibaut, 2014).

As noted above, paraphilias often are accompanied by mental health problems such as anxiety and depression. Treatment of any associated anxiety or mood dis-order is important in such cases, but because few living asphyxiophiliacs have come to the attention of clinicians, there have been limited reports of successful treatment.

RECOMMENDATIONS FOR FUTURE WORK

Although a relatively rare cause of death in the young, asphyxiophilia neverthe-less represents a major concern for educators and counselors (Jenkins, 2000; Saunders, 1989). Studies such as those described above suggest that there are some practical measures that could be recommended, including always having a trusted partner either present or close at hand and using methods of asphyxiation other than hanging. As noted, however, a sizeable number of asphyxiophiliacs are unconcerned about the potential risks, and others, like most paraphiliacs, are reluctant to relinquish their pleasurable activities.

REFERENCES

Abel, G.G., Becker, J.V., Cunningham-Rathner, J., Mittelman, M., & Rouleau, J. (1988). Multiple paraphilic diagnoses among sex offenders. *Bulletin of the American Academy of Psychiatry and the Law*, *16*(2), 153–168.

Alison, L., Santtila, P., Sandnabba, N.K., & Nordling, N. (2001). Sadomasochistically oriented behaviour: diversity in practice and meaning. *Archives of Sexual Behavior*, *30*(1), 1–12.

American Psychiatric Association (2000). *Diagnostic and Statistical Manual of Mental Disorders. DSM-IV-TR, 4th edition Text Revision.* American Psychiatric Publishing Inc.: Washington, D.C.

American Psychiatric Association (2013). *Diagnostic and Statistical Manual of Mental Disorders. DSM-5.* American Psychiatric Publishing Inc.: Washington, D.C.

Assumpção, A.A., Garcia, F.D., Garcia, H.D., Bradford, J.M., & Thibaut, F. (2014). Pharmacologic treatment of paraphilias. *Psychiatric Clinics of North America*, *37*(2), 173–181.

Auden, G.A. (1927). An unusual form of suicide. *British Journal of Psychiatry* 73(302) 428–430.

Bancroft, J., & Marks, I. (1968). Electric aversion therapy of sexual deviations. *Proceedings of the Royal Society of Medicine*, *61*(8), 796.

Behrendt, N., & Modvig, J. (1995). The lethal paraphiliac syndrome: accidental auto-erotic deaths in Denmark 1933–1990. *The American Journal of Forensic Medicine and Pathology*, *16*(3), 232–237.

Blanchard, R. (1993). Varieties of autogynephilia and their relationship to gender dysphoria. *Archives of Sexual Behavior, 22*(3), 241–251.

Blanchard, R., & Hucker, S.J. (1991). Age, transvestism, bondage, and concurrent paraphilic activities in 117 fatal cases of autoerotic asphyxia. *British Journal of Psychiatry, 159*(371), 377.

Bloch, I. (1938). *Sexual life in England, past and present.* London: Alfred Aldor.

Bradford, J.M.W., Boulet, J., & Pawlak, A. (1992). The paraphilias: a multiplicity of deviant behavior. *Canadian Journal of Psychiatry, 37*, 104–107.

Breitmeier, D., Mansouri, F., Albrecht, K., Bohm, U., Troger, H.D., & Kleeman, W.J. (2003). Accidental autoerotic deaths between 1978 and 1997—Institute of Legal Medicine, Medical School Hannover. *Forensic Science International, 137*, 41–44.

Brittain, R.P. (2004). The sexual asphyxias. In *Gradwohl's Legal Medicine* . Camps, F.E. (ed) (3rd ed., pp. 520–522. Baltimore: Williams & Wilkins.

Brownell, K.D., Hayes, S.C., & Barlow, D. (1977). Patterns of appropriate and deviant sexual arousal: The behavioral treatment of multiple sexual deviations. *Journal of Consulting and Clinical Psychology, 45*(6), 1144.

Byard, R.W., Hucker, S.J., & Hazelwood, R.R. (1990). A comparison of typical death scene features in cases of fatal male and female autoerotic asphyxia with a review of the literature. *Forensic Science International, 48*(2), 113–121.

Cesnik, J.A., & Coleman, E. (1989). Use of lithium carbonate in the treatment of autoerotic asphyxia. *American Journal of Psychotherapy, 43*(2), 277–286.

Chivers, M.L., Roy, C., Grimbos, T., Cantor, J.M., & Seto, M.C. (2014). Specificity of sexual arousal for sexual activities in men and women with conventional and masochistic sexual interests. *Archives of Sexual Behavior, 43*(5), 931–940.

Colón, E.A., Popkin, M.K., & Carlson, B. (1989). Non-erotic self-choking in five psychiatric inpatients. *Journal of Clinical Psychiatry, 50*(12), 465–468.

Dietz, P. (1983). Recurrent discovery of autoerotic asphyxia. *Autoerotic Fatalities,* 13–44.

Faccini, L., & Saide, M.A. (2012). "Can you breath?" Autoerotic asphyxiation and asphyxiophilia in a person with an intellectual disability and sex offending. *Sexuality and Disability, 30*(1), 97–101.

Freund, K., Seto, M.C., & Kuban, M. (1995). Masochism: A multiple case study. *Sexuologie, 4*(2), 313–324.

Friedrich, W.N., & Gerber, P.N. (1994). Autoerotic asphyxia: the development of a paraphilia. *Journal of the American Academy of Child & Adolescent Psychiatry, 33*(7), 970–974.

Gosselin, C., & Wilson, G. (1980). *Sexual variations: Fetishism, sadomasochism, and transvestism.* New York: Simon & Schuster.

Gosselin, C., & Wilson, G. (1984). Fetishism, sadomasochism and related behaviours. In K. Howells (Ed.), *The psychology of sexual diversity* (pp. 89–110). Oxford, UK: Basil Blackwell Publisher Limited.

Haydn-Smith, P., Marks, I., Buchaya, H., & Repper, D. (1987). Behavioural treatment of life-threatening masochistic asphyxiation: a case study. *British Journal of Psychiatry, 150*, 518–519.

Hazelwood, R., Deitz, P., & Burgess, A.W. (1982). Sexual fatalities: behavioral reconstruction in equivocal cases. *Journal of Forensic Sciences, 27*, 763–771.

Hazelwood, R., Dietz, P., & Burgess, A. (1983). *Autoerotic fatalities.* Lexington, MA: D.C. Heath and Company.

Hirschfeld, M. (1948). *Sexual anomalies and perversions.* London: Encyclopaedic Press.

Hucker, S., & Blanchard, R. (1992). Death scene characteristics in 118 fatal cases of auto-erotic asphyxia compared with suicidal asphyxia. *Behavioral Sciences and the Law*, *10*(4), 509–523.

Hucker, S.J. (2011). Hypoxyphilia. *Archives of Sexual Behavior*, *40*(6), 1323–1326.

Innala, S.M., & Ernulf, K.E. (1989). Asphyxiophilia in Scandinavia. *Archives of Sexual Behavior*, *18*(3), 181–189.

Innes, R. (1997). Auto-erotic asphyxia and art psychotherapy. In E.V. Welldon & C. Van Velso (Eds.), *A practical guide to forensic psychotherapy* (Forensic Focus, 3rd ed., pp. 172–181). London: Jessica Kingsley Publishers.

Janssen, W., Koops, E., Anders, S., Kuhn, S., and Püschel, K. (2005). Forensic aspects of 40 accidental autoerotic deaths in Northern Germany. *Forenisc Science International*, 147 (Supplement) , S61–64.

Jenkins, A. (2000). When self-pleasuring becomes self-destruction: autoerotic asphyxiation paraphilia. *International Electronic Journal of Health Education*, *3*(3), 208–216.

Kafka, M. (2003). The monoamine hypothesis for the pathophysiology of paraphilic disorders: an update. *Annals of the New York Academy of Sciences*, *989*(1), 86–94.

Kafka, M., & Hennen, J. (2002). A DSM-IV Axis I comorbidity study of males (n= 120) with paraphilias and paraphilia-related disorders. *Sexual Abuse: A Journal of Research and Treatment*, *14*(4), 349–366.

Kim, P.Y. & Bailey, J.M. (1997). Sidestreets on the information superhighway: Paraphilias and sexual deviations on the Internet. *Journal of Sex Education & Therapy*. 22(1), 35–43.

Krafft-Ebing, R. v. (1999). *Psychopathia Sexualis* (B. King. Ed; F. J. Rebman, Trans.). Burbank, CA: Bloat. (Original book published 1903.)

Litman, R.E., & Swearingen, C. (1972). Bondage and suicide. *Archives of General Psychiatry*, *27*(1), 80–85.

Lunetta, P. (2013). Atypical suicides or the first undiagnosed autoerotic deaths in Europe? *Journal of Forensic and Legal Medicine*, 20(8), 1010-1013.

Lunsen, v. H.W. (1991) Auto-erotische asfyxie: Ervaringen met praktikanten van 'wurgseks' en nabestaanden van slachtoffers *Nederlands Forensisch Tijdschrift*, *10*(1), 5–10.

Lykins, A., & Hucker, S.J. (2013). Treatment of sexual masochism. (pp. 102–116). In *Case Studies in Sexual Deviance: Toward Evidence Based Practice*. O'Donohue, W.T. (ed). New York and London: Routledge.

Marks, I., Rachman, S. & Gelder, M. (1965). Methods for the assessment of aversion treatment in fetishism with masochism. Behavioural Research &n Therapy, 3(4), 253–258

Martz, D. (2003). Behavioral treatment for a female engaging in autoerotic asphyxiation. Clinical Case Studies, 2(3), 236–242.

Masand, P.S. (1993). Successful treatment of sexual masochism and transvestic fetishism associated with fluoxetine hydrochloride. *Depression*, *1*, 50–52.

Money, J. (1988). *Lovemaps*. New York: Prometheus Books and Irvington Publishers, Inc.

Moser, C., & Levitt, E.E. (1987). An exploratory descriptive study of a sadomasochistically oriented sample. *The Journal of Sex Research*, *23*(3), 322–337.

Nordling, N., Sandnabba, N., & Santtila, P. (2000). The prevalence and effects of self-reported childhood sexual abuse among sadomasochistically oriented males and females. *Journal of Child Sexual Abuse*, *9*, 53–63.

Ober, W.B. (1984). The sticky end of Frantisek Koczwara, composer of "The Battle of Prague." *The American Journal of Forensic Medicine and Pathology*, 5(2), 145–150.

O'Donohue, W., Letourneau, E., & Dowling, H. Development and preliminary validation of a paraphilic sexual fantasy questionnaire. *Sexual Abuse: A Jouranl of Research and Treatment.* 9(3), 167-178

Paitich, D., Langevin, R., Freeman, R., Mann, K. & Handy, L. The Clarke SHQ: A clinical sex history questionnaire for males. Archives of Sexual *Behavior* 6(5), 421-436.

Pinard, G., & Lamontagne, Y. (1976). Electrical aversion, aversion relief and sexual retraining in treatment of fetishism with masochism. *Journal of Behavior Therapy and Experimental Psychiatry*, 7(1), 71–74.

Rehor, J.E. (2015). Sensual, erotic, and sexual behaviors of women from the "kink" community. *Archives of Sexual Behavior*, 44(4), 825–836.

Resnik, H.L. (1972). Eroticized repetitive hangings: A form of self-destruction. American *Journal of Psychotherapy*, 26(1), 4–21

Roma, P., Pazzelli, F., Pompili, M., Girardi, P., & Ferracuti, S. (2013). Shibari: double hanging during consensual sexual asphyxia. *Archives of Sexual Behavior*, 42(5), 895–900.

Rupp, J.C. (1980). Sex-related deaths. In W.J. Curren, A.L. McGarry, & C.S. Petty (Eds.), *Modern legal medicine, psychiatry and forensic science* (pp. 575–587). Philadelphia, PA: F.A. Davis.

Sandnabba, N.K., Santtila, P., Alison, L., & Nordling, N. (2002). Demographics, sexual behaviour, family background and abuse experiences of practitioners of sadomasochistic sex: a review of recent research. *Sexual and Relationship Therapy*, 17(1), 39–55.

Saunders, E. (1989). Life-threatening autoerotic behavior: A challenge for sex educators and therapists. *Journal of Sex Education and Therapy*, 15(2), 82–91.

Sauvageau, A. (2008). Autoerotic deaths: a seven-year retrospective epidemiological study. *Open Forensic Science Journal*, 1, 1–3.

Sauvageau, A., & Geberth, V. (2009). Elderly victim: an unusual autoerotic fatality involving an 87-year-old male. *Forensic Science, Medicine, and Pathology*, 5(3), 233–235.

Sauvageau, A., & Geberth, V. (2013). *Autoerotic deaths: practical forensic and investigative perspectives.* Boca Raton, FL: CRC Press.

Sauvageau, A., & Racette, S. (2006). Autoerotic deaths in the literature from 1954 to 2004: a review. *Journal of Forensic Science*, 51(1), 140–146. doi: 10.1111/j.1556-4029.2005.00032.x

Seitz, A. (1913). Ein seltener Fall perverser Sexualitat. *Archiv Fur Kriminologie*, 54, 356–362.

Shields, L.B.E. and Hunsaker, D.M. (2005). Autoerotic asphyxia: Part 1. *American Journal of Forenisc Medicine and Pathology* 26(1), 45–52

Shiwach, R.S., & Prosser, J. (1998). Treatment of an unusual case of masochism. *Journal of Sex & Marital Therapy*, 24(4), 303–307.

Thompson, A.R., & Beail, N. (2002). The treatment of auto-erotic asphyxiation in a man with severe intellectual disabilities: the effectiveness of a behavioural and educational programme. *Journal of Applied Research in Intellectual Disabilities*, 15(1), 36–47.

Walsh, F.M., Stahl, C., Unger, H., Lilienstern, O.C., & Stephens, R.G. (1977). Autoerotic asphyxial deaths: a medicolegal analysis of 43 cases. *Legal Medicine Annual: 1977*. New York: Appleton-Century-Crofts.

Williams, A., Phillips, L., & Ahmed, Z. (2000). Assessment and management of auto-erotic asphyxiation in a young man with learning disability: a multidisciplinary approach to intervention. *British Journal of Learning Disabilities, 28*(3), 109–112.

Wilson, G. (1978). *The secrets of sexual fantasy*. London: J.M. Dent & Sons.

Wolfe, R.J. (1984). The hang-up of Frank Kotzwara and its relationship to sexual quackery in late 18th-century London. *Studies on Voltaire and the Eighteenth Century, 228*, 47–66.

Ziemke, E. (1926). Uber zufalliges Erhangen und seine Beziehungen zu sexuellen Perversit. *Archiv fur Kriminologie 78*, 262–264.

Culture-Bound Disorders

12

Koro—A Genital Retraction Syndrome

PETRA GARLIPP ■

... The patients complained of shrinking or retracting of a certain body part (e.g. the penis in men ...). You immediately had to hold the retracting part or have it grasped by several men. Simultaneously gongs and drums had to be beaten. The patients also had to drink ginger soup. Then they were immediately healed. This is a weird disease.

—MO & HEISE, 1997, cited from a local chronicle of the Tang district 1865, p. 106, own translation[1]

VIGNETTE

A 38-year-old German male patient suffering from schizophrenia for 10 years was admitted to the hospital in an acute psychotic state. For years he had relatively good symptom-control taking olanzapine. Due to a concern that he may develop diabetes, a change of medication was made two months prior to admission. Psychotic symptoms returned with the new medication.

The patient reported sleeplessness and auditory hallucinations, sometimes of a commenting character. The voices told him that he had to be punished. He felt threatened and believed that unknown persons wanted him to die. He was afraid his testicles might have been "killed." On examination the genitalia showed no pathological findings. However, the patient insisted he could see the genitals shrinking and asked the doctor, "Can't you also see how they are shrinking?"

The patient was awake and orientated. He reported auditory, visual, and coenesthetic hallucinations. Coenesthetic hallucinations are defined as bodily sensations mainly induced from the outside. They are experienced, for example, as tingling or shrinking sensations. The patient described them as a numb feeling combined with a shrinking sensation. He also suffered from paranoid delusions. Thinking was slowed. Mnestic (i.e., memory-related) functions were subjectively not impaired. The patient presented as friendly, yet suffering. He was also a little distrustful of others and clearly afraid that he might die. There was no hint of acute suicidality or aggressive symptoms. On examination there were no pathological findings. Cranial magnetic resonance imaging (MRI), electroencephalography (EEG), electrocardiography (ECG), and blood tests were all normal. Drug screening was negative.

In a second interview the patient reported that his genital concerns had been persistent for the past 10 years. An autoerotic manipulation had happened before the symptoms started. He also suffered from recurrent erectile dysfunction and eventually consulted an urologist. Testosterone levels were found to be low, and he was given several testosterone injections. When those injections were stopped by the urologist, the patient was convinced he would die and became preoccupied with feelings of guilt because of his past autoerotic sexual experiences. Once, he had tried to ligature his testicles to "cure" himself.

After treating the patient with olanzapine and lorazepam the psychotic symptomatology disappeared, but the koro-like symptoms persisted. A secondary koro in schizophrenia was diagnosed, presenting itself like a psychotic fear; specifically, a coenesthetic hallucination with a delusional background (Garlipp & Machleidt, 2003).

HISTORICAL AND CULTURAL CONTEXT

Koro describes a patient's conviction that his genitals or, rarely, another body part, are shrinking and retracting into the body. This is combined with an intense fear and a conviction that death may be imminent.

Koro epidemics have been reported in South Asia. Koro-like symptoms (or genital-retraction syndromes) have been reported as secondary koro in patients with an organic or mental illness in Western countries, mainly in Europe and North America.

The origin of the word koro is connected to the Malaysian term for the retracting of a turtle's head (Cheng, 1996). Chowdury (1996) related the term to an Indonesian dialect with the meaning "to shrink" (*garring Koro*). In China, koro is termed *suoyang* (*suo* = shrinkage, *yang* = penis) in Mandarin and *suk-yeong* in Cantonese (Bernstein & Gaw, 1990).

The first descriptions of koro-like symptoms (with some similarity to panic disorder symptomatology) can be found in ancient Chinese medical records that are over two thousand years old (Ng & Kua, 1996). Koro epidemics were reported to have occurred as early as 1865 on the Chinese island of Hainan and the Leizhou peninsula (Chowdury, 1996).

Some readers may be surprised that cases of koro-like symptomatology have been described in the West for more than a century. Kraepelin mentioned koro-like symptoms in bipolar patients as early as 1913. Case reports of secondary koro dating from 1954 to 2007 were summarized in detail by Garlipp (2008). Because the history of koro is very much connected to the question of how to best categorize koro in psychiatric classification systems, further historical aspects are discussed in the next chapter.

ROLE IN CURRENT DIAGNOSTIC SYSTEMS

Koro has been noted in the two main psychiatric classification systems used today, but its current role is quite limited. In the *International Classification of Diseases* (ICD-10) (World Health Organization, 1992) it was mentioned in the chapter, "Other Specific Neurotic Disorders." Koro was defined as fear of penis retraction with impending death as a feared result. The disturbance is connected with both cultural beliefs and behavior patterns. It is described as probably not delusional. In the *Diagnostic and Statistical Manual of Mental Disorders* (DSM-5) (American Psychiatric Association, 2013), koro is mentioned in the "Other Obsessive-compulsive and Related Disorders" module. In this context, koro is defined as an intense fear that genitals will retract into the body, which may lead to death. Thus, there is a great deal of overlap with how these systems conceptualize koro, but it is not yet a specific codable disorder and specific diagnostic criteria are not provided.

Koro, originally conceptualized as a culture-bound phenomenon, raises some profound intercultural questions, possibly more so than most mental illnesses that exist worldwide. Some authors have questioned whether it is a disease. Another fundamental issue is whether koro or any other culture-bound phenomenon can be included in a Western-dominated classification system. Some may say that a phenomenon that is originally based on specific cultural beliefs and behaviors must be primarily understood in its cultural and sociological context by research-ers who have an "inside" knowledge of these cultural specificities. In this context, Jilek and Jilek-Aall (2000) discussed the broad spectrum ranging from univer-salism (i.e., mental illnesses are mainly the same all over the world) to cultural relativism (the cultural environment characteristically induces mental distur-bances). Therefore, culturally immanent as well as cross-cultural aspects should be assessed.

In the author's opinion, the epidemic koro is the "real" koro and can be clearly defined. The isolated cases of secondary koro exhibit symptoms that can vary enormously. Although numerous terms have been used in this context, "All clinical phenomena presenting themselves in a wider sense as genital retraction syndromes with the leading symptom of fear should be named as such: genital retraction syndromes. All other nomenclatures, especially koro-like-syndrome, secondary koro, etc. should be dismissed as misleading" (Garlipp 2007, p. 26). Yet, to emphasize the difference between epidemic koro and isolated koro in this chapter, the term "secondary" koro is used for clarification.

In their approach to a conceptual history of koro, Buckle et al. (2007) sum up their findings as follows: "The sociological perspective divides Koro into two broad forms: epidemic and isolated. Isolated Koro, with its sporadic occurrence and association with medical conditions, is best left to medicine. Epidemic Koro, by contrast, is better conceptualized and explained using concepts from the social sciences" (p. 36). The term "mass sociogenic illness" is preferred. The author does not concur with this strict division between epidemic and isolated cases, because the subjective mental suffering of the epidemic koro patients and their need to be treated—a sign of disease—seems to be neglected.

Crozier (2011) presented an extensive and differentiated historical analysis of how the perception of koro developed in intercultural psychiatry. He concluded the following: "This analysis has identified two distinct psychiatric models. On the one hand is the universality of general psychiatric symptoms (as seen in western conceptions of mental illness), and on the other the realisation that different people (in non-western cultures) experience psychiatric trauma and anxieties differently. The history of koro provides a rich example of the tension between these two models, while the fact remains that koro sufferers are found in all groups" (p. 69).

The author concurs with Chowdury (2008) that the reported African epidemics of genital-shrinking differ enormously from koro and should be viewed separately. The main difference is that the affected persons believe that other individuals intend to or have actually stolen their genitals. This does not include the fear of death. The belief of "genital theft" is culturally accepted in the affected regions. Individuals accused of this "genital theft" were subsequently harmed and in some cases even beaten to death. Dzokoto and Adams (2005) investigated epidemics of genital-shrinking or genital-disappearing phenomena in West African countries. In their extensive analysis they show similarities and differences between koro and those African epidemics. They concluded that the West African epidemics should be characterized as "mass psychogenic illnesses." This term is understood to mean that no concrete causality is found, but common beliefs lead to symptoms in a number of community members. Dzokoto and Adams sum up as follows: "Rather than a separate, culture-bound-syndrome, this suggests that genital-shrinking episodes in West African settings are a local manifestation of a universal process: the sociocultural grounding of distress" (p. 72).

SYMPTOMATOLOGY

The general symptomatology that unifies both epidemic koro and secondary koro is the perception that body parts (viz. mostly the penis or testicles in men, vulva or nipples in women, but also other body parts such as tongues) retract into the body. This is accompanied by the patient's intense fear of dying as a consequence.

Males experiencing the epidemic type of koro may try to stop the penis from retracting by manually holding it or by using fixing materials like wire. These attempts may induce additional medical injuries. Deaths have even been reported as a result of these interventions. Cheng (1996) gives the example of a baby who suffocated while its mother tried to rescue the baby's tongue. People known to the koro sufferer will sometimes be asked to assist in trying to keep the penis outside the body. The phenomenon is culturally accepted;, therefore, the patient will feel no fear or shame in presenting his symptoms to others. There have been reports of children being brought to the hospital by parents who suspected koro. Several case reports of a koro *folie à deux* also have been published. Sometimes, people are suspected of having koro and are even treated against their will (Cheng 1996)!

In secondary koro the patient will often shamefully conceal his symptoms, because they are a cultural taboo, and he also may try—in hiding—to manipulate the penis in order to stop the shrinking.

Regarding duration, the symptoms found in epidemic koro are usually short-lived. Cases of secondary koro—as seen in the vignette—can last for a much longer time. In epidemic koro it is mostly young men and those with a prior knowledge of the phenomenon who are affected. In secondary koro the symptomatology varies (e.g., in relation to the intensity of fear). Garlipp (2008) noted: "The 84 case reports cited have two common features: 1. their diversity and 2. fear as a leading symptom. But the clinical pictures vary as much as their psychopathological categories chosen, the underlying mental disorders and the treatment approaches. Fear is the only regularly reported clinical symptom, be it neurotic or psychotic triggered fear. Even the terms chosen to describe the clinical picture vary as mentioned above" (p. 25).

PREVALENCE RATE AND ASSOCIATED FEATURES

Epidemics of koro have been mainly seen in South China, Singapore, Thailand, and India. In typical epidemics, as news and rumors about koro spread, hundreds to thousands of persons become affected. Although koro, both epidemic and secondary, is much more common in males, females also can be affected. Chowdury (2008) names at least 146 female case reports from seven epidemics between 1969 and 1988. There are reports of single cases of epidemic koro as well.

Numerous cases of secondary koro have been described in the literature, including several involving females. At present, it is unfortunately not possible to estimate true prevalence rates. There are a number of reasons why this is likely the case. Firstly, unless patients are directly queried the symptoms associated with koro, especially the genital retraction, will often be concealed due to feelings of shame or a fear of embarrassment. This can be seen in the subjective feelings of guilt described in the vignette. Secondly, patients with genital retraction syndromes may consult primarily doctors other than psychiatrists (e.g., urologists, gynecologists, dermatologists, or general practitioners). Finally, a number of mental health providers are not very aware of koro or its characteristic symptoms and may not consider it as a diagnostic option.

THEORIES OF ETIOLOGY

As with many of the more unusual and frightening disorders, there has been a great deal of theoretical speculation about koro. Etiological explanations range from the mythological to the medical.

In Han Chinese mythology in South China the female fox fairy is believed to be the reason for koro. She is believed to take away human energy. Tseng et al. (1988) explained that, "It is considered vital to maintain the balance of *yin* and *yang* elements, and it is thought that excessive loss of the *yang* element will result in death. As an extension of this concept, many of the elderly in Hainan and Leizhou share the folk belief that ghosts of the dead, who wander in the world of *yin* have no penises (a symbol of the *yang* element). Thus ghosts who are eager to transfer back to human form need penises in order to restore the *yang* element and bring them back to life. Accordingly, many people believe that a ghost, disguised either as a *hu-li-jing* (female ghost fox) or as a fairy lady, would come to collect penises for this purpose" (p. 1539).

Koro epidemics have been documented for centuries and constitute a recurrent phenomenon that is widely known to the respective populations. As the belief is transferred over generations and widely accepted in a community, rumors of koro will form a dynamic base for a "spreading" of the epidemic. Therefore, the disease's dynamic is fueled by a shared conviction of this phenomenon, and it consequently becomes "contagious" in a psychosociological sense. Cheng (1996) argues that persons were even identified by others as "koro-patients," which emphasizes the necessity of a culturally implemented and widely known common belief as a base for such an epidemic. Cheng supports the relevance of a "social process" for developing a koro epidemic: "The fact that relatives and neighbours are eager to help rescue the sex organ suggests that koro is not something which is only experienced by the victim, but there is a social reality defined by cultural meanings attached to the koro phenomenon so that those who live together in a community share similar expectations" (p. 70).

Along with these folk psychological theories, there have been various psychological hypotheses about koro's etiology and predisposing factors. These include certain cultural and religious backgrounds (which may possibly lead to feelings of guilt and shame), local seclusion with transferred beliefs, poor education, social crisis, and a general knowledge of koro.

Further, Chowdury (2008) discussed the relation of koro to body dysmorphic disorder. For both epidemic and secondary koro, fear of castration (in the classic psychoanalytical sense) and psychosexual conflicts have been named. Garlipp and Machleidt (2003) argue that epidemic koro is a form of bodily sensation related to panic attacks. They rated the symptomatology of secondary koro in a patient with schizophrenia as delusional. There is no clear connection to a somatic cause, especially for secondary koro, but an organic illness, especially neurological, with consecutive psychiatric symptoms, also can lead to genital retraction syndromes.

ASSESSMENT OPTIONS

The most important factor for detecting/assessing genital retraction syndromes is the simple knowledge that they do, in fact, exist. Unfortunately, rare and unusual syndromes and symptoms—as summarized in this book—are often not properly taught in medicine and psychiatry. The psychologist/psychiatrist will only correctly identify, interpret, and treat symptomatology that is known.

In epidemic koro, the patient will likely name the problem and look for help. In secondary koro, or in genital retraction syndromes more generally, it is important that patients can talk in an atmosphere of confidence and trust if they are to reveal their specific problems. In the vignette, for example, the patient disclosed the problem. Yet, it is necessary that the assessor always ask the patient if bodily changes (or strange sensations in general) are experienced; this approach creates a solid foundation for speaking about a patient's fears and symptoms.

Differential diagnosis can, perhaps not surprisingly, be difficult. This is especially the case when it is necessary to exclude somatic illnesses. Urologists and other physicians confronted with these symptoms should know about the relevant psychiatric syndromes. It is recommended that they transfer the patient to a psychiatrist prior to starting a somatic treatment that may not target the problem.

DIFFERENTIAL DIAGNOSIS

Isolated cases of koro can have a multitude of causes. The symptomatology itself has been variously described as delusional, an overvalued idea, fear, hypochondriacal, somatoform, obsessive-compulsive (as in DSM-5, American Psychiatric Association, 2013), depersonalization, and coenesthetic. It has been identified as a somatoform disorder, as a delusional disturbance, as panic disorder, as a neurotic (including histrionic) disorder, and as an obsessive-compulsive disorder. It is recommended that a substantial somatic examination, including cranial MRI, EEG, and blood analysis, as well as a drug test should be administered in order to rule out physical and neurological causes. Psychiatric diagnostics should identify any underlying mental illnesses. In case reports, the following illnesses were mentioned as concurring with secondary koro: schizophrenia and other psychotic syndromes, drug use (cannabis, amphetamines), depression, anxiety disorders, and bipolar disorder.

TREATMENT OPTIONS

Traditionally, an assortment of rituals are used to "treat" epidemic koro. Mo and Heise (1997) described that the main emergency treatment used is to attempt to keep the genital organ outside of the body by holding it, ligating it with a string, and holding it with a special clamp. Additionally, the patient may be instructed to drink soup made from peppers or ginger and the skin may be treated with oils (e.g., menthol). Other general recommendations are: "1. Participation in taoistic rituals; 2. parading with other people in the street; 3. beating gongs and drums; 4. setting off fire crackers; 5. loud shouting to threaten the devil; 6. covering the body with fishing nets; 7. beating the patient with peach tree branches; 8. pressing the patient's left hand's middle finger with two crossed chop sticks" (Mo & Heise, 1997, p. 109, own translation).

Garlipp (2008) reviewed the various published medical methods used to treat singular cases of koro. The following were used for treatment in connection with the underlying disorders: psychopharmacology (e.g., antipsychotics, antidepressants, tranquillizers, and mood stabilizers), electroconvulsive therapy, psychotherapy, and psychoeducation. The effects of treatment ranged from successful to not successful, but no large-scale randomized controlled trials (RCTs) were reported

Generally speaking, the most important treatment factor is to determine the underlying disorder, be it neurological, mental, or other—and to treat that appropriately first. Secondary koro may improve as a result. Psychotherapy should be offered if necessary. The specific symptomatology and recovery-hindering feelings (e.g., guilt, shame) should be addressed in order to help the patient better cope with the symptoms. An atmosphere of trust is needed so that the patient will be able to talk freely about real or imagined difficulties (e.g., sexual concerns). A clinical sexologist's approach may be helpful if the sexual problems are of greater concern.

Immediate relief can be given to the patient by prescribing a benzodiazepine like lorazepam. If delusional aspects are present, antipsychotics with a mood stabilizing potency, such as olanzapine, can be helpful. Selective serotonin reuptake inhibitors have also proven helpful in several cases. Antidepressants in general may be used if the symptomatology is of longer duration and the patient has concurrent depressive symptomatology. Psychoeducation with the patient and any relevant partners/family members should be offered in order to inform and relieve their intimate social network. If a *folie à deux* is present, the relative should be included in therapeutic sessions.

In general, the most effective way to prevent epidemics of koro is through providing a thorough and effective sex education program for adolescents, so that false beliefs can be eliminated across whole communities.

RECOMMENDATIONS FOR FUTURE WORK

In a globalized world, the knowledge of koro and genital retraction syndromes is more important than ever. For those providers who regularly treat patients from different cultural backgrounds, this knowledge can be very helpful. Research on epidemic koro is relatively extensive and has been undertaken during several epidemics. Various approaches, be they psychosocial, biological, or sociological are currently used and should be continued.

In secondary koro, or, more correctly, the genital retraction syndromes, it is necessary to learn more about isolated cases and their circumstances. Therefore, an interdisciplinary approach (e.g., urologists and psychiatrists) with a prospective study design could investigate its occurrence as well as identify possible causal factors. Further, discussions of whether to include culture-related disorders in the main classification systems must be critically reviewed in historical, sociological, intercultural, and ethical contexts.

The author does not see epidemic or secondary koro as an obsessive-compulsive disorder, but original koro appears to be related to panic disorder (Garlipp & Machleidt, 2003). Genital retraction syndromes have to be evaluated individually regarding their psychopathological expression and context.

As Garlipp (2008) described, many patients who presented with secondary koro had an immigrant background. In a globalized world the challenges for contemporary psychology and psychiatry include intercultural aspects, and it is necessary to have a working knowledge of culture-related syndromes. Being culturally sensitive, and having knowledge of rare and unusual syndromes, can lead to a more individualized treatment approach, which will likely result in an earlier detection of these symptoms as well as the development of more optimum treatment methods. This will ultimately be of benefit to patients.

ANNOTATION

(1) "Die Kranken zeigten eine Schrumpfung oder ein Zurückziehen eines bestimmten Körperteils, zum Beispiel des Penis bei Männern, (. . .). Man mußte sofort den zurückgezogenen Teil mit der Hand festhalten oder von mehreren Männern zurückziehen lassen. Gleichzeitig mußte man Gongs und Trommeln schlagen. Die Kranken sollten auch Ingwer-Suppe trinken. Dann wurden sie sofort geheilt. Das ist eine komische Krankheit."

REFERENCES

American Psychiatric Association. (2013). *Diagnostic and statistical manual of mental disorders, fifth edition.* Arlington, VA: American Psychiatric Association.

Buckle, C., Chuah, Y.M.L., Fones, C.S.L., & Wong A.H.C. (2007). A conceptual history of Koro. *Transcultural Psychiatry, March,* 27–43.

Cheng, S.T. (1996). A critical review of Chinese Koro. *Culture, Medicine and Psychiatry, 20,* 67–82.

Chowdury, A.N. (1996). The definition and classification of Koro. *Culture, Medicine and Psychiatry, 20,* 41–65.

Chowdury, A.N. (2008). Cultural Koro and Koro-Like Symptom (KLS). *German Journal of Psychiatry, 11,* 81–82.

Crozier, I. (2011). Making up Koro: Multiplicity, psychiatry, culture, and penis-shrinking anxieties. *Journal of the History of Medicine and Allied Sciences, 67,* 36–70.

Bernstein, R.L., & Gaw, A.C. (1990). Koro: Proposed classification for DSM-IV. *American Journal of Psychiatry, 12,* 1670–1674.

Dzokoto, V.A., & Adams, G. (2005). Understanding genital-shrinking epidemics in West Africa: Koro, Juju, or mass psychogenic illness? *Culture, Medicine and Psychiatry, 29,* 53–78.

Mo, G.M., & Heise, T. (1997). Die Koroepidemie in Südchina. In: K. Hoffmann & W. Machleidt (Eds.), *Psychiatrie im Kulturvergleich* (pp. 105–111). Berlin: VWB.

Garlipp, P. (2008). Koro—a culture-bound phenomenon. Intercultural psychiatric implications. *The German Journal of Psychiatry, 11*, 21–28.

Garlipp, P, & Machleidt, W. (2003). Koro—Erörterung eines transkulturell psychopathologischen Phänomens. *Fortschritte Neurologie Psychiatrie, 71*, 1–5.

Jilek, W. G., & Jilek-Aall, L. Kulturspezifische psychische Störungen. In: H. Helmchen, F. Henn, H. Lauter, & N. Sartorius (Eds.), *Psychiatrie der Gegenwart, Band 3* (pp. 379–423). New York: Springer.

Kraepelin, E. (1913). *Psychiatrie, ein Lehrbuch fuer Studierende und Aerzte* (8. Edition, Vo. 3). Leipzig: Johann Ambrosius Barth.

Ng, B.Y., & Kua, E.H. (1996). Koro in ancient Chinese history. *History of Psychiatry, 7*, 563–570.

Tseng, W.-S., Mo, K.-M., Jing, H., Li, L.-S., Ou, L.-W., Chen, G.-Q., & Jiang, D.-W. (1988). A sociocultural study of Koro epidemics in Guangdong, China. *American Journal of Psychiatry, 145*, 1538–1543.

World Health Organization. (1992). *The ICD-10 classification of mental and behavioural disorders. Clinical descriptions and diagnostic guidelines.* Geneva, Switzerland: World Health Organization.

13

Taijin Kyofusho

BRIAN A. SHARPLESS, AMY L. BALKO,
AND JESSICA LYNN GROM ∎

VIGNETTE

Valeria was a 24-year-old Hispanic female who presented for assessment at the first author's lab. She volunteered for the study in order to acquire research participation credit for her introductory psychology class. She had a medium build, was fairly nondescript in her appearance, and would not have attracted any unusual degree of attention in terms of her dress or personal style on any college campus. She was, however, notable for being quite anxious throughout all aspects of the procedure (i.e., informed consent, administration of questionnaires, clinical interview) in a way that was clearly apparent to study personnel.

Valeria reported struggling in college. She felt that she should be doing much better and reported attentional difficulties while on campus in general and during classes in particular. Her grades were suffering and she found herself becoming increasingly anxious and isolated. Her most consistent source of comfort was her church (i.e., Church of Latter-Day Saints). She was fairly symptomatic during the clinical interview and reported symptoms consistent with social anxiety disorder (SAD) and major depressive disorder (mild).

Though SAD was her principal diagnosis per overall clinical severity, her specific anxiety symptoms did not map neatly onto standard SAD diagnostic criteria. She endorsed the paradigmatic fear of embarrassment in front of others and avoidance of typical social situations, but also reported symptoms that fell outside of the "standard" SAD symptoms. Specifically, Valeria was preoccupied with a fear that she would offend/upset/alienate others due to the many unpalatable aspects of herself. As will be seen, this fear was quite pervasive and generalized.

Valeria always anticipated negative reactions to conversations. She found herself unable to relax even when conversing with friends. Not only did she fear that she would "bore" people, but she also worried that she might inadvertently hurt their feelings due to careless statements. Valeria also worried about eye contact, and what her eyes looked like to others. She found herself wondering where "the best place to look" was when talking so as to avoid making others uncomfortable. She was also afraid to laugh due to a belief that her face would stiffen and negatively impact upon her conversation partner. Not surprisingly, her discomfort often led to blushing, another focus of her fear. Valeria believed that blushing would be seen as offensive, and would make others want to discontinue conversations.

She also believed that she was "ugly," and that her appearance would lead to observer discomfort. This fear was not focused on one small perceived defect, but was more general. For example, it was almost intolerable for her to have stylists look at her face during haircuts. She also feared that her body odor was offensive. It is unclear whether she engaged in excessive cleaning rituals, but she was preoccupied with this belief regardless.

Clearly, Valeria suffered from a number of social fears and inhibitions. She believed that something was so fundamentally wrong with her that her mere presence caused negative impacts in others. She felt sorry others had to be with her, and these beliefs were powerfully experienced. Because she presented in the context of a research study, no treatment was offered, although she was provided with referrals. It is unclear whether she commenced psychotherapy.

HISTORICAL AND CULTURAL CONTEXT

Anxiety in social situations is presumably found in every culture (e.g., Dinnel, Kleinknecht, & Tanaka-Matsumi, 2002; Good & Kleinman, 1985; Mesquita & Frijda, 1992). However, there may be differences *across* cultures in the specific ways that this anxiety manifests itself and is subjectively experienced by the sufferer (e.g., Woody, Miao, & Kellman-McFarlane, 2015). For example, *taijin kyofusho* has been thought to be an Asian variant of social anxiety that is uniquely situated within that cultural context. Though little known in the West, it has been recognized in Japanese diagnostic systems for almost a century (Kleinknecht, Dinnel, Kleinknecht, Hiruma, & Harada, 1997).

Taijin kyofusho (TK) can be translated as fear (*kyofu*) of interpersonal relations (*taijin*) disorder (*sho*) (Takahishi, 1989). Some scholars believe that TK is culture-bound and limited to the East, especially Japan and Korea (e.g., Tarumi, Ichimiya, Yamada, Umesue, & Kuroki, 2004). Therefore, and perhaps not surprisingly, TK has often been discussed in terms of individualism and collectivism. Such cultural differences are thought to contribute to the putative social anxiety variations found between Easterners and Westerners (Kleinknecht et al., 1997). For instance, it is widely held that individualistic cultures emphasize independence and individual success. Thus, Western conceptualizations of social anxiety tend to have an egocentric focus (i.e., fear of embarrassing *oneself*) (e.g., Heimberg et al., 2014). In contrast, collectivist cultures, which place more emphasis on the group and group harmony/cohesion, may focus social fears on offending or upsetting *others* (a core feature of TK). TK has even been described as an "altruistic phobia," given that the individual's distress resides in the fear of making others uncomfortable (Kasahara, 1970, as cited in Russell, 1989). Although this viewpoint is intuitively appealing and, at least in some ways, quite elegant, the matter may be more complex than the individualistic–collectivist dichotomy may imply. Further, empirical work has recently challenged these more global claims (e.g., Oyserman, Coon, & Kemmelmeier, 2002). Moreover, given the complexity of humans and how they can experience themselves in many different, and sometimes even logically incompatible ways, it seems reasonable to conclude that individuals can possess both independent and interdependent self-construals that vary according to time, place, and situation. As noted by Kleinknecht et al. (1997), "the extent that these two types of self-construal relate to different forms of social anxiety, some of each should be identifiable in each culture, although one form should predominate in a given culture (p. 159)." As will be shown in a subsequent section, this may be the case.

ROLE IN CURRENT DIAGNOSTIC SYSTEMS

TK was first described in the early 1920s by Shoma Morita (Kirmayer, 1991; Takahashi, 1989). Morita used the term to indicate a more specific form of "*shinkeishitsu*" or nervous weakness (Kirmayer, 1991). *Shinkeishitsu* bears a strong resemblance to Western neurasthenia (i.e., a combination of anxious, depressive, and somatic symptoms as in Beard, 1881). Although the term taijin kyofusho was used for a number of years in Japan, diagnostic criteria were not formalized in any way until 1995 (Maeda & Nathan, 1999), and some questions remain.

TK has a very interesting, and somewhat unusual role in contemporary diagnostic systems. At present, it is not a diagnosis in either the *Diagnostic and Statistical Manual of Mental Disorders* (DSM-5) (American Psychiatric Association [APA], 2013) or the *International Classification of Mental and Behavioral Disorders* (ICD-10) (World Health Organization, 1992). It was included, however, in the DSM-5's *Glossary of Cultural Concepts of Distress* (APA, 2013) and, previously, had been in DSM-IV's (APA, 1994) category of social phobia under *Specific Culture, Age, and Gender Features*. TK is also mentioned in ICD-10's Diagnostic Criteria for Research under *Culture-Specific Disorders*. Suggested ICD-10 codes for TK are social phobia and other phobia anxiety disorders (Essau, Sasagawa, Chen, & Sakano, 2012; World Health Organization, 1992).

As demonstrated in the next section, the scope of TK symptoms is quite broad. This may lead to some conceptual confusion in those who are unfamiliar with it. Though it is not a stand-alone diagnosis in the West, TK symptoms can be captured using several contemporary diagnoses. First, a core aspect of TK (viz., evaluative social concerns) can be found in social anxiety disorder (SAD) (APA, 2013). Although fears of negative evaluation are common to both disorders, the fears found in TK (especially the "offensive" subtypes) are usually focused on making *others* uncomfortable. Second, the particular subtype of TK that includes a fear of having a deformed or offensive body (*shubo-kyofu*) bears a strong phenomenological resemblance to body dysmorphic disorder (APA, 2013). A third feature of TK could be found in the "*Other Specified Obsessive-Compulsive and Related Disorders*" section of the DSM-5. Specifically, the *shubo-kyofu* (fear of having a bodily deformity) and *jiko-shu-kyofu* (fear of having an offensive body odor) subtypes of TK are listed as examples of more obsessive presentations. Although not in the DSM-5 or ICD-10, olfactory reference syndrome also possesses overlapping symptoms with the *jiko-shu-kyofu* subtype of TK (e.g., Suzuki, Takei, Kawai, Minabe, & Mori, 2003). Finally, at a level of symptom *severity*, TK can resemble a delusional disorder (e.g.,Lee & Oh, 1999) if an individual's concern reaches a psychotic level of intensity (i.e., the patient manifest deficits in consensual reality).

Thus, TK manifestations are currently nested within a variety of Western categories and there is acknowledgement of possible cultural contributions. There are, however, no Western constructs that capture even the majority of TK's many features (APA, 2013; Essau et al., 2012; World Health Organization, 1992).

Interestingly, evidence exists that some Western diagnoses, which roughly correspond to TK subtypes, are often comorbid with SAD. For example, a recent review found that body dysmorphic disorder is the fourth most common SAD comorbid condition, with rates ranging from 8% to 12% (Asakura et al., 2012). Additionally, Phillips and Menard (2011) found that 65% of individuals with olfactory reference syndrome also had lifetime SAD, with 60% experiencing it at the time of their study. In our reading of the literature, findings such as these raise interesting questions about the overall relationships between TK and Western disorders. In concert with Suzuki et al. (2003), we believe that the scattered presence of TK across the Western classification systems seems to be an argument against a simple culture-bound conception. Further, the particular nosological values that one holds (i.e., lumping vs. splitting) likely impact upon opinions as to whether the field should: (1) add a specific TK diagnosis to existing systems, (2) collapse TK symptoms into existing Western categories, or (3) reduce the number of current diagnoses on the basis of shared and overlapping features.

SYMPTOMATOLOGY

At present, no consensus yet exists on the precise diagnostic definition of TK or the number of subtypes (if any). Instead, our literature review identified several sets of proposed criteria (e.g., see Kobayashi et al., 2003; Lee & Oh, 1999). A good amount of heterogeneity was found in terms of symptom specificity and specific diagnostic focus. Our two preferred sets of criteria can be found in Table 13.1. Both include a range of symptoms as well as minimum symptom durations. Thus, they may be particularly useful for empirical research as well as clinical diagnosis. Subtypes have also been proposed.

Table 13.1. Diagnostic Criteria for *Taijin Kyofusho* from Matsunaga et al. (2001) and Nagata et al. (2011)

MATSUNAGA ET AL. (2001)[1]
A. A marked and persistent fear of social or performance situations in which the person is exposed to unfamiliar persons or to possible scrutiny by others. The individual fears that he or she will offend or embarrass others (e.g., by having an offensive odor).
B. Exposure to the feared social situation almost invariably provokes anxiety, which may take the form of a situationally bound or situationally predisposed panic attack.
C. The person recognizes the fear is excessive or unreasonable. Note: In children, this feature may be absent.
D. The feared social or performance situations are avoided or else are endured with intense anxiety or distress.
E. The avoidance, anxious anticipation, or distress associated with the feared social or performance situation(s) interferes significantly with the person's normal routine, occupational (academic) functioning, or social activities or relationships; or, there is marked distress about having the phobia.
F. In individuals under age 18 years, the duration is at least six months.
G. The fear or avoidance is not due to the direct physiological effects of a substance (e.g., a drug of abuse, a medication) or a general medical condition and is not better accounted for by another mental disorder (e.g., panic disorder with or without agoraphobia, separation anxiety disorder, body dysmorphic disorder, a pervasive developmental disorder, or schizoid personality disorder).
H. If a general medical condition or another mental disorder is present, the fear in criterion (A) is unrelated to it (e.g., the fear is not of stuttering or of trembling in Parkinson's disease, or of exhibiting abnormal eating behavior in anorexia nervosa or bulimia nervosa).
NAGATA ET AL. (2011)[2]
A. At least one of the following features:
1. Fear of blushing in the presence of others
2. Fear of stiffening of facial expression; of trembling of the head, hands, feet, or voice; of sweating while facing others
3. Fear of physical deformities being noticed
4. Fear of emitting body odors
5. Fear of line-of-sight becoming uncontrollable
6. Fear of uncontrollable flatus in the presence of others
B. Either of the following two, because of the above fear(s)*
1. Tension subtype: Fear of being looked at (noticed) by others
2. Offensive subtype: Fear of offending or embarrassing others

(continued)

Table 13.1. CONTINUED

NAGATA ET AL. (2011)[2]
C. At most points during the course of the disorder, the person recognizes that the fear is excessive or unreasonable.
D. The fear(s) interfere(s) significantly with the person's normal routing, occupational (academic) functioning, social activities, or social relationships; or, there is marked distress about having the fear(s).
E. The symptoms must have been present for at least one year. In individuals under age 18 years, the duration should have been at least six months.

NOTES: [1] = Matsunaga, H., Kiriike, N., Matsui, T., Iwasaki, Y., & Stein, D. J. (2001). Taijin kyofusho: a form of social anxiety disorder that responds to serotonin reuptake inhibitors? *The International Journal of Neuropsychopharmacology, 4*, 231–237.
[2] = Nagata, T., Matsunaga, H., van Vliet, I., Yamada, H., Fukuhara, H., Yoshimura, C., & Kiriike, N. (2011). Correlations between the offensive subtype of social anxiety disorder and personality disorders. *Psychiatry and Clinical Neurosciences, 65(4)*, 341–348.

*In this study, a diagnosis of the offensive subtype required the patient to meet criterion B(2).

Taijin Kyofusho Subtypes

Some researchers have dichotomized TK into nonoffensive (or "sensitive") and offensive types. The former is very similar to Western SAD; fears tend to be fairly egocentric in nature and are focused on embarrassment arising from social/performance situations (e.g., APA, 2013; Lee & Oh, 1999) and the sufferer's putative shortcoming or physical manifestations of anxiety. In contrast, *offensive* TK is characterized by allocentric fears. In other words, the individual fears that he/she will cause others to suffer offense, displeasure, or embarrassment (e.g., Nagata, Wada, Yamada, Iketani, & Kiriike, 2005). When this nonoffensive–offensive dichotomy is superimposed onto an individualistic–collectivistic dichotomy, it is easy to see the intuitive appeal of relegating offensive TK to a culture-bound, or at least culturally influenced, disorder. Apart from this broad offensive/nonoffensive distinction, two other classifications of TK phenomena have been made upon the basis of specific fears and overall severity, respectively.

SUBTYPES BASED ON THE FOCUS OF FEARS
Subcategories of TK include the fear of blushing (*sekimen-kyofu*), fear of a deformed body (*shubo-kyofu*), fear of eye contact (*jiko-shisen-kyofu*), and fear of one's own body odor (*jiko-shu-kyofu*) (Iwata et al., 2011; Suzuki et al., 2003; Takahasi, 1989). It is worth noting that Lee and Oh (1999) offered a slightly different interpretation of *jiko-shisen-kyofu*. Specifically, they noted that there may be a belief that one's eyes are too sharp or hostile and, therefore, cause distress to others. This type of fear can also be subdivided into a fear of offending through

one's side gaze or by staring at valuables (i.e., watches, jewelry) and/or defective body parts (Lee & Oh, 1999).

The presence of at least four specific subtypes also raises the issue of whether multiple manifestations are often present in the same patient. Iwata et al. (2011) suggested that individuals typically have only one fear at a time. However, case reports (e.g., Ono et al., 2001) indicate that multiple fears (e.g., bodily odors and physical deformities) can coexist. Further, Lee and Oh (1999) suggested that individuals have a variety of fears, but usually focus on one (i.e., the most clinically distressing), which can change over time (Lewis-Fernández et al., 2010). Thus, when assessing TK it may be helpful to inquire beyond the principal area of fear.

It is important to note that there are research discrepancies on the most common presenting symptoms of TK. Whereas some studies reported a fear of blushing as most common (James, 2006; Takahashi, 1989), others found eye contact to be most common (Lee & Oh, 1999). Further, some researchers conceptualize blushing as a symptom that typically remits with age and is only infrequently a presenting complaint (Iwata et al., 2011).

SUBTYPES BASED UPON SEVERITY

TK has also been divided into four presentations based upon severity (Kirmayer, 1991). These are: (1) a transient form of social anxiety typically manifested during adolescence, (2) a neurosis very similar to social anxiety disorder, (3) a "borderline" form of phobia with ideas of reference, and (4) a delusional form with fixed beliefs (Choy, Schneier, Heimberg, Oh, & Liebowitz, 2008; Kasahara, 1987, as cited in Kirmayer, 1991). The borderline form can be considered a "severe social phobia," given that individuals often believe that they are manifesting something that is causing others to avoid them (Kirmayer, 1991, p. 20). The delusional form is most severe, with the specific symptoms and beliefs remaining even when the patient is outside of social situations (Kirmayer, 1991). It is believed that the borderline and delusional subtypes typically fall within the offensive classification. As noted above, the offensive symptoms found in the third and fourth presentations encompass fears such as having a physical defect or unpleasant body odor. Other, milder fears (i.e., fear of blushing or trembling) are believed to be common in the nonoffensive types (Choy et al., 2008). Scholars who view TK as *not* culturally bound tend to adopt this graduated symptom classification (e.g., Kim, Rapee, & Gaston, 2008).

There is also a sense that TK progresses in severity over time. For example, a fear of blushing is thought to be the first fear experienced after the onset of heightened overall anxiety. Fears are then thought to expand to eye contact, odor, etc. (Lee & Oh, 1999; Takahashi, 1989).

PREVALENCE RATE AND ASSOCIATED FEATURES

Although the prevalence rates for SAD are relatively well-known, even in international samples, this is not the case for TK. We were unable to locate rates for the general population, but some limited data suggest that it is fairly common in clinical settings. Although some have speculated that this scarcity of prevalence data may be due to the concealment of TK symptoms from others and seeking treatment in secret (Takahashi, 1989), there are likely other factors involved (e.g., lack of research investment, lack of uniform diagnostic criteria).

Prevalence rates among Japanese psychiatric patients ranged from 7% to 36% (Chang, 1984; McNally, Cassiday, & Calamari, 1990). Although TK is thought to be more prevalent in East Asia (Essau et al., 2012; Iwata et al., 2011), symptoms of offensive TK have been documented in the United States and Australia (e.g., Grom & Sharpless, 2014; Iwata et al., 2011; Kim et al., 2008).

Regarding SAD more generally, a recent review of the literature suggested that it is much more prevalent in North America and parts of South America (6.4%–9.1%) than in East Asia (0.2%–0.8%, as in Hofmann, Asnaani, & Hinton, 2010). Another review, however, suggested that symptoms of SAD are endorsed more frequently in East Asian countries than in the Unites States and Europe (e.g., Lewis-Fernández et al., 2010). Additionally, Woody et al. (2015) combined data from 31 studies and found that individuals of Asian descent endorsed more social anxiety symptoms (per self-report measures) than did Europeans. The discrepancy between SAD rates and symptom frequency may be due to the more collectivist nature of East Asian cultures; thus, there may be more acceptance of putative SAD behaviors and higher endorsements on self-report measures, but also a lower likelihood of meeting diagnostic criteria given a lack of reported impairment (e.g., Lewis-Fernández et al., 2010). Additionally, Krieg and Xu (2015) found that higher levels of social anxiety in Asians may be partially accounted for by a lower independent self-construal. Interestingly, increased social anxiety was not associated with acculturation, suggesting that symptoms were not elevated due to factors associated with being an ethnic minority (Krieg & Xu, 2015).

Unlike the Western conceptualization of SAD, TK may be more frequent in males than females, with a 3:2 ratio (Essau et al., 2012; Lewis-Fernández et al., 2010; Russel, 1989; Takahashi, 1989). Some studies, however, suggested that rates among females are increasing (Takahashi et al., 1996, as cited in Maeda & Nathan, 1999). TK also seems to be more common in adolescents/young adults (Russel, 1989; Lewis-Fernández et al., 2010), typically decreases after age 30, and is rare past age 40 (Maeda & Nathan, 1999; James, 2006). It is possible, however, for the disorder to become chronic and quite severe (Maeda & Nathan, 1999; Russel, 1989).

Symptoms of TK appear most acutely during interactions with *acquaintances* (Maeda & Nathan, 1999). Anxiety may be lowered around close friends and family members because they will presumably forgive faults or mistakes. Similarly, it is believed that strangers also may overlook or not notice faults and imperfections (Lee & Oh, 1999).

Insight into the veracity of fears is not a requirement for TK diagnosis in most systems, but is included in some (e.g., Table 13.1). Regardless of insight, fear and anxiety often result in avoidance and social withdrawal (Ono et al., 2001).

Avoidance (e.g., limiting interactions and avoiding attention as in Kelly, Walters, & Phillips, 2010) likely maintains symptoms.

TK has been found to co-occur with SAD, depression, body dysmorphic disorder, obsessive-compulsive disorder, and various personality disorders (Matsunaga, Kiriike, Matsui, Iwasaki, & Stein, 2001). Ono et al. (1996) found that six out of eight individuals with avoidant personality disorder (APD) also presented with TK symptoms. They also concluded that APD is conceptually similar to TK.

THEORIES OF ETIOLOGY

A number of etiological theories have been proposed (e.g., temperament, neurobiology, and family/cultural factors). Morita's original formulations attributed TK to temperamental predispositions toward hypochondria and certain environmental experiences. These factors led TK individuals to overinterpret events, fear interpersonal situations, focus excessive attention on bodily sensations, and overinterpret bodily sensations (e.g., Maeda & Nathan, 1999). Morita thought this a cyclical process (termed "psychic interaction") such that increases in both attention and sensations exacerbated the problem (Maeda & Nathan, 1999). Consistent with Morita, Simard and Nielsen (2005) found that individuals who feared blushing had a greater number of negative learning experiences than those who did not fear blushing.

Familial/cultural factors have also been proposed. For example, Essau et al. (2012) found that parental care predicted social anxiety involving fear of negative evaluation in English samples whereas parental overprotection predicted both anxiety in social interactions and TK symptoms in Japanese samples (Essau et al., 2012). Further, family sociability contributed to all variations of social anxiety in both samples (Essau et al., 2012).

Other aspects of East Asian child-rearing and/or family practices have been implicated in TK. For example, Japanese mothers have been reported to foster dependency in their children and to emphasize group membership in forms of punishment (e.g., threats of ridicule and abandonment, and a focus on mothers as victims of behaviors, as in Kirmayer, 1991). This is thought to evoke guilt in children and highlight the emotional effect of their actions on others (Kirmayer, 1991). Additionally, although eye contact is valued in the West, Japanese children are socialized to not engage in *direct* eye contact and to focus their gaze elsewhere (e.g., the throat, Kirmayer, 1991).

Other theories combine neurobiological and cultural factors. These suggest that cultural factors influence the ways in which universal disorders are expressed. Although this is clearly a complex issue, and there remains a great deal to be learned about the neurobiology of SAD and TK, individuals with TK have been shown to respond to medications used to treat SAD (see Treatment Options). Although we do not want to succumb to a *post hoc, ergo propter hoc* fallacy, these empirical findings may suggest the presence of common neurobiological underpinnings to the surface symptom topographies of both (Matsunaga et al., 2001).

Additionally, a recent review of the literature suggested that many of the afore-mentioned factors that are thought to contribute to the development of TK (e.g., temperament, negative interactions, and cognitive processes) are also believed to play an etiological role in SAD and body dysmorphic disorder (i.e., a disorder similar to the *shubo-kyofu*, Kelly et al., 2010).

Making the matter more complicated, Krueger, Chentosova-Dutton, Markon, Goldberg, and Ormel (2003) argued that there are universal forms of psychopathology that are deemed syndromes (or not) depending upon the cultural frame. This idea is reflected in the fact that behaviors classified as pathological in one culture can be valued or encouraged in another. For example, verbal reticence, emotional restraint, social introversion, and shyness are not unusual in Asian cultures, but are characteristics of SAD in the West (Woody et al., 2015).

Consistent with the above, some TK behaviors seem to be encouraged, and even valued, in East Asian females (Kirmayer, 1991). Although purely speculative, the emphasis on these behaviors may play a role in the lower rates of female TK, given that females may be less likely to view their symptoms as pathological/problematic. Thus, they would neither report their symptoms nor seek treatment. Evidence suggests, however, that the percentage of females with TK symptoms may be increasing (Takahashi, 1996, as cited in Maeda & Nathan, 1999). It is interesting to speculate whether this reported shift, if accurate, is the result of shifting gender mores.

ASSESSMENT OPTIONS

Several assessment instruments for TK exist, but none has yet reached predominance. This is likely due to outstanding questions about the best way to define TK, disagreement over the presence/number of subtypes, and the relatively young state of the empirical research base.

Self-report Measures

The most widely used measure is the *Taijin Kyofusho Scale* (TKS) (Kleinknecht et al., 1997, available in article). It contains 31 items and uses a 7-point scale ranging from 1 (exactly true) to 7 (totally false). Thus, lower scores indicate higher TK levels. Item content reflects offensive and nonoffensive fears. Regarding psychometrics, the TKS has demonstrated excellent internal consistency (α's ranging between 0.92 and 0.96) in Japanese, American, and British samples (Essau et al., 2012; Kleinknecht et al., 1997). A factor analysis of the TKS by Tarumi et al. (2004) identified five factors that accounted for 58.4% of the variance.

The *Taijin Kyofu Sho Questionnaire* (TKSQ) (Choy et al., 2008, available in article) includes 30 items rated on a 4-point scale (i.e., 0 = not fearful at all to 3 = extremely fearful). Specifically, the questionnaire has 10 core items that are repeated to assess for one egocentric (i.e., embarrassing oneself) and two allocentric concerns (i.e., making others uncomfortable and offending others). The TKSQ has six subscales containing five items each. Internal consistencies ranged from questionable to good (α = .65 to α = .83) for each of the subscales in an American sample and from poor to good (α = .57 to α = .87) in a Korean sample (Choy et al., 2008).

The *Social Anxiety/Taijin-Kyofu Scale* (SATS) was developed by Asakura et al. (2012) to address perceived weaknesses of the TKSQ (viz., the degree to which patients actually believe they are offending another person). It contains 12 items answered using a 5-point format (i.e., 0 = no symptoms to 4 = extreme symptoms). Internal consistencies were excellent (α = .97) for the measure and acceptable for the three subscales (α = .72 to α = .78) (Asakura et al., 2012).

In general, we recommend the TKS for most clinical applications based upon its ease of scoring, comprehensiveness, and use in prior studies (e.g., Essau et al., 2012; Kim et al., 2008).

Clinical Interview

Ono et al. (2001) developed a five-question instrument to target core TK symptoms (e.g., fears of appearance, body odor) within the context of more encompassing diagnostic interviews. The questions are quite broad in scope compared to self-report measures. Nakamura, Kitanishi, Miyake, Hashimoto, and Kubota (2002) also reported the use of clinical interviews. Unfortunately, details about the nature of these interviews were not provided in the article. Interrater agreement (two raters) was high for TK diagnosis (100%) and the three TK subtypes (0.83).

DIFFERENTIAL DIAGNOSIS

Caveats

At the present time, recommendations for the differential diagnosis of TK are difficult to make for at least three reasons. First, the field lacks uniform diagnostic criteria for TK. In the absence of reliable and widely used definitions, differential diagnosis—an already complicated task—becomes even more complicated (and possibly arbitrary). Of course, this also depends upon the pragmatic aim that is attached to differential diagnosis (e.g., clinical description or research).

Second, TK has an unusual connection to SAD, given that it is mentioned in DSM-5's SAD section, but the two are not clearly delineated. Interestingly, it would have been much easier to provide differential diagnostic advice using DSM-IV criteria (APA, 1994, pp. 416–417) than using DSM-5 criteria (APA, 2013). This is because the later edition amended the previous edition's SAD criteria by including fear of offending others as a means to meet criterion B (pp. 202–203). We feel that this inclusion of TK symptomatology was good for the sake of symptomatic coverage (because we believe that SAD and TK are not fundamentally distinct disorders), but makes differential diagnosis more challenging.

Third, and related to the previous points, there is a great deal of symptom overlap between TK and other disorders. Points of rarity between them, if they indeed exist, are not yet known. For example, it remains an open question as to whether the fear of emitting offensive odors is best characterized as olfactory reference syndrome or *jiko-shu-kyofu*, or if the answer to this question is largely a semantic one. More generally, we are not yet sure whether TK and these other disorders are better conceptualized as separate entities, separable in principle, or more overlapping than their distinct terminologies would imply. In the absence of firm answers, we now will attempt to provide some practical guidance.

Recommendations

In general, we recommend the use of broad semistructured interviews as a basis for diagnosis whenever possible. Given the murky symptomatic overlap between TK and other disorders, we believe this will help ensure that the full breadth of symptom topography is assessed. Of course, deviations from DSM-5 constructs will be needed, and this could be facilitated through use of the criteria in Table 13.1 and/or use of one or more self-report or interview measures. Further:

- It is important to assess for TK in non-East Asian individuals.
- Those with delusional TK should be assessed for other psychotic symptoms, the pervasiveness of delusionality, and degree of impairment in consensual reality testing.
- Those with TK may experience the most anxiety with acquaintances rather than close friends, family, or strangers (Maeda & Nathan, 1999).
- The *shubo-kyofu* subtype of TK is difficult to distinguish from body dysmorphic disorder. The fear and discomfort seen in the latter may be more pervasive, whereas *shubo-kyofu* fears appear with the greatest intensity in the presence of acquaintances (Lee & Oh, 1999). *Shubo-kyofu* patients are more preoccupied with how perceived defects will cause difficulties with others than with the perceived defects themselves. Further, *shubo-kyofu* does not typically result in a desire for surgical interventions (Tarumi et al., 2004).
- *Jiko-shu-kyofu* is difficult to differentiate from olfactory reference syndrome, but there may be differences. First, individuals with olfactory reference syndrome may manifest egocentric fears surrounding their putative odors as opposed to the allocentric fears thought to epitomize TK, but we are not aware of data suggesting that this is an actual difference. Second, those with olfactory reference syndrome often engage in compulsive checking/cleaning behaviors (Feusner et al., 2010) whereas those with TK engage in repetitive behaviors that are avoidant in nature

and not focused on resolving the *source* of their fears (Kleinknecht et al., 1997).

- TK may be able to be distinguished from APD on the basis of interpersonal impairment. Those with APD demonstrate impairment in intimate relationships (APA, 2013) whereas those with TK typically only experience this difficulty in intermediate relationships (Lee & Oh, 1999).
- It is important to distinguish TK from shyness and culturally appropriate behaviors.

TREATMENT OPTIONS

Various psychopharmacological and psychotherapeutic interventions have been used to treat TK. To date, however, no large-scale randomized clinical trials have taken place.

Psychopharmacology

ANTIDEPRESSANTS

Several antidepressants appear promising, but the results require replication. For instance, Matsunaga et al. (2001) examined the effectiveness of either clomipramine (25–200 mg per day) or fluvoxamine (50–250 mg per day) in an uncontrolled study. Approximately half of the sample improved (i.e., lower *Clinical Global Impression* [CGI] scores) after six months or more of treatment. Therapeutic action was unfortunately difficult to determine because most participants were also prescribed benzodiazepines, and nearly one third received adjunctive antipsychotics. However, Asakura, Tajima, & Koyama (2007) noted that fluvoxamine has been effective in treating SAD and would likely be similarly helpful for TK.

The effectiveness of paroxetine (10–40 mg x day) was tested in an uncontrolled study by Kobayashi et al. (2003). Its use reduced TK severity in two of the three cases. Paroxetine (10–40 mg per day) was also investigated in an open trial of 22 patients with offensive TK (Nagata et al., 2006). Of the 19 completers, all but one showed improvement from baseline on CGI scores.

In Nagata et al.'s (2003) first open-trial study of milnacipran (50–150 mg per day) for TK, 10 out of 11 completers demonstrated improvement, and more than half were either very much or much improved per the CGI. In their second milnacipran study (50–150 mg per day), there was a high (37.5%) dropout rate, but the results appeared promising (Nagata et al., 2005).

OTHER PHARMACOLOGICAL AGENTS AND COMBINED TREATMENTS

Other psychopharmacological treatments for TK have included phenelzine, moclobemide, and clonazepam (e.g., case studies in Clarvit, Schneier, &

Liebowitz, 1996). Four case studies described by Iwata et al. (2011) treated patients with Morita therapy and/or a combination of anxiolytics, antidepressants, or antipsychotics. The patients experienced mixed outcomes such that some experienced symptom relief but either discontinued treatment prematurely or needed significantly more improvement to be considered a success.

It is also possible that certain TK symptoms may be more responsive to medication than others. For instance, Iwata (2011) reported that "fear of one's own glance" and fear of having distorted facial features cannot be treated with medication, but this awaits additional evidence.

Psychotherapeutic Approaches

The main psychotherapeutic approaches for TK have been group therapy (i.e., a social/treatment club described in Takahishi, 1975), psychoanalysis (Russel, 1989), cognitive behavioral therapies, and Morita therapy. Limited data exist for the last two approaches.

Cognitive behavioral therapies (CBT), which are effective treatments for SAD, have been applied to TK. McNally et al. (1990) discussed the treatment of a patient who believed that she uncontrollably stared at genitalia and that this behavior embarrassed others. Treatment consisted of graduated *in vivo* exposure to the feared stimuli. Although the treatment was an initial success, the client refused follow-up treatment, and therapeutic gains were not maintained. Lee and Oh (1999) reported that group therapy involving cognitive restructuring among offensive social phobia patients was successful. In a study by Kim et al. (2008), a treatment consisting of CBT, self-help, or relaxation-skill training was provided to SAD patients. Results indicated that offensive TK symptoms also responded to treatment.

A culturally indigenous form of psychotherapy for TK is Morita therapy. As originally conceived, Morita therapy took place over the course of 40 days in inpatient hospitalization settings, involved a hierarchy of activities starting with isolation from others and bed rest, and gradually increased the patient's activity level and socialization (Maeda & Nathan, 1999; Morita, 1998). During the last stage of treatment, patients learned how to be more productive and accepting of their symptoms. Today, Morita therapy is employed in outpatient settings for a variety of mental disorders (Maeda & Nathan, 1999). In line with current trends toward psychotherapy integration, Dinnel et al. (2002) recommended that Morita therapy include aspects of CBT in order to more successfully treat any TK symptoms that may be present in individuals diagnosed with SAD. However, Russell (1989) noted that the lengthy and highly directive nature of traditional Morita therapy may not be well-tolerated by all patients.

From this review, it is clear that no well-established treatments yet exist for TK. Future studies should utilize appropriate comparison groups and examine psychopharmacological and psychological interventions with larger sample sizes and under greater control.

RECOMMENDATIONS FOR FUTURE WORK

Important basic questions remain. First, and perhaps most fundamentally, how should the field conceptualize TK? There are several options: (1) include TK as a new (and very broad) Western diagnosis, (2) emphasize the offensive features of TK and formulate them into a specific SAD subtype or possibly a specific standalone diagnosis, (3) "split" TK into several different versions and/or relegate specific symptom sets to existing diagnostic categories (e.g., relegate *shubo-kyofu* symptoms to body dysmorphic disorder), or (4) "lump" TK and other closely related disorders (e.g., SAD, body dysmorphic disorder) into a broad category closer to the original vision of Morita. More empirical and conceptual work is needed to answer the question of how to best conceptualize TK. In particular, the identification of "points of rarity" between TK symptoms and other disorders, if they exist, is of primary importance. At this point in time, it appears reasonable to maintain TK's position as a category worthy of further study, but we imagine that some degree of categorical lumping may be necessary in the future.

Even in the absence of clear diagnostic categories, good empirical work on TK can still commence. Isolating individual symptoms, their relations with other syndromes, and their clinical impacts could be very useful for our understanding of general psychopathology as well as the ways in which symptoms may manifest differently across individuals and cultures.

Existing data are clear that TK symptoms are not limited to one particular culture, but this does not mean that differences in emphasis may not be present or important. Regardless, as noted above, human self-construals are quite nuanced, and we wonder whether a strict reliance on the egocentric/allocentric and individualist/collectivist dichotomies might actually be problematic for understanding TK. For instance, when TK sufferers are interviewed (whether East Asian or not), allocentric concerns are at the forefront (e.g., "I'm afraid X will offend the group"). With additional questioning, however, egocentric fears are just as present and powerful, but discussed less (e.g., "if X offends the group, I will feel bad, guilty, and less adequate"). Thus, allocentric fears seem explicit, but egocentric fears are implicit. If this hypothesis is empirically supported, it would provide additional evidence that TK and SAD are not so distinct.

Other specific recommendations:

- In order to make study comparisons and interpretations of research findings easier, subtypes of TK should be reported if they are assessed.
- Additional psychometric evaluation is needed for existing TK measures.
- New measures, both self-report and interview-based, would be useful for research.
- Evidence suggests that existing SAD treatments may be helpful for TK patients. This should be further assessed with randomized controlled trials (RCTs) and effectiveness studies.

- Psychotherapy researchers should explore whether or not components of Morita therapy could potentially augment cognitive behavioral or other therapy approaches.

REFERENCES

American Psychiatric Association. (1994). *Diagnostic and statistical manual of mental disorders: DSM-IV* (4th ed.). Washington, DC: American Psychiatric Association.

American Psychiatric Association. (2013). *Diagnostic and statistical manual of mental disorders: DSM-V* (5th ed.). Arlington, VA: American Psychiatric Association.

Asakura, S., Tajima, O., & Koyama, T. (2007). Fluvoxamine treatment of generalized social anxiety disorder in Japan: a randomized double-blind, placebo-controlled study. *The International Journal of Neuropsychopharmacology, 10*, 263–274. doi:10.1017/S1461145706006602

Asakura, S., Inoue, T., Kitagawa, N., Hasegawa, M., Fujii, Y., Kako, Y., . . . Nakagawa, S. (2012). Social Anxiety/Taijin-Kyofu Scale (SATS): development and psychometric evaluation of a new instrument. *Psychopathology, 45*, 96–101.

Beard, G.M. (1881). *American nervousness: Its causes and consequences.* New York: G.P. Putnam's Sons.

Chang, S.C. (1984). Review of 1. Yamashita "Taijin-Kyofu." *Transcultural Psychiatric Research Review, 21*, 283–288.

Choy, Y., Schneier, F.R., Heimberg, R.G., Oh, K.S., & Liebowitz, M.R. (2008). Features of the offensive subtype of Taijin-Kyofu-Sho in U.S. and Korean patients with DSM-IV social anxiety disorder. *Depression and Anxiety, 25*, 230–240. doi:10.1002/da.20295

Clarvit, S.R., Schneier, F.R., & Liebowitz, M.R. (1996). The offensive subtype of Taijin-kyofu-sho in New York City: the phenomenology and treatment of a social anxiety disorder. *The Journal of Clinical Psychiatry, 57*, 523–527.

Dinnel, D.L., Kleinknecht, R.A., & Tanaka-Matsumi, J. (2002). A cross-cultural comparison of social phobia symptoms. *Journal of Psychopathology and Behavioral Assessment, 24*, 75–84.

Essau, C.A., Sasagawa, S., Chen, J., & Sakano, Y. (2012). Taijin Kyofusho and social phobia symptoms in young adults in England and in Japan. *Journal of Cross-Cultural Psychology, 43*, 219–232. doi:10.1177/0022022110386372

Feusner, J.D., Phillips, K.A., & Stein, D.J. (2010). Olfactory reference syndrome: issues for DSM-V. *Depression and Anxiety, 27*, 592–599. doi:10.1002/da.20688

Good, B., & Kleinman, A. (1985). Culture and anxiety: Cross-cultural evidence for patterning of anxiety disorders. In A. Tuma & J. Maser's (Eds) *Anxiety and the Anxiety Disorders* (pp. 297–324). Hillside, NJ: Lawrence Erlbaum Associates.

Grom, J.L., & Sharpless, B.A. (2014, August). *Symptoms of taijin kyofusho in a Western sample.* Poster presented at the 122nd annual meeting for the American Psychological Association, Washington, DC.

Heimberg, R.G., Hofmann, S.G., Liebowitz, M.R., Schneier, F.R., Smits, J.A., Stein, M.B., . . . Craske, M.G. (2014). Social anxiety disorder in DSM-5. *Depression and Anxiety, 31*, 472–479. doi:10.1002/da.22231

Hofmann, S.G., Asnaani, A., & Hinton, D.E. (2010). Cultural aspects in social anxiety and social anxiety disorder. *Depression and Anxiety, 27,* 1117–1127. doi:10.1002/da.20759

Iwata, Y., Suzuki, K., Takei, N., Toulopoulou, T., Tsuchiya, K.J., Matsumoto, K., ... Mori, N. (2011). *Jiko-shisen-kyofu* (fear of one's own glance), but not taijin-kyofusho (fear of interpersonal relations), is an east Asian culture-related specific syndrome. *Australian and New Zealand Journal of Psychiatry, 45,* 148–152.

James, R., (2006). Culture-bound syndromes: Taijin-kyofusho. In Y. Jackson (Ed.), *Encyclopedia of multicultural psychology* (pp. 145–146). Thousand Oaks, CA: SAGE Publications.

Kasahara, Y. (1970). Fear of eye-to-eye confrontation among neurotic patients in Japan. In T.S. Lebra and W.P. Lebra (Eds.): *Japanese culture and behavior.* Honolulu: University of Hawaii Press.

Kasahara, Y. (1987, February 13–14). Social phobia in Japan. Paper presented at the First Cultural Psychiatry Symposium between Japan and Korea, Seoul, South Korea

Kelly, M.M., Walters, C., & Phillips, K.A. (2010). Social anxiety and its relationship to functional impairment in body dysmorphic disorder. *Behavior Therapy, 41,* 143–153.

Kim, J., Rapee, R.M., & Gaston, J.E. (2008). Symptoms of offensive type Taijin-Kyofusho among Australian social phobics. *Depression and Anxiety, 25,* 601–608. doi:10.1002/da.20345

Kirmayer, L.J. (1991). The place of culture in psychiatric nosology: Taijin kyofusho and DSM-III-R. *The Journal of Nervous and Mental Disease, 179,* 19–28.

Kleinknecht, R.A., Dinnel, D.L., Kleinknecht, E.E., Hiruma, N., Harada, N. (1997). Cultural factors in social anxiety: A comparison of social phobia symptoms and Taijin Kyofusho. *Journal of Anxiety Disorders, 11,* 157–177.

Kobayashi, N., Kurauchi, S., Sawamura, T., Shigemura, J., Sano, S.Y., & Nomura, S. (2003). Case study: The effect of paroxetine on Taijinkyofusho: A report of three cases. *Psychiatry, 66,* 262–267.

Krieg, A., & Xu, Y. (2015). Ethnic differences in social anxiety between individuals of Asian heritage and European heritage: A meta-analytic review. *Asian American Journal of Psychology, 6,* 66–80.

Krueger, R.F., Chentsova-Dutton, Y.E., Markon, K.E., Goldberg, D., & Ormel, J. (2003). A cross-cultural study of the structure of comorbidity among common psychopathological syndromes in the general health care setting. *Journal of Abnormal Psychology, 112,* 437–447. doi:10.1037/0021-843X.112.3.437

Lee, S., & Oh, K.S., (1999). Offensive type of social phobia: Cross-cultural perspectives. *International Medical Journal, 6,* 271–279.

Lewis-Fernández, R., Hinton, D.E., Laria, A.J., Patterson, E.H., Hofmann, S.G., Craske, M.G., ... Liao, B. (2010). Culture and the anxiety disorders: Recommendations for DSM-V. *Depression and Anxiety, 27,* 212–229.

Maeda, F., & Nathan, J.H. (1999). Understanding taijin kyofusho through its treatment, Morita therapy. *Journal of Psychosomatic Research, 46,* 525–530.

Matsunaga, H., Kiriike, N., Matsui, T., Iwasaki, Y., & Stein, D.J. (2001). Taijin kyofusho: a form of social anxiety disorder that responds to serotonin reuptake inhibitors? *The International Journal of Neuropsychopharmacology, 4,* 231–237.

Mesquita, B., & Frijda, N. (1992). Cultural variation in emotions: A review. *Psychological Bulletin, 112*, 179–204. doi:10.1037/0033-2909.112.2.179

McNally, R.J., Cassiday, K.L., & Calamari, J.E. (1990). Taijin-kyofu-sho in a black American woman: Behavioral treatment of a "Culture-bound" anxiety disorder. *Journal of Anxiety Disorders, 4*, 83–87.

Morita, S. (1998). *Morita therapy and the true nature of anxiety-based disorders (shinkeishitsu).* (A. Kondo, Trans; P. Levine, Ed.). Albany, NY: SUNY Press.

Nakamura, K., Kitanishi, K., Miyake, Y., Hashimoto, K., & Kubota, M. (2002). The neurotic versus delusional subtype of taijin-kyofu-sho: Their DSM diagnoses. *Psychiatry and Clinical Neurosciences, 56*, 595–601.

Nagata, T., Oshima, J., Wada, A., Yamada, H., Kiriike, N., & Iketani, T. (2003). Open trial of milnacipran for Taijin-Kyofusho in Japanese patients with social anxiety disorder. *International Journal of Psychiatry in Clinical Practice, 7*, 107–112. doi:10.1080/13651500310000690

Nagata, T., Wada, A., Yamada, H., Iketani, T., & Kiriike, O. (2005). Effect of milnacipran on insight and stress coping strategy in patients with Taijin Kyofusho. *International Journal of Psychiatry in Clinical Practice, 9*, 193–198. doi:10.1080/13651500510029228

Nagata, T., van Vliet, I., Yamada, H., Kataoka, K., Iketani, T., & Kiriike, N. (2006). An open trial of paroxetine for the "offensive subtype" of taijin kyofusho and social anxiety disorder. *Depression and Anxiety, 23*, 168–174. doi:10.1002/da.20153

Nagata, T., Matsunaga, H., van Vliet, I., Yamada, H., Fukuhara, H., Yoshimura, C., & Kiriike, N. (2011). Correlations between the offensive subtype of social anxiety disorder and personality disorders. *Psychiatry and Clinical Neurosciences, 65*, 341–348. doi:10.1111/j.1440-1819.2011.02224.x

Ono, Y., Yoshimura, K., Sueoka, R., Yamauchi, K., Mizushima, H., Momose, T., . . . Asai, M. (1996). Avoidant personality disorder and taijin kyoufu: Sociocultural implications of the WHO/ADAMHA international study of personality disorders in Japan. *Acta Psychiatrica Scandinavica, 93*, 172–176.

Ono, Y., Yoshimura, K., Yamauchi, K., Asai, M., Young, J., Fujuhara, S., & Kitamura, T. (2001). Taijin Kyofusho in a Japanese community population. *Transcultural Psychiatry, 38*, 506–514. doi: 10.1177/136346150103800408

Oyserman, D., Coon, H.M., & Kemmelmeier, M. (2002). Rethinking individualism and collectivism: Evaluation of theoretical assumptions and meta-analysis. *Psychological Bulletin, 128*, 3–72.

Phillips, K.A., & Menard, W. (2011). Olfactory reference syndrome: demographic and clinical features of imagined body odor. *General Hospital Psychiatry, 33*, 398–406.

Russell, J.G. (1989). Anxiety disorders in Japan: A review of the Japanese literature on Shinkeishitsu and taijinkyōfushī. *Culture, Medicine and Psychiatry, 13*, 391–403.

Simard, V., & Nielsen, T.A. (2005). Sleep paralysis-associated sensed presence as a possible manifestation of social anxiety. *Dreaming, 15*, 245–260. doi:10.1037/1053-0797.15.4.245

Suzuki, K., Takei, N., Kawai, M., Minabe, Y., & Mori, N. (2003). Is taijin kyofusho a culture-bound syndrome? *The American Journal of Psychiatry, 160*, 1358.

Takahashi, T. (1975). A social club spontaneously formed by ex-patients who had suffered from anthropophobia (taijin kyofu (sho)). *International Journal of Social Psychiatry, 21*, 137–140. doi:10.1177/002076407502100209

Takahashi, T. (1989). Social phobia syndrome in Japan. *Comprehensive Psychiatry*, *30*, 45–52.

Takahashi, T., Watanabe, N., Watanabe, T., Fukushima, T., Udagawa, I., Onodera, A., Okuyama, N. (1996). Sei-mariana-ikadaigakubyouin-seishinryohosenta ni okeru tai-jin kyofusho no rinshoteki-kento [A clinical study of anthropophobia in the Center of Psychotherapy, St. Marianna University School of Medicine]. *Moritaryoho-gakkai-zasshi [J Morita Ther]* 7,109–116 [in Japanese].

Tarumi, S., Ichimiya, A., Yamada, S., Umesue, M., & Kuroki, T. (2004). Taijin Kyofusho in university students: Patterns of fear and predispositions to the offensive variant. *Transcultural Psychiatry*, *41*, 533–546. doi:10.1177/1363461504047933

Woody, S.R., Miao, S., & Kellman-McFarlane, K. (2015). Cultural differences in social anxiety: A meta-analysis of Asian and European heritage samples. *Asian American Journal of Psychology*, *6*, 47–55.

World Health Organization. (1992). *The ICD-10 classification of mental and behavioural disorders: clinical descriptions and diagnostic guidelines*. Geneva, Switzerland: World Health Organization.

14

Brain Fag Syndrome

PETER O. EBIGBO, CHIMEZIE LEKWAS ELEKWACHI, AND FELIX CHUKWUNENYEM NWEZE ■

VIGNETTE

Case 1

Mr. A., a 19-year-old male medical student, was referred to the clinic by one of his supervisors. He described his main complaints in the following terms: "Recently I have been having poor concentration, weak memory and heat sensations in my head. This has led to my having low scores on exams. When I noticed that this persisted, I went home to my parents. My mother then quickly took me to a prayer house where they gave me some prayers and they told me that some people, who did not want me to be relevant (i.e., helpful) to my parents, were responsible for my low performance in school" (Ebigbo, Elekwachi, & Nweze, 2015, pp. 315–316). *About a year earlier Mr. A had been performing reasonably well. The problem started, however, as he was approaching his second professional examinations, because these required extensive reading.*

Mr. A. was the second son of three male siblings who were students and doing well. He described his relationship with his mother and father as cordial. Both parents were well educated. As the second child in his family, and considering that his siblings were all doing fine academically, he felt he ought to also be successful in his academic work, and this was a means to help the family. Additional exploration showed he had heard frightful stories about how tough the mock second professional exams were. He was, therefore, afraid to look at all the questions at once, and would instead cover all questions other than the one he was currently answering. In the process of doing this, his mind would go totally blank (i.e., "blackout"). When results were posted, he found that he indeed performed poorly. At this point he became suspicious of what was happening to him and returned home. Mr. A. subsequently was referred to the clinic by his supervisors.

Case 2

U. U. is a 22-year- old, male, Nigerian, single, medical student who was referred to the clinic by his supervisor. His complaint was as follows: "It's happening in my mind. It started as arguments going on in my mind about issues related to God. I subsequently started having a sensation like sharp worms trying to pierce my brain. When these feelings come I attribute them to a spiritual attack and start praying since I cannot concentrate anymore on my studies or read. One day I started notic-ing something like rays of light coming to my body. I also felt as if my clothes were noisy. I feel like a furnace is trying to melt my brain. My brain feels like a stone and a rod are being used to press my brain together. At times I feel like barbed wire is being used to cover my body. Later, I started feeling that my mind was hanging out-side in the air, taken away from me such that I cannot think. Sometimes when I see the breasts of a woman I am attracted to, I look at them, but I struggle with myself whether to continue looking or to stop. If I insist I usually have this sharp pain in my heart and that is the only time I stop looking."

The client reported that these symptoms began approximately one year ago when he was writing a second test during a festive period. Since then his symptoms pro-gressively worsened. The client's complaints of heat in the head, crawling sensations, and dizziness made studying difficult and led to his recent low academic perfor-mance. At the time of assessment his concentration was limited, as was his ability to retain information.

U. U. came from a polygamous family and his parents were both alive. At the time of assessment his father was 85 years old and his mother was 40 years younger. The first wife of his father had three children (two males and one female), but died approximately 10 years ago. The second wife (i.e., the client's mother) had nine chil-dren (seven males and two females). The patient was the eighth child in birth order and the last of the seven males. He described a cordial relationship with his mother and siblings, but there was tension reported between the step-siblings. Because of this, U. U. and his siblings resolved to be independent and successful and not rely on their elder stepbrothers for assistance. The patient also reported a strict religious upbringing. On campus he belonged to one of the charismatic groups (i.e., Roman Catholics whose mode of worship is similar to Pentecostal Christians).

HISTORICAL AND CULTURAL CONTEXT

Brain fag is a form of psychological distress first described in Nigeria by Raymond Prince (1960). The colorful name was created by the students who experienced it. This syndrome was initially believed to be a result of a general brain fatigue (Prince, 1960) with the original symptoms described as: intellectual impairment, sensory impairment (mainly visual), and somatic complaints usually in the form of pain or burning sensations in the head and neck. Other accompanying symp-toms such as lack of concentration or forgetfulness often impeded the student's ability to study. The symptoms occur continuously, which may make patients iso-late themselves from intellectual activities (Prince, 1989). These symptoms also were identified more recently by Ola and Igbokwe (2011).

Although initially observed among the southern tribes of Nigeria (i.e., the Yoruba, Igbo, and other ethnic groups), brain fag syndrome has been reported in other societies (Prince, 1959; 1960). More specifically, it has been found in Uganda (German, German, & Assael, 1971; Minde, 1974), Liberia (Thebaund & Rigamer, 1976), the Ivory Coast (Parin, 1984), and Malawi (Peltzer, 1987). Symptoms of brain fag also have been reported among African students study-ing abroad in Britain (N. Malleson, 1973, personal communication as cited in Minde, 1974). This indicates that brain fag is not peculiar to Africans in Africa, but also found in the African diaspora. The fact that brain fag has been so widely reported supports the notion that the syndrome may not be culture-bound (Prince, 1985). Others have argued, however, that the manifestation of brain fag syndrome among Africans in diaspora indicates that their culture is strong enough to influence them even outside of their original locales (Ebigbo et al., 2015).

Brain fag has been perceived as a very common psychoneurotic syndrome occurring among students and other people in academic settings (Prince, 1960). Jegede (1983), however, observed symptoms among illiterate workers and, there-fore, suggested that theirs did not directly relate to "strain of their brains." Ebigbo et al. (2015) presented cases of brain fag syndrome among nonstudents. They sug-gested that it may not just be a disease entity of its own, but could be a kind of defense mechanism that prevented individuals from full mental breakdown.

ROLE IN CURRENT DIAGNOSTIC SYSTEMS

Globalization has highlighted the potential need for universal diagnostic catego-ries. These categories are important because they help to provide a basis for com-paring similar symptoms of mental illness across different cultures. The *Diagnostic and Statistical Manual of Mental Disorders* (DSM) (American Psychiatric Association, 2013) and *The International Statistical Classification of Diseases and Related Health Problems* (ICD) (World Health Organization, 1992) are the most popular diagnostic systems that have evolved to satisfy this need.

The effort to produce a universal classification of mental illness is of great value. The culture-specific understanding of symptomatic manifestations is of great importance as well, however. Brain fag syndrome instantiates this need because some somatic complaints that accompany brain fag are indeed culture-specific. It is, therefore, important to understand these cultural idioms of dis-tress in order to enable a clear diagnosis (and treatment) of brain fag. We will argue later that brain fag should be placed in the *Glossary of Cultural Concepts of Distress* in the DSM.

The comorbidity of brain fag syndrome with somatization, anxiety, and depres-sion has been documented (Ebigbo et al., 2014). This led to the conceptualization that brain fag may be a variant of one or more of these disorders. Consequently, successful medical treatment using antidepressants and anxiolytics has been reported based on this diagnostic impression (Neki & Marinho, 1968). This common co-occurrence of somatic complaints with depression, anxiety, and brain fag symptoms in Nigeria may lead to some confusion when attempting to diagnose it (Ebigbo et al., 2014). For example, it was noted in ICD-10 (World Health Organization, 1992) that the search for clear distinguishable symptom characteristics of culture-specific disorders such as brain fag have failed. As noted earlier, however, somatization does not predict core symptoms of depression among Nigerians (Okulate et al., 2004; Gureje, et al., 1997). Brain fag, from our understanding, is an entity of its own, but this awaits additional empirical verification. The accompanying somatization communicates the person's worry/problem, anxiety and/or depression are possible consequences of this worry if it is not addressed.

SYMPTOMATOLOGY

The main features of the syndrome as originally described by Prince are: crawling sensations in the head and body, unpleasant cranial symptoms (pain, burning, heat in the head, feelings of vacancy), visual disturbances (dimness of vision, pain in the eyes, and tearing), cognitive impairment (inability to grasp the meaning of written and/or spoken words, inability to concentrate, poor retention) and a variety of other symptoms such as weakness, dizziness, writer's cramp, and migrating pains (Prince, 1960; 1989). Notably, all these symptoms occur when, or are exacerbated by, reading and/or listening to lectures. The symptomatic onset is quite gradual, with the initial somatic symptoms in the head typically occurring prior to the feelings of intellectual impairment. The patient may notice burning sensations in the head while reading. Later, symptoms occur with intellectual activity of any kind. Finally, the symptoms may be present continually and patients may isolate themselves from intellectual activities altogether.

Although infrequent, brain fag symptoms may be found in nonstudents whose work requires regular mental calculations (Ebigbo et al., 2014). Thus, the symptoms appear to function more generally as an expression of psychological distress that reflects pressures emanating from individual or societal expectations. These pressures are perceived to exceed the coping capacities of the individual. The characteristic symptoms may constitute a defensive process, which helps prevent a full-fledged decompensation (i.e., the psychological result of a failure to generate effective coping mechanisms in response to overwhelming stressors as in Ebigbo et al., 2015).

Patients with brain fag syndrome often present with unhappy, tense facial expressions and may demonstrate repetitive gestures. For example, they may frequently pass their hand over the surface of their scalp or rub the vertex of their skull, especially when discussing a question that requires concentration.

PREVALENCE RATE AND ASSOCIATED FEATURES

Brain fag syndrome has been reported to affect 6 to 54 adolescents out of 100 (Ola, Morakinyo, & Adewuya, 2009). There are, however, a wide range of results from other studies, which assessed the prevalence of brain fag symptoms using various symptomatic measures. For example, Fatoye and Morakinyo (2003) found a rate of 22.9% among secondary school students; Morakinyo and Peltzer (2002) found a rate of 13.7% among apprentices; Fatoye (2004) found a rate of 38.9% among university students, and Ola found a rate of 40.2% among senior secondary school students.

Brain fag appears to be more common in males (Prince, 1960; Broffka & Marinho, 1963; Neki & Marinho, 1968; German & Arya, 1969; German & Assael 1971). Ola, Morakinyo, & Adewuya (2009) suggested that the reason for male predominance was that potential female brain fag patients had already been removed from the Nigerian educational system prior to secondary school. Thus, a healthier population of girls than boys remained in higher institutions of learning.

Somatic symptoms are usually comorbid with brain fag (Prince, 1989), depression, and anxiety (Gureje, Ustun, & Simon, 1997). This frequent comorbidity may have prompted earlier clinicians in Africa to view brain fag as a variant of depression (Jegede, 1979). For example, Binitie (1975) extracted items from the *Present State Examination* (Coleman, 2003). The *Present State Examination* is a semistructured interview similar to the *Hamilton Depression Rating Scales* (Hamilton, 1983) designed to provide objective evaluation of symptoms associated with mental disorders (Coleman, 2003). These selected items were administered to patients attending the *Nervous Disease Clinic* Uselu, Benin, Nigeria. These patients had received a prior diagnosis of affective disorder. The same items were administered to a sample of London patients with affective diagnoses. When comparing their scores, Binitie (1975) found a higher factor loading on the somatic items of the *Hamilton Scale* in the Nigerian sample compared with the British sample. This finding led him to conclude that depression among the Benin people of Nigeria presented in a more somatized form. This study supported the view that somatic complaints may indicate depression.

In a recent study by Okulate, Olayinka, and Jones (2004) conducted in Lagos, Nigeria, the researchers set out to determine the diagnostic contributions of somatic complaints to depression. In other words, they wanted to determine to what extent somatic complaints could predict depression. In order to be more culturally specific, they included somatic complaints that have been described as common in Africa. These were heat or "peppery" sensations in the head or body; heaviness or tension in the head; pain; emptiness; feeling of fluid within the head; and/or crawling sensations. Using the *Patient Health Questionnaire* (Spitzer, Kroenke, & Williams, 1999) they made use of the somatic and depression subscales of the questionnaire and omitted the others. A principal component analysis and multiple regressions were used to analyze data collected from 829 participants. The findings of their study suggested that somatic complaints, including the culturally unique ones, did not load with core depressive symptoms. Their study tended to support a multicenter study conducted by the World Health Organization (WHO) in Ibadan, Nigeria, which showed that somatic symptoms were not significantly associated with depression (Gureje, Ustun, & Simon, 1997). In conclusion, Okulate et al. (2004) noted that, given no strong diagnostic weight of somatization to depression among Africans, perhaps the somatic complaints may have more weight with generalized anxiety disorders, panic disorder, obsessive-compulsive disorder, and somatization disorder. The Okulate et al. (2004) study opposed Binitie's (1975) study which studied a similar group of participants. Based on this finding, it is important to follow the recommendation of Ola and Igbokwe (2011) that the diagnosis of brain fag be made on the basis of (a) the presence of the unpleasant sensations around the head/neck and (b) study/concentration difficulties.

THEORIES OF ETIOLOGY

The etiology of brain fag has been somewhat controversial. Prince (1960) made some early speculations linking the disturbance to Westernization. He noted that, prior to the 19th century (when significant European influence began), the written word and student life (which are so intimately bound up with brain fag syndrome) were unknown to the inhabitants of Southern Nigeria. Second, brain fag was rarely seen in Europe among the indigenous Europeans. Prince posited that the illness was related in some way to the fusion of European learning techniques with the Nigerian personality. That meant that the African, not accustomed to a more rigid upbringing, felt overwhelmed when he or she came into contact with grammar schools and their regimented rules (e.g., time to eat, sleep, study, or play). Coupled with the expectations of community members who may have contributed money to send children to school, the children felt pressure to study hard and pass exams in order to pay back the villagers. When taken together, these expectations were hypothesized to result in brain fag.

German et al. (1971) proposed the following etiological factors: isolation from parents, distress over power hierarchies in school between teachers and students, a necessity to communicate in a second language, borderline intelligence, and faulty study habits. Minde (1974) and Morakinyo (1980), however, reported that brain fag syndrome appeared to be unrelated to intelligence and intellectual capacity (Morakinyo, 1985). Furthermore, Guiness (1992) linked five additional factors to the etiology of brain fag: (a) the financial implications of education in terms of a change from subsistence to cash economies; (b) fear of envy and bewitchment; (c) parenting in the pre-school years; (d) academic ability; and (e) attributes of the school.

As noted earlier, it has been suggested that brain fag syndrome may prevent individuals who have it from decompensating into full-fledged psychosis (Ebigbo et al., 2014). This is supported by Durst et al. (1993), who suggested that brain fag may be a coping reaction to immigration and transcultural stress, both of which required massive adaptation.

Other individual characteristics may relate to brain fag. For example, trait neuroticism has been linked to it (Morakinyo, 1980). Some have speculated that a delayed entrance into adulthood (i.e., greater dependency and an external locus of control) may be a developmental background for brain fag. Another developmental contributor could be the internalization of family/community expectations for success. If the student/apprentice is high in neuroticism and/or low in self-esteem, this could lead to feelings of overwhelming pressure, which may result in fear, a lack of concentration, subsequent exam failure, and with the ensuing distress being communicated somatically (heat in the head or crawling sensations, etc.). Depending once again on the personality of the person, symptoms of mild depression and anxiety (e.g., a loss of appetite, palpitations, profuse sweating in the palms, dry mouth) may set in.

If this whole culturally determined constellation is not understood holistically, and if attempts instead are made to classify it using a Western diagnostic category, its diagnosis may be missed and/or an improper treatment may be applied (Ebigbo, 1986).

ASSESSMENT OPTIONS

There are currently limited options for the assessment of brain fag symptoms. The *Brain Fag Syndrome Scale* (BFSS) was developed by Prince (1962) and Morakinyo (1980). The BFSS screens for and diagnoses brain fag syndrome using a 3point scale (0–2, corresponding to never, sometimes, and often). Scores range from 0–14 and a score of 6 or above indicates brain fag. For a diagnosis of brain fag to be made, however, the respondent must obtain a score of 1 or above in either items 1 or 2 and a score of 1 or above in items 4 and 5. Recent psychometric data obtained by Ola and Igbokwe (2011) indicated poor internal consistency (Cronbach's alpha = 0.52) and relatively weak convergent validity with the *State Trait Anxiety Inventory Y1* (r = 0.29; Spielbeger, 1983) and with *State Trait Anxiety Inventory Y2* (r = .28; Spielbeger, 1983). The mean for the BFSS is 6 (Ola & Igbokwe, 2011). The BFSS was predominantly used to assess the manifestation of brain fag symptoms in student populations (Ola & Igbokwe, 2011).

DIFFERENTIAL DIAGNOSIS

In discussing brain fag in Nigeria some authors (e.g., Savage & Prince, 1967) described it as a depressive equivalent or a masked depression. As noted above, brain fag is accompanied by somatic reactions to studying (Prince, 1960), and the context in which these symptoms manifest is important for differential diagnosis. Further, the diagnosis of brain fag should be made after proper medical examinations have ruled out a biological basis for the symptoms.

The proper diagnosis of brain fag is dependent on understanding the somatic complaints. Brain fag symptoms can be differentiated from other, similar conditions (e.g., anxiety disorders, major depressive disorder, and somatization disorder) through cognitive (e.g., lack of concentration, poor retention and understanding of written and spoken language, poor academic performance, momentary "blackouts" in examinations), behavioral (e.g., unpleasant cranial sensations when in intellectually challenging situations, which may result in holding a hand up to the forehead while head is bent forward), and social cues (i.e., an individual with high expectations imposed by the self, the family, or community members).

TREATMENT OPTIONS

Psychopharmacology

Some pharmaceutical options are available for the treatment of brain fag. For example, in Lagos, Nigeria, Neki and Marinho (1968) treated their cases with either antidepressants or tranquilizers (anxiolytics). Although patients in both groups made progress, the group treated with antidepressants had a better outcome. Despite the fact that the group who received antidepressants evidenced a better treatment outcome, it has been noted by many authors in Africa that anxiety is often an important accompaniment of brain fag (Minde, 1974; Thebaud & Rigamar, 1976).

Psychotherapeutic Approach Using Harmony Restoration Therapy/Theory

There is a paucity of research publications regarding using the popular psychotherapy models for managing brain fag. However, presented here is the Harmony Restoration Therapeutic (HRT) framework. This provides a rubric for applying various other forms of psychotherapy in the management of psychological distress (Ebigbo, Elekwachi, & Nweze, 2015).

Harmony Restoration Therapy (HRT; Ebigbo et al., 1995) posits that illness is a result of dysfunctional relationships in one's *cosmos*. The cosmos is an individual's world of relationships and comprises the endocosmos (mind and body relationship), mesocosmos (relationship with animate and inanimate objects of importance such as family members, colleagues, and friends), and exocosmos (one's relationship with beings outside of oneself such as God, gods, ancestors, or spirits). Treatment using HRT aims at repairing dysfunctional relationships through using various psychotherapeutic measures (Ebigbo et al., 1995). HRT is an approach to treatment developed in Nigeria and is based on a particularly Nigerian set of values and world presuppositions. Randomized controlled trials (RCTs) on HRT have yet to be conducted.

APPLYING HARMONY RESTORATION TO BRAIN FAG

Various methods of psychotherapy can be eclectically applied in HRT, such as behavior therapy, psychoanalysis, client-centered therapy, psychodrama, music therapy, or family therapy (Ebigbo, 1995). Further, principles derived from salutogenesis (Antonovsky, 1976), which emphasize what builds health rather than what makes one ill, can also be used. A search for the causes of illness is also important, especially during the stage of mapping out the *cosmogram*. If the dysfunctional relationship is at the *endocosmic* area, cognitive behavior therapies, psychodrama, family therapy, and psychodynamic approaches can be applied. If it is in the *mesocosmic* area, communication therapy (Watzlawick, Beavin, & Jackson, 1967; Watzlawick, Weakland & Fisch, 1974) and psychodynamic therapy (or other interpersonal approaches) can be applied. If there is a lack of harmony in the *exocosmic* area, existential therapies (e.g., logotherapy) could be applied or traditional healers can be sought.

ASSESSMENT AND TREATMENT OF CASE II

The following psychological tests were administered to Case II: *Enugu Somatization Scale* (ESS; Ebigbo, 1982), *Neurotic Illness Questionnaire* (NIQ; Janakiramaiah & Kolkar, 1981), and the *Eysenck Personality Questionnaire* (EPQ; Eysenck & Eysenck, 1975). Results indicated high levels of somatization, anxiety, and depression, and the EPQ indicated that the patient was introverted with high levels of neuroticism. The various relationships in his world were then mapped out (cosmogram). His cosmogram indicated that there was a distortion in the endocosmic/intrapsychic domain (e.g., "it is bad to look at a woman's breasts"). In the mesocosmos, it was discovered that the process of adjustment to campus life was difficult. Not wanting to rely on his elder stepbrother because of a quarrel the two had experienced (i.e., a dysfunctional relationship), he decided to be more independent, work hard, and help his siblings. His expectations for himself were high. His restricted and controlled family environment sharply contrasted with the freedom he found on campus. In the exocosmic area, he experienced a conflict between being a member of a charismatic society (which was consistent with his rigid religious training) and desiring the secular freedoms offered on campus. This resulted in guilty feelings. More specifically, he was unable to resolve the conflict between religious demands for sexual abstinence and his sexual drives. We conceptualized his subsequent crawling sensation as a manifestation of his sexual ambivalence and the barbed wire sensations as indicative of restriction. These symptoms all occurred within the context of a serious determination to succeed in order to defy the negligence of his elder stepbrother. Put simply, these experiences were overwhelming, and led to the development of brain fag syndrome, which served the purpose of giving him some momentary relief from his distress.

Cognitive therapy techniques were applied in order to help him realize that the various sexual urges he experienced were normative. It also was emphasized that he must choose and accept his decision for sexual expression based on maintaining harmony in his own particular world. Second, the patient was encouraged to re-evaluate his personal expectations (e.g., whether or not he would attempt to secure his elder stepbrother's financial help for his studies).

Thus, changes were made to the endocosmic and mesocosmic levels of functioning for this patient.

RECOMMENDATIONS FOR FUTURE WORK

The inclusion of culture-bound syndromes in DSM-IV marked an unprecedented milestone in the history of diagnosis. It also highlighted the need for more studies focusing on syndromes such as brain fag and resulted in better positioning for those who wish to develop research agendas on such syndromes. This was an improvement over previous classifications, which had tended to focus on subsuming the culture-bound syndromes into existing categories (Guarnaccia & Rogler, 1999). The present DSM-5 has no place for brain fag, and it is only mentioned briefly in the entries for *shenjing shuairuo* and *kufungisisa* (APA, 2013). We, therefore, suggest that subsequent editions include an entry on brain fag in the *Glossary of Cultural Concepts of Distress*.

Much more basic research is needed. For example, efforts should be undertaken to determine the actual prevalence rates in clinical and community samples in West Africa and abroad. Furthermore, longitudinal and cross-sectional studies are needed to better understand the relationship of brain fag to other forms of psychopathology, as well as to clarify etiology. There is also a clear need to develop reliable and valid assessment measures. Finally, more work needs to be done to establish empirically supported treatments for this condition.

REFERENCES

American Psychiatric Association. (2013, May 12). *Cultural concepts in DSM -5*. Retrieved from www.psychiatry.org/.../practice/dsm/dsm.../cultural-concepts-in-dsm-d.p

Antonovsky, A. (1993, August–September). A salutogenic orientation. The sense of coherence and psychosomatic medicine. *Paper presented at the World Congress of Psychosomatic Medicine*. Bern, Switzerland.

Binitie, A. (1975). A factor analytical study of depression across cultures (African and European). *British Journal of Psychiatry, 127*, 559–563.

Borrofkka, A., & Marinho, A. (1963). Psychoneurotic syndromes in urbanized Nigerians. *Transcultural Psychiatric Research*, 15 44–46.

Coleman, A.M. (2003). *Oxford dictionary of psychology*. New York: Oxford University Press.

Durst, R., Minuchin-Itzigsohn, S., Jabotinsky-Rubin,K. (1993). "Brain-fag" syndrome: Manifestation of transculturation in an Ethiopan Jewish immigrant. *Israel Journal of Psychiatry and Related Sciences, 30*, 223–232.

Ebigbo, P.O. (1982). Development of a culture specific (Nigeria) screening scale of somatic complaints indicating psychiatrc distrubance. *Culture Medicine and Psychiatry, 6*, 29–43.

Ebigbo, P.O., & Ihezue, U.H. (1981a). "Ogbe-Nje" phenomenon and its meaning for psychotherapy in Nigeria. *Psychosomatische Medizin und Psychoanalyse, 27*, 84–91.

Ebigbo, P.O., & Ihezue, U.H. (1981b). Some psychodynamic observations on the symptom of heat in the head. *African Journal of Psychiatry, 7,* 25–30.

Ebigbo, P.O., & Ihezue, U.H. (1981d). Uncertainty in the use of Western diagnostic illness categories for labelling mental illness in Nigeria. *Psychopathologie Africaine, 18,* 59–74.

Ebigbo, P. O. (1986). A cross sectional study of somatic complaints of Nigerian females using Enugu Somatization Scale. *Culture Medicine and Psychiatry, 10,* 167–186.

Ebigbo, P. O. (1995, July). Harmony restoration therapy: An African contribution to psychotherapy. Paper presented at the annual meeting of the Royal College of Psychiatrists, Riviera Centre Torquay, UK.

Ebigbo, P.O., Elekwachi, C.L., & Nweze, C.F. (2015). Brain fag: New perspectives from case observations. *Transcultural Psychiatry, 52*(3), 311–330. doi:10.1177/1363461514557064

Ebigbo, P.O., Elekwachi, C.L., & Nweze, F.C. (2012). Challenges in the treatment of drug abuse in a Nigerian female health worker: A case study applying the Wawa technique. *Journal of Contemporary Psychotherapy, 42,* 257–264.

Ebigbo, P.O., Elekwachi, C.L., & Nweze, F.C. (2014). Brain fag: A case study showing the diagnosis and therapy in Nigeria. *Jounal of Contemporary Psychotherapy, 44*(4), 263–271. doi:10.1007/s10879-014-9273-0

Ebigbo, P.O., Oluka, J., Ezenwa, M., Obidigbo, G., & Okwaraji, F. (1995). Harmony restoration therapy—An African contribution to psychotherapy. In *The practice of psychotherapy in Africa* (pp. 10–32). Lagos, Nigeria: Chumez.

Eysenck, H.J., & Eysenck, S.B. (1975). *Manual of the Eysenck Personality Questionnaire (adult and junior).* London: Hodder & Stoughton.

Eysenck, H.J., & Eysenck, S.B. (1975). *Manual of the Eysenck Personality Questionnaire.* London: Hodder & Stoughton.

German, G., & Arya, P. O. (1969). Psychiatric morbidity amongst a Ugandan student population. *British Journal of Psychiatry, 115,* 1323–1329.

German, G.A., & Assael, M.I. (1971). Achievement stress and psychiatric disorders amongst students in Uganda. *Israel Annals of Psychiatry and Related Disciplines, 9,* 30–38.

Guarnaccia, P.J., & Rogler, L.D. (1999). Research on culture bound syndromes: new directions. *American Journal of Psychiatry, 158,* 1322–1327.

Guiness, E. A. (1992). Profile and prevalence of brain fag syndrome: psychiatry morbidity in school population in Africa. *British Journal of Psychiatry, 16,* 42–52.

Gureje, O., Simon, G. E., Tevfik, B., Ustun, P. D., & Goldberg, D. P. (1997). Somatization in cross-cultural perspective a World Health Organization Study in primary care. American Journal of Psychiatry, 154, 989–995.

Hamilton, M. (1983). Symptoms and assessment of depression. In E.S. Paykel (Ed.), *Handbook of affective disorders* (pp. 3–11). New York: Guildford Press.

Janakirahmiah, H., & Kolkar, D. (1981). Neurotic illness questionnaire: A brief report. *Indian Journal of Psychological Medicine, 1,* 33–38.

Jegede, R.O. (1983). Psychiatric illness in African students—Brain fag syndrome revisited. *Canadian Journal of Psychiatry, 28* (3), 188–192.

Jegede, R. (1979). Depression in Africans revisited. *African Journal of Medical Science, 8,* 125–132.

Minde, K. (1974). Study problems in Ugandan secondary school students: A controlled evaluation. *British Journal of Psychiatry, 25,* 131–137.

Morakinyo, O. (1980). Psychophysiological theory of a psychiatric illness (the Brain fag syndrome) associated with study among Africans. *Journal of Nervous and Mental Disease, 168*(2), 84–88.

Morakinyo, O. (1985). The brain-fag syndrome in Nigeria: Cognitive deficits in an illness associated with study. *British Journal of Psychiatry, 146*, 209–210.

Neki, J., & Marinho, A.A. (1968, March 5–9). A reappraisal of the brain fag syndrome. Paper presented at 2nd Pan-African Psychiatric Conference. Dakar, Senegal.

Nweze, F.C. (2015). *Personality trait and family and family academic expectation as predictors of brain fag among students.* Anambra, Nigeria: Department of Psychology Nnamdi Azikiwe University Awka.

Okulate, G.T., & Olayinka, M.O. (2004). Somatic symptoms in depression: Evaluation of their diagnostic weight in an African setting. *British Journal of Psychiatry, 184*, 422–427.

Ola, B.A., & Igbokwe, D.O. (2011). Factorial validation and reliablility analysis of the brain fag syndrome scale. *African Health Sciences, 3*, 334–340.

Ola, B.A., Morakinyo, O., & Adewuya, A.O. (2009). Brain fag syndrome—A myth or a realtiy. *African Journal of Psychiatry, 12*, 135–143.

Parin, P. (1984). A case of "brain-fag" syndrome: Psychotherapy of the patient Adou A. In a village of Yosso, Ivory Coast Republic. In W. Muensterberger, B.L. Boyer, & S.A. Grolnick (Eds), *Psychoanalytic study of society* (Vol. 10pp. 1–52). New Jersey: Analytic Press.

Peltzer, K. (1987). *Some contributions of traditional healing practices towards psychosocial health care in Malawi.* Eschborn, Germany: Fachbuchhandlung fur Psychologie.

Prince, R. (1989). The brain fag syndrome. In K. Peltzer & P.O. Ebigbo (Eds.), *Clinical psychology in Africa* (pp. 276–296). Enugu: Working Group for African Psychology.

Prince, R. (1959). The brain-fag syndrome in Nigeria. Review and newsletter. *Transcultural Research in Mental Health Problems, 6*, 40–41.

Prince, R. (1960). The "brain fag" syndrome in Nigerian students. *British Journal of Psychiatry*, 559–570.

Prince, R. (1985). The concept of culture-bound syndromes: Anorexia Nervosa and brain-fag. *Social Sciences and Medicine, 21*(12), 197–203.

Prince, R.H.,(1962). Functional symptoms associated with study in Nigerian students. *West African Medical Journal, 11*, 198–206.

Savage, C., & Prince, R. (1967). Depression among the Yoruba. In W. Muensterberger, & S. Axelrad (Eds.), *The psychoanalytic study of society* (Vol. 4, pp. 83–98).

Spielbeger, C.D. (1983). *Manual for the State Trait Anxiety Inventory: STAI (Form Y).* Palo Alto, CA: Consulting Psychology Press.

Spitzer, R.L., Kronenke, K., & Williams, J.B. (1999). Validation and primary care study. *Journal of American Medical Association, 282*, 1737–1744.

Thebaund, E., & Rigamer, E.F. (1976). Some considerations on student mental health in Liberia. *African Journal of Psychiatry, 1*, 227–232.

Watalawick, P., Weakland, J.H., & Fisch, R. (1974). *Change principles of problem formation and resolution* . New York: Norton.

Watzlawick, P., Beavin, J.H., & Jackson, D.D. (1967). *Pragmatics of human communication: a study of interactional patterns, pathologies and paradoxes.* New York: Norton.

World Health Organization. (1992). *The ICD 10 classification of mental and behavioural disorders.* Geneva: WHO.

15

Jerusalem Syndrome and Paris Syndrome

Two Extraordinary Disorders

ELIEZER WITZTUM AND MOSHE KALIAN ■

VIGNETTE

Jerusalem Syndrome

Maria was a schoolteacher in her mid-thirties, who had come to Jerusalem by herself from the European country where she lived. She had been married for several years, but had no children. Maria was known to suffer from bipolar disorder with recurrent manic or hypomanic episodes, and with long remissions between them. She was regularly on maintenance-treatment pharmacotherapy but stopped medications each time she got pregnant. So far, however, every pregnancy ended in spontaneous abortion. This situation was quite a tragedy for the couple, and her husband tried to convince her to consider adoption. Yet, Maria was worried that the social-service agencies would deny their appeal for adoption because of her psychiatric history. Being a religious woman, she wondered why God punished her repeatedly, denying her the bliss of motherhood. In one of her moments of deep agony, a sudden vision of solace entered her mind. She became convinced that God had destined her to be the mother of the new baby Jesus. She stopped medications again and, without confiding in him about her sudden divine reflection, told her husband she was taking a tour of the Holy Places. On her third day in Jerusalem, she felt some pain in her abdomen and was alarmed by the idea that another miscarriage was impending. She rushed to an emergency room, where she was checked and told that she was not suffering any miscarriage and was not pregnant at all. She could not accept this "verdict," became furious, paranoid and even aggressive, and eventually was referred to psychiatric hospitalization in an acute manic state.

Pharmacotherapy stabilized her condition dramatically and she could establish good rapport with the staff, to whom she revealed her tragic story. After about 10 days she was ready to return for treatment in her country. Yet she insisted on another gynecological check-up and only then she agreed to travel back home.

Paris Syndrome

A 30-year-old Japanese student arrived in September 1994 to study fine arts in Reims. Instead, he remained isolated for two months in Reims, then moved to Paris, where he stayed in a hotel near the Gare du Nord. After a short time, the hotel management contacted the Japanese embassy because of behavioral problems and hallucinatory activity associated with insomnia, anorexia, severe anxiety, and depressed mood, as well as threats to kill both his family and himself. It turned out that he had no prior psychiatric history. He was an only child, attended school until the age of 18, studied in a sewing school for two years, and then worked in a cosmetics company for another two years. He took French lessons in Japan and was keen for a change of atmosphere by studying arts in romanticized France. Since his arrival, however, he had lived in isolation, not communicating, unable to continue his studies or to integrate into the surrounding student milieu. He returned back to Japan escorted by his father.

HISTORICAL AND CULTURAL CONTEXT

Psychogeography and the Role of "A Significant Place"

The affinity of people to a meaningful geographical area is a well-known behavioral phenomenon in the history of human civilization. Some scholars labeled this complex mental relationship with a significant space as "psychogeography." The term was introduced by the psychoanalyst William Niederland, who since the early 1950s published several articles dealing with the symbolism of tunnels and bridges (Stein, & Niederland, 1989).His approach concentrated mainly on associations among unconscious fantasies including sexual fantasies. In a broader sense, this approach was rephrased by Stein (1986) as "psychoanalytic approach of spatial representations." The main idea in this approach is that there are schemes in our mind that represent reality, influenced by various factors such as culture, religion, symbolic systems and fantasies, combined with unconscious elements. Our approach, in turn, reflects an attempt to understand unusual overt behavioral expressions observed in some specific sites, especially in places of unique significance (Witztum & Kalian, 2013).

Sigmund Freud documented one of the earliest professional observations relating to the impact of a significant geographical site on specific mental symptomatology. Being an enthusiastic admirer of Hellenistic culture and a keen self-observer, Freud documented his personal experience of derealization upon arriving at a unique place, referring to his visit to the Acropolis in 1904. Writing home he exclaimed that the experience there had surpassed anything he had ever seen or could imagine (Jones, 1955). The emotional impact of that single incident was so deep, that more than 30 years later in a letter to Romain Roland (Freud, 1964) Freud still remembered in detail his overwhelming psychological experience. It was a peculiar disbelief in the reality of what was before his eyes. He had puzzled his brother by asking him if it was true that they were on the Acropolis. He felt himself being divided into two persons, one who was, in fact, on the Acropolis and another who could not believe that it was so. Another skilled and self-observant traveler was the famous 19th-century French writer Stendhal (Marie Henri Bayle), who gave a vivid description of his sudden "fainting" upon observing a painting by Giotto at the church of Santa Croce in Florence.

Magherini and Zanobini (1987) described a particular form of acute mental reaction arising in art-loving tourists who are overwhelmed by the sight of Renaissance paintings upon visiting Florence. They named this the "Stendhal Syndrome" after the famous French writer. Magherini and Zanobini studied the cases of 107 visitors who required psychiatric hospitalization between the years 1978 and 1986. The analysis of the data revealed that most of them came from European countries and were between 20 and 40 years of age. They were mainly single people who had undertaken an individual journey as opposed to an organized tour. There was no relevant difference between males and females; prognosis was benign and the holiday was only temporarily interrupted. In recent years there have been reports of peculiar mental breakdown observed in Japanese tourists visiting Paris, and possibly in Chinese tourists, too. Their symptoms included anxiety attacks as well as feelings of estrangement and dissociative reactions.

Another striking phenomenon is the so-called White House Syndrome, observed in Washington DC. This relates to psychotic tourists, mainly schizophrenics, who demand to meet the American president or who claim they are presidents themselves. About one hundred of them are hospitalized each year (Sebastiani & Foy, 1965; Shore et al., 1985).

Odd behavior labeled as "Jerusalem syndrome" was observed in tourists and pilgrims who upon arriving at the Holy City began to perceive themselves as biblical or prominent figures with special messianic missions (Kalian & Witztum, 1998; Witztum, Kalian, & Brom, 1994).

There are noticeable differences among these site-related "syndromes" derived from the symbolic significance of each site. Florence is perceived as the shrine of Renaissance arts, exhibiting an overwhelming wealth of colossal classical works, which symbolize a turning point in the history of Christian humanism. The 15th-century Renaissance works reflect a religious philosophy that no longer views life as a vale of tears but as a quest for enlarging man's powers, and likewise his awareness of God. Paris is perceived by some Japanese tourists, who have long anticipated their visit, as a destination of romanticized fantasy, expected to be almost the ultimate representation of candid yet profound Western civilization, a beautiful city of culture and fashionable good-mannered inhabitants. With such mounting expectation regarding their visit to the city, and the clash with reality upon their arrival, emerges an acute form of inevitable culture shock. The White House in Washington, DC is regarded by some generations as a symbol of the mightiest earthly powers. It symbolizes a modern political philosophy, wherein a mortal is elected by the people for the people and is granted the power to influence global affairs. The building is a symbol of human superpower; thus, becoming a magnet for those peculiar visitors who aspire to influence major local or global affairs.

The significance of Jerusalem as a unique symbol is totally a spiritual one. It is embedded in both Jewish and Christian religious history as well as messianic traditions, and its uniqueness is derived from being perceived as "the center of the world"—a place where the last episode of doomsday will occur at the end of times. The so-called Jerusalem Syndrome is thus considered to be related to the spiritual significance of the city.

City Syndromes

Another attempt to formulate psychological reactions of visitors to significant urban settings was labeled as "city syndromes" (Halim, 2010). This theory claims that over the last few decades a cluster of psychiatric syndromes has emerged in several of the world's most revered travel destinations. "These disorders strike tourists, usually shortly after their arrival in a city, and appear to be triggered by the historical, aesthetic, or spiritual intensity of the place. Symptoms range from anxiety and panic attacks, through visual and aural hallucinations, to full-blown psychotic episodes." Halim claims that newspapers around the world periodically run "News of the Weird" stories about them, with headlines like "Visiting Jerusalem Can Spark a Psychotic Reaction" or "Florence's Art Makes Some Go to Pieces" (Halim, 2010).

The Phenomenology of Tourist Experience

Eliade (1971) pointed out that every religious "cosmos" possesses a "center" that is preeminently the zone of the sacred, the core of absolute reality, "where the *axis mundi* penetrates the earthly sphere." Cohen (1979, 1984) developed a phenomenological typology of tourist experiences based on Eliade's concept of "the quest for the center." The "center" may not be geographically central to the life space of the community of believers, and according to Turner (1973) an *ex-centris* location "may give direction and structure to pilgrimage"—a sacred journey of spiritual ascension to "the center out there." Cohen's typology of tourist experience seems to be most compatible with our approach. He describes five modes of tourism: The recreational—typical of modern man whose trip is akin to other forms of modern entertainment, and represents a movement away from the center. The diversionary—representing an escape from the boredom and emptiness of everyday routine—characterized by alienated tourists who merely enjoy their holiday or "have a good time." The experiential—expresses a desire to experience vicariously the authentic life of others. The experimental—in which tourists actually try out various other lifestyles in an effort to discover which one they would like to adopt. The fifth mode—the existential—involves travel to an elective spiritual center and is regarded as analogous to pilgrimage. Cohen concluded that tourism is principally a modern metamorphosis of pilgrimage, yet secularization has destroyed the deep structural themes and much of their symbolic significance and mystical powers. This has transformed their loci to "places of attraction" or mere destinations.

Historical and Cultural Background of "Jerusalem Syndrome"

The Judeo-Christian tradition is constructed around messianic aspirations in which the *axis mundi* of faith—the holy city of Jerusalem—is perceived as the arena where great dramatic events are about to occur. This eschatological core element is at times exploited in a broader sense in the service of a public or an individual, to the extent where boundaries between reality and imagination are blurred. Discussing the spiritual magnetism of Jerusalem from an anthropological point of view, Bowman (1992) stressed that "the visions of pilgrims, as presented in the massive body of their writings, provide a glass through which we can clearly trace transformations of European beliefs and perceptions. Jerusalem, the Holy City, is regarded a sacred space for all three monotheistic religions" (in our study we focus on Judaism and Christianity).

Jewish pilgrimage to Jerusalem goes back as a custom since the era of the first temple, and exists in Christianity since its earliest days. It became an established model of worship by Christians in the fourth century. Turner defined this phenomenon as a "prototypical" pilgrimage, in which the spiritual content of the act is directly related to the life of the founder of the faith and to geographical sites where major events in the history of the religion took place (Turner, 1978).

The Messianic Idea and Millenarianism

The messianic idea was originated and is still embedded in the Jewish faith. It is based on the belief that the Messiah—a descendent of King David—will be revealed and usher in a series of events. The Messiah shall break the regime of foreigners, revive the kingdom of Israel, and gather its children from the Diaspora. In addition, the temple in Jerusalem will be rebuilt and the work of sacrifice reestablished. Messianism was born during the post-biblical era, and it reappears repeatedly throughout history with each generation, reflecting a new set of ideas. The practice of defining the Messiah as an eschatological figure originates from the apocalyptic literature of the second temple contemporaries. Calculations and speculations regarding the date of redemption have been part of Jewish culture since the Middle Ages and continue into modern times. A central theme in Christian eschatology is the expectation of the Second Advent of Christ and the establishment of the kingdom of God on earth, based on interpretations of the book of Daniel and the book of Revelation to John. According to this somewhat mythological approach, the rule of the Antichrist will inflict upon earth a set of disasters. Yet, finally, redemption will occur, with its climax in the fall of the Great Babel and the overthrow of Satan and his aids, who will be doomed to incarceration in Hell for a thousand years ("the millennium"). At the end of the millennium, there shall be the war of Gog and Magog with the triumph of Good over Evil. The results shall lead to the resurrection of the dead and the establishment of the new Jerusalem (Witztum, 1987). Millenarian movements have been known to appear since the Middle Ages (Cohn, 1970). Millenarians tend to adopt the "method" of attaching biblical quotations to contemporary events, thus "confirming" current events as significant "markers" of the approaching redemption.

Historical and Cultural Background of "Paris Syndrome"

"Paris syndrome" is regarded as a type of cultural shock affecting some Japanese tourists who visit the city. In general, international tourists are the largest group of people exposed to cross-cultural experiences, and their number is steadily increasing. Research has confirmed that being a tourist can be a stressful experience. Additional consideration is given to the consequences of "culture shock" for intercultural relations, including the attitudes and perceptions of tourists and members of the host society. The culture-shock hypothesis or "concept" implies that the experience of visiting or living in a new culture is an unpleasant surprise or a shock, partly because it is unexpected, and partly because it may lead to a negative evaluation of one's own and/or the other culture (Furnham, 1997, Ward, Bochner, & Furnham, 2001). The anthropologist Oberg (1960) was the first to use the term and mentions at least six aspects of culture shock:

1. Strain due to the effort required to make necessary psychological adaptations.
2. A sense of loss and feelings of deprivation in regard to friends, status, profession, and possessions.
3. Being rejected by and/or rejecting members of a new culture.
4. Confusion in role, role expectations, values, feeling, and self-identity.
5. Surprise, anxiety, even disgust and indignation, after becoming aware of cultural differences.
6. Feelings of impotence due to not being able to cope with he new environment.

Bock (1970) described culture shock as primarily an emotional reaction resulting from inability to understand, control, and predict another's behavior. When customary experiences no longer seem relevant or applicable, peoples' usual behavior becomes "unusual." Lack of familiarity with the local milieu (etiquette, ritual) has this effect, as well as experiences related to the use of time.

Culture shock is regarded nowadays as a temporary stress reaction wherein salient psychological and physical rewards are generally uncertain, and hence, difficult to control or predict. Thus a person is anxious, confused, and apparently apathetic until he or she has had time to develop a new set of cognitive constructs to understand and enact the appropriate behavior.

Many Asian tourists regard Paris with an mixture of idealization and fantasy. They perceive the city as a highly romanticized destination—the cobblestone streets as seen in the film *Amelie*, the beauty of French women, or the high culture and art at the Louvre. Given such idealization, facing reality may yield disappointment, frustration, and shock. Since the 19th century, the Japanese have idealized France, and especially Paris, as a cultural symbol. From 1860 to 1930, mostly students traveled there to experience European culture and a visit to Paris was a status symbol. After World War II, when Japan was under U.S. occupation, the trip symbolized the assimilation of Westernization, with the idea that Europe was the origin of American culture. In the 1970s, economic prosperity led to the democratization of travel, first mainly for business purposes and then extending to vacations by couples and families, either in organized tours or just individually. The number of Japanese travelers continued to grow (Viala et al., 2004) and several surveys revealed that Western destinations were highly popular among them. Even now, Paris remains a magic attraction and the symbol of European culture—an image amplified by the multitude of modern media channels. The main sources of its attraction are the arts and the culture, as well as local history, cooking, and fashion (Viala et al., 2004). Only a few Japanese speak French and the ensuing communication difficulties may be a source of gross errors, displacement, anxiety, and feelings of isolation. It should be noted that contrary to Japanese mentality, the Latin culture of France allows mood swings and attitudes to interfere with interpersonal behavior. Such direct interventions, sometimes excessive, even eccentric and disconcerting, can be generators of misunderstanding and misinterpretation. Japanese sociability is based on group membership. Isolated from their community, they can take refuge in silence or display a fixed smile as a means of protection, up to the point of isolation or prostration. In such a context, disappointment derived from contact with the daily local reality could yield disillusionment and depression, as well as fear and misunderstanding (Viala, et al., 2004).

The first afflicted Japanese tourists were recognized in 1988 by Professor Hiroaki Ota (1988), a Japanese psychiatrist working in France. His findings soon resulted in media curiosity and attention. Newspapers, as well as the British Broadcasting Corporation (BBC) (Wyatt, 2006), vividly described the sort of "shocking experiences," encountered by Japanese tourists, experiences that might merely elicit a laugh from a Western tourist; for example, an encounter with a rude local taxi driver or a Parisian waiter who shouts at customers who cannot speak fluent French. It seemed that for some Japanese tourists, arriving from a civilization characterized by significant politeness, where angry voices are seldom raised, "the experience of their dream-city turning into a nightmare can simply be too much." (Ota, 1988).

An Emerging Chinese "Paris syndrome"?

It appears that Chinese tourists are now walking down the path already trod-
den by the Japanese. The growing number of Chinese tourists arriving in Paris
armed with wads of cash, typically unable to speak French and still somewhat
naïve about the ways of the West after decades of China's relative isolation, are
falling victim to their unrealistic expectations of the city, while also being vic-
timized by brazen thieves who target them because they are easily identifiable
as Asians. Chinese tourism industry officials warned that the risk to Chinese
tourists from Parisian bandits is so acute that the Chinese government recently
considered sending police officers to Paris to help protect them. Parisian tourism officials said the proposal was shelved amid concerns over how such officers
would operate. Psychologists warned that Chinese tourists shaken by thieves,
and with their expectations dashed, were at risk for Paris Syndrome. Chinese
newspapers recently reported that like their Japanese counterparts—an epidemic
is gripping Chinese tourists visiting the French capital when they confront the
clash between their romanticized image of Paris and the crude reality. "They
know about French literature and French love stories," said Jean-Francois Zhou,
president of the Chinese association of travel agencies in France. But some of
them end up in tears, swearing they "ll never come back." No serious study or
survey of psychiatric morbidity among Chinese tourists in Paris has been published yet; however, it appears as though they are about to be or already are the
new victims of Paris syndrome.

ROLE IN CURRENT DIAGNOSTIC SYSTEMS

Neither Jerusalem syndrome nor Paris syndrome are included in the *Diagnostic
and Statistical Manual of Mental Disorders* (DSM-5; American Psychiatric
Association, 2013) or the *International Classification of Diseases* (ICD; World
Health Organization, 1992). We, the authors, see these syndromes as culture-
bound syndromes. The DSM-5 prefers another formulation—"cultural conceptualizations of distress," which describes cultural constructs that influence the
way in which an individual experiences, understands, and communicates his
or her symptoms or problems to others. "These constructs may include cultural
syndromes, idioms of distress, and explanatory models or perceived causes." We
believe that the formulation chosen in the DSM-5 includes the cultural and symbolic elements of these syndromes and their explanatory models. However, the
symptoms could be coded only as a type of *Unspecified Mental Disorder*.

Disagreement about city syndromes tend to hinge on whether they fit into
our psychiatric taxonomy, or whether it is more appropriate to read them
as cultural phenomena. Based on secondary sources, Halim (2010) tried to
generalize city syndromes "as acute and short-lived disorders that share similar symptoms and common patterns of onset and recovery, seen in popular
tourist-destination cities and diagnosed by local psychiatrists." These include

Paris syndrome, Stendhal syndrome (Florence), and Jerusalem syndrome. We prefer a broader approach, based mainly on the concept of psychogeography (Witztum, Kalian, 2013).

SYMPTOMATOLOGY

Jerusalem Syndrome

Examination of the behavior of the patients before admission shows that deviant behavior, including excessive preaching and vagrancy, was found in 33%. Manifestations of aggression, such as physically attacking people or threatening them with a weapon, led to the admission of 11%; another 11% were walking around naked when apprehended and referred to hospital. Some 13% were admitted after attempting suicide. The psychiatric diagnoses were: schizophrenia—49 cases, acute psychosis—14 cases, affective psychosis—11 cases, personality disorder—7 cases, dementia—2 cases, and "other"—6 cases (some patients had more than one psychiatric diagnosis; Bar-El, Witztum, & Kalian et al., 1991).

Paris Syndrome

Paris syndrome is a mental condition in which foreigners suffer depression, anxiety, feelings of persecution, and even hallucinations, when their rosy images of champagne, majestic architecture, and Monet paintings clash with reality and are upended by local stresses.

A decade after Ota's intriguing findings, Katada (1998) gave a vivid description of a single case. It concerned a manic-depressive patient who suffered symptoms of insomnia, mood swings, aggression, irritation, and increased sex drive shortly after visiting Paris. Katada claimed that the broken fantasy and idealization of Paris played a major role in this patient's abnormal behavior, as did his separation from his family, and his solitude in Paris, where he was no longer regarded as a father or a professor.

DSM-IV diagnoses of patients with "Paris syndrome" were (according to Viala et al., 2000): schizophrenia = 23, schizophreniform disorder = 4, schizoaffective disorder = 9, acute delusional state = 11, induced psychotic disorder toxic substance = 1, major depressive state = 4, manic state = 6, disorder due to a general medical condition = 4, anxiety disorders: social phobia = 1.

PREVALENCE RATE AND ASSOCIATED FEATURES

"Jerusalem syndrome" and "Paris syndrome" are two rare phenomena, named after the loci where psychiatric clinical pictures of afflicted tourists are revealed and related directly to the city, at times leading to hospitalization.

Jerusalem Syndrome

Approximately 40 years after the first psychiatric observations of the so-called Jerusalem syndrome were published by Dr. Heintz Herman (1937), Kfar-Shaul Psychiatric Hospital started to admit all foreign tourists in the Jerusalem area in need of psychiatric hospitalization. This was an administrative arrangement designed by the ministry of health, because residents of Jerusalem at that time were referred to three other local psychiatric hospitals in the vicinity. In the first year, only 25 tourist-patients were admitted. With the increased influx of tourists, however, the average number of admissions climbed to 50 patients per annum.

For several years, comprehensive statistical data have been gathered regarding the hospitalized tourists. The most extensive data, on which our findings are based, were collected during 1986 and 1987 from a group of 89 tourists (Bar-El et al., 1991). Data from this group were compared with the demographic data of an earlier study of 177 tourists hospitalized in the same hospital between 1979 and 1984 (Kalian, Eisenberg, & Bar-El, 1985). No differences were found regarding age, sex, marital status, religion, country of origin, method of referral, and number of previous visits to Israel. The group studied in 1986–1987 comprised 32 women and 57 men whose mean age was 32.4 years; 74% were single, 15% were divorced, and only a minority—11%—were married. Some 52% had received 13 or more years of education, 36% had between 8 and 12 years of education, while 7% had received less than five years of education. Most tourists came from North America (40%) and Western Europe (44%); the remainder came from Eastern Europe, South America, South Africa, or elsewhere. Recreational tourism was the mode for 38% of our group. Some 26% came for reasons of a mystical/religious nature. About 15% were visiting relatives and 7% came to do volunteer work. The experiential mode, that is, trying out a new lifestyle, provided the chief impetus for 11% of our group. These people came to learn and considered staying.

To bring the nexus between religion and their illness into sharper focus, patients were asked to describe the nature of their experience at the time of their admission. Forty percent reported mystical experiences, and the majority of these believed they were a mystical/religious figure. Twenty-four patients (27%) thought they were the messiah, four patients felt they were God, three patients identified with Satan, and another seven patients identified with biblical figures. Although the overlap was not perfect, most of the people who reported a mystical experience were the ones who identified with these figures. An interesting phenomenon is that mystical experiences were more frequent in patients with a Roman Catholic background than in Jewish or Protestant patients.

Our assumption that people suffering an acute psychotic episode during a journey had previous psychiatric problems was confirmed: 82% of the patients in our survey had a psychiatric history dated and documented before they set out for their journey to Jerusalem. For 18% of the patients, however, there was no clear previous documentation dating from before their odd behavior emerged in Jerusalem. Still, no differences appeared in the demographic variables, purpose of their journey, religious involvement, or the nature of their religious delusions.

Paris Syndrome

A group of French psychiatrists in collaboration with Dr. Ota (a consultant to the Japanese embassy) published in 2004 the only significant work regarding Paris syndrome. According to their study, 63 Japanese tourists were hospitalized between 1988 and 2003. Of these, 34 were women, 29 men, aged 20 to 65 years (50% were between 20 and 30 years of age). The presenting symptoms included wandering; psychomotor agitation; car breakdown; trying to jump from trains; aggression against themselves or others; suicide attempts; delusions—often with persecutory content; at times megalomaniacal, maniacal, erotomanic, or mystical delusions. Other prominent clinical findings were anxiety states—often in connection with a state of strangeness, as well as derealization, depersonalization, or dissociation. Not surprisingly, many showed reluctance to cooperate, a response obviously increased by the cultural gap and the comprehension difficulties experienced in the hours or days before hospitalization.

Viala and his group named two types of pathological reactions: the "Classic Travel Reaction" ("type 1") and the "Delayed Expression" ("type 2"; Viala et al., 2004). "Type 1" relates to exacerbation of an underlying psychotic disease, such as schizophrenia or mood disorder, with current content linked directly to the trip. A medical history often reveals previous psychiatric diagnoses as well as hospitalizations. Symptoms may be triggered by the trip itself and occur upon arrival at the airport or in the following days; for example, a 39-year- old woman, hospitalized in an acute psychotic state with megalomaniacal delusions claiming to be the Queen of Sweden, Finland, and Denmark. In this case, the initiating trigger was an advertising poster on the walls of the Tokyo subway announcing, "France is waiting for you." She believed it was a sign directed personally toward her, so she set out for the trip. While hospitalized in Paris, it was discovered that she had a history of psychiatric hospitalizations since the age of 19. After two weeks in a psychiatric ward in Paris, she returned home accompanied by her family to continue treatment in Tokyo.

"Type 2" individuals demonstrate their initial pathological manifestations at least three months after their arrival. The motivation for the trip is not necessarily unusual or weird, and there is typically no previous psychiatric history. The affected individuals often are considered fragile personalities trying to flee integration problems in their homeland, or seeking liberation from traditional or conservative family ties (e.g., work, marriage). They usually manifest an identity crisis, searching for an "ideal elsewhere." Once hospitalized, their condition often makes their treatment, as well as their return, most complicated (e.g., see case vignette).

THEORIES OF ETIOLOGY

The two syndromes demonstrate a set of differences; however, there is one striking similarity regarding the clinical background of the affected individuals. In Jerusalem, the afflicted individuals are either regular tourists or pilgrims of various nationalities as well as religions, and the syndrome is related directly to the historical and religious significance of the city. Since the Middle Ages, well-documented travel literature regarding Jerusalem has included vivid descriptions of the syndrome. In Paris, the afflicted are Japanese tourists (and recently perhaps Chinese, too).Their breakdown is related mainly to culture shock resulting from the clash between two entirely different cultures. Culture shock is considered to be a product of the massive increase in global travel since the 20th century. It also has been suggested that a major contribution to the emergence of "Paris syndrome" is the clash between reality and the romanticized image of Paris in the eyes of the Japanese visitor.

Therefore, while Jerusalem syndrome represents an idiom of distress by a visitor who came to the city because of its deep spiritual significance, Paris syndrome is mainly a psychological breakdown enhanced by culture shock, disappointment, and the collapse of an illusion.

Interestingly, for groups in both Paris and Jerusalem, there was clear evidence of psychiatric history prior to arrival. This finding is not surprising, however, given that one can expect fragile individuals to be more vulnerable in extreme affect-laden situations. In recent years, apart from the syndromes already mentioned, there have been a considerable number of publications relating to psychopathology demonstrated in a specific geographical space (e.g., "Honeymoon psychosis" in Hawaii; "Airport wanderers" in Kennedy airport; "Death in Venice" by suicidal Europeans (Stainer et al., 2001); "Eilat syndrome" in Israel (Belhassen, 2012). It seems that none of these syndromes are purely medical entities. People who demonstrate these "syndromes" basically suffer from well-known psychiatric clinical entities; however, the narrative and the content of their thoughts and actions are clearly related to the cultural, historical, religious, or political significance of the place where the "syndrome" appeared, as well as to the patient's personal background. It has been suggested that these breakdowns were due to feelings of incompatibility in those who felt alienated, ridiculed, and incompetent—a shameful experience in the face of intimidating strangers.

ASSESSMENT OPTIONS

Assessment options include a standard psychiatric interview and examination. In our study, we used questionnaires that included a demographic section and a section designed to reveal cultural and religious components (e.g., mystical experiences; identification with religious figures), as well as semistructured interviews (e.g., in Florence, concerning Stendhal syndrome, we asked questions such as, "What kind of art and artists do you admire?" "What was your most exciting experience in the city?" and "To which work of art do you feel especially attached?").

DIFFERENTIAL DIAGNOSIS

Clinicians who are likely to encounter these "syndrome" phenomena should be aware of the historical and the culturally symbolic background of the content expressed by the patient. Assessing the basic psychopathology behind the colorful and idiosyncratic mask is, however, essential. The clinician should remember that the patients could be diagnosed as suffering from paranoid schizophrenia, yet concerning the content of their delusions, hallucinations, and their explanatory model, patients could be included within the framework of culture-bound syndromes like Jerusalem syndrome as well as city syndromes such as Paris syndrome.

TREATMENT OPTIONS

Jerusalem Syndrome

Basically, treatment options are not grossly different from standard psychiatric approaches. Once diagnosis is established, psychopharmacology should be prescribed in accordance with the basic clinical picture (antipsychotics, anxiolytics, and mood stabilizers, when indicated). Once hospitalized, it is essential to maintain contact with the hospital staff, to inform the local consulate of the patient's condition as well as any legal complications, and to establish contact with the patient's family and psychiatrist (if applicable). Coordinated visits are advised in order to reduce feelings of estrangement and isolation. Of course, verbal communication with professionals who understand the patient's language is highly recommended. Having gained some initial insight, patients are encouraged to continue therapy upon their return home.

Paris Syndrome

The standard pharmacological approach is universal and basically the same, including antipsychotics, anxiolytics, and mood stabilizers, when indicated. Dr. Ota assisted with verbal interviews, allowing patients to express themselves in their own language, as well as to be reassured about the treatment plan set up for them, with the possibility of psychotherapeutic interviews as soon as the patient's condition allowed. Because most patients did not benefit from insurance coverage in France, it was advised that their stay should be as short as possible. The average length of stay was about two weeks.

It is advised that people with formal psychiatric history should travel only in periods of good remission of their illness, and not travel solitarily. They should be furnished with medical insurance, a letter from their doctor, and prescribed medications sufficient to maintain their good psychiatric remission. Long-distance flights, as well as rapid time-zone changes, should be minimized if not avoided. An accompanying responsible adult is essential. If traveling in a tour group, the tour leader should be made aware of the patient's condition. It also is advised that the group leader be made aware of pertinent local medical and psychiatric services. The utilization of a local psychiatrist is recommended once exhilaration is spotted to be accompanied by clear disturbance of sleep, odd behavior, or odd verbal content. In such cases, it is never too early for psychiatric consultation, which could avoid further deterioration and undesirable hospitalization, an event that is always perceived as traumatic by the patient.

RECOMMENDATIONS FOR FUTURE WORK

Several "syndromes" have been named after a major city or a significant place. As stated in our study, the historical–religious uniqueness of Jerusalem was a powerful factor contributing to the emergence of the "syndrome," as opposed to the "culture shock" that characterizes "Paris syndrome." Culture shock has been studied around the globe. Psychological reactions by tourists and pilgrims at significant destinations deserve further study. We believe that preliminary caution and early guidance could serve as valuable preventive factors for those at risk for breakdown. Such an assumption, however, deserves further study. There is also too little attention paid to factors yielding breakdown of pilgrims and tourists visiting other significant religious places, such as Mecca or Vatican City in Rome. It is recommended that further studies regarding such significant places be carried out, as well as a multinational study comparing the various sites, with emphasis on clinical pictures, etiological and epidemiological issues, and modes of prevention and treatment.

REFERENCES

American Psychiatric Association. (2013). *Diagnostic and statistical manual of mental disorders, DSM-5*. Arlington, VA: American Psychiatric Association.

Bar-El, Y., Witztum, E., Kalian, M., & Brom, D. (1991). Psychiatric hospitalization of tourists in Jerusalem. *Comprehensive Psychiatry, 32*, 238–244.

Belhassen, Y. (2012). Eilat Syndrome: deviant behavior among temporary hotel workers. *Tourism Analysis, 17*, 673–677.

Bock, P. (Ed.) (1970). *Culture shock: A reader in modern psychology.* New York: A. A. Knopf.

Bowman, G. (1992). Pilgrim narrative of Jerusalem and the Holy Land: A study in ideological distortion. In A. Morinis (Ed.), *Sacred journeys: The anthropology of pilgrimages* (pp. 149–168). Westport, CT: Greenwood.

Cohn, N. (1970). *The pursuit of the millennium.* Oxford: Oxford University Press.

Cohen, E.A. (1979). Phenomenology of tourist experiences. *Sociology, 12*, 179–201.

Cohen, E. (1984). The sociology of tourism: Approaches, issues, and findings. *Annual Review of Sociology, 10*, 373–392.

Eliade, E. (1971). *The myth of eternal return.* Princeton, NJ: Princeton University Press.

Furnham, A. (1997). Culture shock, homesickness, and adaptation to a foreign culture. In M. van Tilburg & A. Vingerhoets (Eds.), *Psychological aspects of geographical moves: homesickness and acculturation stress* (pp 17–35). Amsterdam: Amsterdam University Press.

Halim, N. (2010). *Mad Tourists: The Vectors and Meanings of City-Syndromes.* Retrieved from www.interisciplinary.net/ptb/persons/madness/m1/halim%20paper.pdf

Herman, H. (1937). Psychiatrisches aus Palastina, *Folia Clinica Orientalia, 1,* 232–237 .

Freud, S. (1964). A disturbance of memory on the Acropolis. In *Standard edition of the complete psychological works of Sigmund Freud, Vol. 22* (pp. 239–248). London: Hogarth.

Jones, E. (1955). *The life and work of Sigmund Freud, Vol. 2,* New York: Basic Books.

Kalian, M., Eisenberg, M., & Bar-El, Y. (1985). Tourists who need psychiatric hospitalization: Population characteristics and treatment principles. *Proceedings of the First International Congress on Hospital Laws,* Tel Aviv, Israel.

Kalian, M., & Witztum, E. (1998). Facing a holy space: Psychiatric hospitalization of tourists in Jerusalem. In B.Z. Kedar & R.J.Z.W. Werblowsky (Eds.), *Sacred space: shrine, city, land* (pp. 316–330). NewYork: New York University Press.

Katada, T. (1998). Reflections on a case of Paris syndrome. *Journal of the Nissei Hospital, 26(2),* 127–132.

Magherini, G., & Zanobini, A. (1987). "Eventi e psicopatologia: Il perturbante turistico: nota preleminare," *Rassegna Studio Psichiatrici, 74,* 1–14.

Oberg, J. (1960). Culture shock: Adjustment to new cultural environments. *Practical Anthropology, 7,* 177–182.

Ota, H. (1988). Voyages et déplacements pathologiques des japonais vers la France. *Nervure, 6,* 12–16.

Sebastiani, J.A., & Foy, J.L. (1965). Psychotic visitors to the White House. *American Journal of Psychiatry, 122,* 679–686.

Shore, D., Filson, C.R., Davis, T.S., Olivos, G., Delisi, L., & Wyat, G.R. (1985). "White House Cases": Psychiatric Patients and the Secret Service. *American Journal of Psychiatry, 142(3),* 308–312.

Stainer, D., Ramacciotti, F., & Colombo, G. (2001). Death in Venice: Does a laguna syndrome exist? *Minerva Psichiatrica, 42,* 125–140.

Stein, H.F. (1986). The influence of psychogeography upon the conduct of international relations: Clinical and metapsychological considerations. *Psychoanalytic Inquiry,* 6,193–222.

Stein, H.F., & Niederland, W.G. (1989). *Maps from the mind: Readings in psychogeraphy.* Norman, OK: University of Oklahoma Press.

Turner, V. (1973). The center out there: The pilgrim's goal. *History of Religion, 12,* 191–210.

Turner, V. (1978). *Image and pilgrimage in Christian culture.* Oxford: Blackwell.

Viala, A., Ota., H., Vacheron, M.N., Martin, P., & Caroli, F. (2004). Les Japonais en voyage pathologique à Paris: un modèle original de prise en charge transculturelle. *Nervure Supplément 5,* 31–34.

Ward, C.A., Bochner, S., & Furnham, A. (2001). *The psychology of culture shock.* East Sussex: :Routledge.

Wyatt, Caroline. (2006). *Mastering French manners, the hard way.* BBC News. Retrieved April 19, 2015.

Witztum, E., Kalian, M., & Brom, D. (1994). Pilgrims' perils: Breakdown in Jerusalem. In *Medical and health annual.* Chicago, IL: Encyclopedia Britannica.

Witztum, E. (1987). Doomsday prophets, millenarians, and messiahs in Jerusalem of the 19th and early 20th century [Hebrew]. *Teva va Aretz,* 30:36–39.

Witztum, E., & Kalian, M. (2013). *Jerusalem of holiness and madness.* Ramot Hshavim: Aryeh Nir Publishers [Hebrew.].

16

Dhat Syndrome

ROCÍO MARTÍN-SANTOS, RICARD NAVINÉS,
AND MANUEL VALDÉS ∎

VIGNETTE

SAP, a 23-year-old male, came to the local Community Health Center and requested an urgent visit with his general practitioner (GP). He explained that he was very preoccupied with several episodes of semen loss in the last few weeks. These losses occurred in the morning, when urinating, and while masturbating. Since this started, he had felt distressed, less energetic, and downcast. His appetite decreased and he had the impression that something was wrong with him. He complained of "feeling unwell." The patient had discussed his symptoms with relatives and some Pakistani friends he had made in the city, all originally from the area of Punjab. He explained to the doctor that some of these people had stressed the importance of the loss of dhat and its association with vital energy, fatigue, and distress symptoms.

SAP is a single man from Pakistan, the third of five brothers and sisters. He used to live with his family and work with his father, a tailor, in the city closest to his home. However, three months previously he moved to Europe to work in a shop owned by one of his mother's brothers in Barcelona, Spain. He did not mention any personal or family history of mental illness. SAP completed his secondary studies in Pakistan and was able to speak English and some Spanish. He was engaged to a girl from his town, and they planned to marry in the next two years; he thought that traveling to Spain would be a good opportunity for him to earn money and gain life experience before the marriage. SAP described himself as an ambitious and responsible person, albeit, slightly perfectionistic. He reported good relationships with his friends and relatives. He was young and healthy and had no significant previous history of physical illness or drug use.

The GP examined him for symptoms of a urinary tract infection and sexual dysfunction, but all examinations were negative. Nevertheless, he asked the patient to take a urine test (to officially rule out an infection) and to come back in a few days. During the next visit, the patient was accompanied by his uncle and increasingly distressed and worried about the passage of dhat. He explained that he still had episodes of semen loss, together with sleeping difficulties, fatigue, anxiety, and sadness, along with an inability to concentrate at work. His uncle confirmed the patient's change of mood and behavior in the last two months. The doctor explained that the results of the urine test were normal, and that the symptoms did not appear to be due either to an infection or to a sexual dysfunction. Because the patient presented with a moderate-to-high level of emotional distress, low mood, and insomnia, however, the GP referred him for a psychiatric assessment at the same Community Health Center.

The liaison-psychiatrist examined the patient and found him distressed, hypothymic, and anhedonic. He also reported asthenia, slight appetite loss, sleeping difficulties, and excessive guilt related to masturbation and semen loss. The patient's score on the Hamilton Depression Rating Scale (Hamilton, 1960) was 14. These symptoms started just one month after arriving from Pakistan. SAP told the psychiatrist that coming to Europe had represented a great change for him; he had had to cope with so many new things. Moreover, before the start of the dhat loss, he had had a single episode of premature ejaculation, which worried him greatly. The psychiatrist diagnosed adjustment disorder with mixed anxiety and depressed mood and dhat syndrome, according to the Diagnostic and Statistical Manual of Mental Disorders (DSM-IV-R; American Psychiatric Association [APA], 2004). He treated SAP with supportive psychotherapy (including psychoeducation) and reassured him about masturbation and sexual practices, at all times taking into account the patient's cultural background. Two months later, the patient experienced a complete recovery from both dhat syndrome and adjustment disorder.

HISTORICAL AND CULTURAL CONTEXT

The term *dhat* derives from the Sanskrit word "*dhatus*," which, according to the classical texts of Ayurvedic medicine (*Sushruta Samhita*), means "elixir that constitutes the body" (Mehta et al., 2009). In traditional Hindu culture it is believed that it takes 40 drops of blood to create a drop of bone marrow, and 40 drops of bone marrow to create a single drop of sperm. For this reason, semen is considered to be a "vital fluid" in some cultures (Sumathipala et al., 2004). Historically, dhat syndrome was thought to be a culture-bound sexual neurosis of the East, because it was mainly described in countries of southern and southeast Asia, especially on the Indian subcontinent (Malhotra & Wig, 1975). Although there are few epidemiological studies on the prevalence of the syndrome, it appears to be common in India (Dhikav et al., 2007; Khan, 2005). Similar clinical manifestations also are found in Sri Lanka, Nepal, Pakistan, Bangladesh, and some parts of China and southeast Asia (Khan, 2005; De Silva & Dissanayake, 1989; Cheng, 1989).

Some authors also argued that extended forms of semen-loss anxiety existed in Western countries in the 19th century, and probably until the mid-20th century, but disappeared almost entirely in response to social, economic, and cultural changes (Sumathipala et al., 2004; Raguran, 1994). Certain beliefs in Western countries still harken back to tradition and religion, even though today they have far less impact in the West than on the Indian subcontinent (Prakash et al., 2014). For example, a study of British patients suffering from neurotic depression disorder (International Classification of Diseases [ICD-9]) found that some of them reported a link between semen loss or retention and psychological problems (Jadhav, 2007).

ROLE IN CURRENT DIAGNOSTIC SYSTEMS

The latest version of the *Diagnostic and Statistical Manual of Mental Disorders* (DSM-5; APA, 2013) lists dhat syndrome under the section *Glossary of Cultural Concepts of Distress*. It describes dhat syndrome as anxiety and distress about the loss of dhat in the absence of any identifiable physiological dysfunction. This description indicates that, in spite of the name, it is not a discrete syndrome, but rather a cultural explanation of distress. The new description is very different from the one found in the DSM-IV-R, in which the syndrome had been classified in the section *Glossary of Culture-Bound Syndromes* as a "folk diagnostic term used in India to refer to severe anxiety and hypochondriacal concerns associated with discharge of semen" (APA, 2000, p. 900). Moreover, the 10th revision of the World Health Organization's (WHO) International Clinical Diagnostic criteria (or International Classification of Diseases; ICD-10) classified the syndrome as a separate entity under *Neurotic Disorders, Others*, noting, nevertheless, that it is of uncertain etiology and nosological status (WHO, 1992).

The phrase *cultural concept of distress* (CCD) refers to "ways that cultural groups experience, understand and express suffering, behavioural problems, or troubling thoughts or emotions" (APA, 2013, p.758). For some clinicians and researchers, the introduction of this new term in the DSM-5 represented an advance in nosology, because it was intended to categorize psychological distress with a demonstrable cultural influence that did not conform to the standard Western notions of mental disorder (Kohrt et al., 2014).

However, other authors (Prakash & Mandai, 2014) challenged the assumption that there was sufficient evidence to suggest that, rather than a culture-bound syndrome, dhat syndrome should be viewed as a cultural explanation of distress. They contended that the main reasons for supporting the change in the DSM-5—the historical presence of similar beliefs in other cultures (Jadhav, 2007; Sumathipala et al., 2004; Ranguran, 1994), the high prevalence of depression in dhat syndrome (Rajkumar & Bharadwaj, 2014; Udina et al., 2013; Dhikav et al., 2007; Mumford, 1996), and finally, that all disorders have cultural influences and are not just culture-bound syndromes (Balhara, 2011)—were still too weak.

It is the opinion of the authors that the changes in the status of dhat found in DSM-5 are positive. These changes are also indicative of the necessity for taking cultural expressions of distress seriously, given that this syndrome is mainly observed in people originally from the Indian subcontinent. Future research into this topic over the next decade may lead to better understandings of the syndrome and its characteristic psychopathology across cultures and continents.

SYMPTOMATOLOGY

Most studies establish a diagnosis of dhat syndrome when a patient complains of semen loss, in any form, accompanied by vague symptoms or discomfort ("I lose semen when passing urine," "My urine is cloudy," "I feel weakness because I am losing semen," "I feel exhausted," "I have lost vitality," "I feel unwell," "I feel distress due to the passage of dhat"). However, slightly different diagnostic criteria seem to have been used in the various studies. In some, dhat syndrome was clearly the main symptom of focus (along with the accompanying belief that this caused discomfort), whereas in others it may only have been a secondary complaint. In addition to the passage of dhat, a systematic review of dhat syndrome ($N = 805$ cases) showed that fatigue and weakness were the most common symptoms and affected approximately 75% of surveyed patients (Udina et al., 2013). Other symptoms such as sleepiness, loss of concentration, heart palpitations, headache, and stomach pain also were frequently described in patients with dhat syndrome. The results of a large, nationwide multicenter study of dhat syndrome in India ($N = 780$) supported these results and demonstrated similar accompanying psychological and somatic symptoms (Grover et al., 2015b; 2015c).

Semen loss may occur under various circumstances: with urine during or at the end of micturition, during sleep, while passing stools, spontaneously during the day, during masturbation, and during hetero- and homosexual intercourse (Grover et al., 2015a; Menéndez et al., 2013; Dewaraja & Sasaki, 1991; Bhatia & Malik, 1991; De Silva & Dissanayabe, 1989; Behere & Natraj, 1984). In the nationwide multicenter study (Grover et al., 2015b), the most common situations in which patients experienced passage of dhat were "night falls" (60.1%) and "while passing stools" (59.5%). More than 90% of the patients reported multiple situations. The frequency of dhat loss varied from less than once a month to more than once a day. Some 14% of patients described a frequency of more than once a day, and another 40% described two to three times per week (Grover et al., 2015a).

PREVALENCE RATE AND ASSOCIATED FEATURES

There are few epidemiological studies of the prevalence of dhat syndrome in the general population. A study in Pakistan of 1,777 patients (assessed by 70 outpatient health professionals of various specialties in Lahore using ICD-10 criteria) estimated its one-month prevalence to be 16% (Khan, 2005). Most of the data came from clinical settings such as outpatient psychiatry units (Grover et al., 2015a), urology clinics (Menéndez et al., 2013), or sexual health clinics (Kendurkar et al., 2008). These were conducted on the Indian subcontinent (Kendurkar et al., 2008; Grover et al., 2015a) and elsewhere (Menéndez et al., 2013; Dewaraja & Sasaki, 1991; De Silva & Dissanayake, 1989). Please see Table 16.1 for results and sample characteristics.

According to its standard definition, dhat syndrome affects males only. However, some authors (Chaturvedi et al., 1993) have argued that there also may be a female variant. Chaturvedi et al. described both healthy women (13%) and psychiatric patients with predominantly somatic complaints (53%) who believed that passing nonpathological whitish discharge *per vaginum* was harmful to their health. Some case reports of the syndrome in women also have been published (Grover et al., 2014b; Singh et al., 2001; Trollope-Kumar, 2001; Chaturvedi, 1988).

These possible exceptions aside, however, dhat syndrome is most commonly found in young adult men. The Lahore study found a mean age of 24 years (SD = 8.5) with a range of 12–65 years (Khan, 2005). Another systematic review reported an estimated mean age of 26 years (Udina et al., 2013) and a recent cross-sectional, multicenter study of 780 subjects with dhat syndrome using ICD-10 criteria at 15 Indian centers (Grover et al., 2015c) found a mean age of 28.1 years (SD = 8.7). Thus, these reports corroborated previous data. The mean age of onset was 23.9 years (SD = 8.5) and the mean duration of symptoms was 4.3 years (SD = 4.4).

Dhat syndrome also may be related to other sociodemographic variables such as marital status, income, and level of education. Some studies argued that the condition was more common among unmarried patients and among those with low incomes and lower educational levels (Khan, 2005). Not all studies reached this conclusion, however, and other variables such as age, place of origin, and year of the study also were found to exert an influence (Udina et al., 2013). The results from the Indian nationwide multicenter study of 780 patients with dhat syndrome found that three fifths of the population were from rural backgrounds, half of them were single, and two thirds belonged to a family of average socioeconomic status. With regard to education, the patients had a mean of 10.4 (SD = 4.3) years of schooling (Grover et al., 2015c). We cannot rule out a selection bias, however, due to the differences in the clinical environments in which the studies were performed, given that the settings ranged from rural clinics to urban teaching hospitals (see Table 16.1).

No studies of dhat syndrome mention the personality traits which, together with coping strategies, may jointly contribute to the development of the condition. Nor do many studies or case reports discuss the respective contributions of family history, childhood events, or more recent life events (Rajkumar & Bharadwaj, 2014).

Premature ejaculation and other forms of sexual dysfunction were also common accompanying problems in patients with dhat syndrome, and may be related to certain common beliefs and attitudes towards sex. In Udina's (2013) review of six studies (Bhatia & Malik, 1991; Chadda & Ahuja, 1990; Dewaraja & Sasaki, 1991; Dhikav et al., 2008; Singh, 1985; Udina et al., 2012), approximately 50% of patients suffered from either impotence or premature ejaculation. A similar frequency (60%) was found in the large study conducted by Grover et al. (2015a). The most commonly reported reasons for suffering dhat syndrome seemed to be bisexual dreams, excessive sexual desire, excessive masturbation, urinary infection, problems in the urinary tract, or constipation (Grover et al., 2015b). The two most commonly described consequences of passage of dhat were weakness in sexual ability and poor erection (Grover et al., 2015b). The presence of masturbatory guilt also should be explored, given that it is not always spontaneously reported (Prakash, 2013).

Table 16.1. RESULTS OF A SYSTEMATIC REVIEW OF DHAT SYNDROME (DS): CHARACTERISTICS OF STUDIES AND SAMPLES

Author/ Year/ Country	Design	Aims of study	Setting	N %	Age Mean (SD) range	Single %	Rural %	Socio-economic status %	Years education Mean (SD) Range %	Age onset Mean (SD) Range	Years DS Mean (SD) Range %
Behere 1984 India	CS	Phenomenology of DS	OPD TCH	50	16–45	48	>Rural	58 Lower/ middle	–	–	>1 68
Singh 1985 India	CS	Revised DS	OPD TCH hospital	50	25.9 (5.8) 18–45	30	–	–	10 0–15	21.8 (4.0) 16–25	4.1 (1.8)
Chadda 1990 India	CS	DS & psychiatry comorbidity	OPD TCH	52	–	50	–	64 Middle	12	–	>1 54
Dewaraja 1991 Sri Lanka	CS	DS comparison between Sri Lanka & Japan	OPD TCH	35	25	91	–	–	–	–	–
Bhatia 1999 India	CS	Analysis of culture=bound syndromes	OPD TCH	46/60 76.7	24	–	–	–	–	–	1
Khan 2005 Pakinstan	CS	One-month prevalence of DS at different professional health clinics	OPD 75 health community professionals**	284/1777 16	24 (8.5) 12–65	75	–	55.7 Low	10th 67	–	<1 60
Dhikav 2008 India	CS	Depression in DS	OPD TCH	30	29 20–40	64.2	–	–	5th 70%	19	1***

Study	Design	Aim	Setting	n	Age						
Gautham 2008 India	CS	Sociocultural, Infectious, & psychosexual correlates	Rural health care (Agra landscape)	269/368 73.5	28	38	100	44.6 Middle	8–10	–	1
Kendurkar 2008 India	CS	Pattern sexual dysfunction	Sexual/Marriage unit TCH	78/1242 12.3	<20	80	–	–	–	–	–
Menéndez 2013 Spain	CS	Prevalence of DS in patients attending a urology service	Urological unit Community	32/170	35.4 18–54	37.5	–	–	–	33	2
Verma 2013 India	CS, r	Nature of sexual disorders	Sexual/Marriage unit TCH	126/698 18.1	<20 (58%)	54	8.3	51 Middle	10 0–15	–	–
Grover 2015 India	CS	Phenomenology & comorbidity in DS	OPD, nationwide multicenter (15 centers) TCH	780	28.1 (8.7) 17–68	47	59.2	61.5 Middle	10.4 (4.3) 0–20	23.9 (8.5) 12–63	4.6
Chadda 1995 India	CC	To compare illness behavior in DS & controls	OPD TCH	50/50	23/28 15–45	–	–	–	–	–	–
Sukla 2000 India	CC	Supportive psychotherapy in DS	OPD	40/40	25	–	–	–	–	–	–
Perme 2005 India	CC	Illness behavior characteristics of DS	OPD TCH	32/33	25.4/33.9	76/23	–	–	15 y 24.1/68.7	–	–
Rajkumar 2014 India	CC	Genetic link DS & depression	Sexual/Marriage unit TCH	19/27 F+/F-	26.5 (5.9) 18–45	84.8	–	–	11.7 (4.2)	–	2.9 (2.6)

(continued)

Table 16.1. CONTINUED

Author/ Year/ Country	Design	Aims of study	Setting	N %	Age Mean (SD) range	Single %	Rural %	Socio-economic status %	Years education Mean (SD) Range %	Age onset Mean (SD) Range	Years DS Mean (SD) Range %
Bhatia 1989 India	C	Sociodemographics, clinical findings, & comparison of DS treatments	OPD TCH	31	24	–	>Rural	Lower/middle	–	–	–
Bhatia 1991 India	C	Sociodemographics, clinical findings, & comparison of DS treatments	OPD TCH	93/144	23.5 (3.3) 20–38	54	>Rural	Lower/middle	–	20.6 (4.5) 16–24	3.1 (1.2)
Grover 2015 India	C, r	Sex, attitudes, & prevalence of comorbidity in DS	Sexual/Marriage unit TCH	264	26.7	71.2	60.2	Middle 49.6	11.2 (3.7) 0–26	21.1 (6.6)	5.7 (4.4)

NOTE: Original studies published until July 2015 in PubMed database, using key words: "Dhat syndrome" OR "Dhat syndrome" OR "Semen-loss" OR "Semen-loss anxiety." *Inclusion criteria* (N = 18): Design: CS: cross-sectional; C: cohort; CC: case-control studies. Diagnostic criteria: ICD-9 or 10 (WHO criteria), DSM-III-R, IV, or V (APA criteria). *Exclusion criteria* (N = 37): Samples fewer than 30 cases; Reviews, case reports, and series of case report articles. We collected *author, year, and country of the study data; sociodemographic data* (age, age of onset, marital status, level education, locality); *setting* (OPS: outpatients psychiatry units, sexual /marriage clinics; rural; *TCH:* tertiary care hospitals; community); *Dhat symptomatology* (1: semen loss on urine, or 2: any other circumstance: night emission, masturbation, . . .); and other symptoms; *comorbidity* (sexual dysfunction, depression disorders, anxiety, stress-related, or somatization disorders; and both sexual dysfunction and mental disorders); and *assessment tools: ADI: Amritsar Depressive Inventory: self-report instrument for depression symptomatology; HAMD: Hamilton Depression Rating Scale; GHQ: Global Health Questionnaire; DSQ: Dhat Syndrome Questionnaire; ICD-10: International Classification of Diseases (World Health Organization, 1992); SSI: Somatization Screening Index; SIBQ: Screening Version of Illness Behaviour Questionnaire; CFS: Chalder Fatigue Scale; SKAQ-II: Sex Knowledge and Attitude Questionnaire; IBQ: Illness Behaviour Questionnaire.*

**Hakim (49.7%), Homeopath (23.6%), Physician (18.6%), Psychiatrist (1.6%), Psychologist (0.7%), Urologist (0.3%), Infertility specialist (5.6%) (p < 0.001)

***11 months

Several patients presented with comorbid psychiatric symptoms, especially anxiety and depression, although it should be noted that the diagnostic criteria used to define psychiatric conditions varied widely among studies (Udina et al., 2013). In some cases, the standardized diagnostic criteria were not specified, whereas other studies used the DSM or ICD classifications. In general, most studies reported a high rate of associated psychiatric symptoms. Approximately 50% of patients had depressive disorders and 22% had anxiety disorders. However, findings from the large nationwide multicenter study in India (Grover et al., 2015a) should be considered fairly reliable, because they were based on the ICD-10 criteria administered by a trained psychiatrist using a semistructured clinical interview. This study found that 20% of patients with dhat syndrome had comorbid depressive disorders and another 20% had comorbid neurotic, stress-related, and somatoform disorders.

THEORIES OF ETIOLOGY

From the etiological point of view, the "a priori" atheoretical discussion of dhat syndrome as a discrete culture-bound syndrome or as a cultural explanation of distress (DSM-5) is relatively unhelpful (Keshavan, 2014; Balhara, 2011). It is also at odds with the current ICD-10 classification, which assigns dhat syndrome a separate status under the section *Neurotic Disorder, Others*. The syndrome also has been explained as an expression of a major depression disorder, because some authors have found it to have a strong association with depression (Dhikav et al., 2008; 2007) or functional somatic illness (Ranjith & Mohan, 2006; Perme et al., 2005). The most recent evidence in the field, however, does not support this high comorbidity with depression. Again, the results of the nationwide multicenter study of dhat syndrome showed that the most prevalent comorbid disorder was not depression (20%) but sexual dysfunction, with the latter present in 51.3% of the study sample (Grover et al., 2015a). These results corroborated the findings of Prakash et al. (2013; quoted in Prakash & Mandai, 2015, p. 108) showing that the prevalence of depression was much lower (see Table 16.2).

The recent conceptions of dhat syndrome underscore the importance of cultural beliefs that regard the passage of semen as a loss of vitality that affects sexual knowledge and practices. Grover et al.'s (2015) nationwide multicenter study in India found that 60.5% of patients believed dhat to be semen, supporting previous reports in the field (Deb & Balhara, 2013; Udina et al., 2013), although 29.5% did not report any explanation. Moreover, dhat syndrome patients had poor levels of sexual knowledge, not only of dhat/semen but of other areas of overall sexuality as well (Grover et al., 2015b). Cultural background and beliefs appear to play an important role in both sexuality and the subjective expressions of emotional distress. Beliefs of this kind can be found worldwide, but they are particularly strong in the traditional Hindu culture found on the Indian subcontinent and in south Asian countries, as well as among those who have emigrated from these areas (Menéndez et al., 2013; Udina et al., 2012).

Table 16.2. Results of Systematic Review of Dhat Syndrome (DS): Clinical Assessment and Comorbidity

Author/ Year	N %	Clinical tools	Semen loss	Dhat Syndrome Symptomatology							Sexual dysfunction %	Dhat Syndrome Comorbidity		
				Fatigue Weakness %	Low mood %	Anxiety %	Loss of appetite %	Loss of concentration %	Insomnia %	Pain Headache Hypochondriasis %		Depressive disorder %	Anxiety, stress-related, somatization disorder %	Both (sexual dysfunction & mental disorder) %
Behere 1984	50	Clinician Interview	2	68	–	38	–	–	–	46	26	–	–	–
Singh 1985	50	Clinician ADI	2	73.8	62.5	51.6	43.8	18.8	31.3	68.0	35.5	48	16	–
Chadda 1990	52	Clinician	1	–	50	72	–	–	–	80	80	40	50	–
Dewaraja 1991	35	Clinician	1	40	–	–	–	–	–	50	33	–	–	–
Bhatia 1999	46/60 76.7	Clinician Interview ICD-9	1	–	–	–	–	–	–	–	–	23.9	19.5	–
Dhikav 2008	30	Clinician HAMD DSM-IV	1	–	–	–	–	–	–	–	39.3	66	–	–
Gautham 2008	269/368 73.5	Clinician One item GHQ-12	2	40	–	–	–	–	–	15	–	**	**	–
Kendurkar 2008	78/1242 12.3	Clinician ICD-9 & 10	2	–	–	–	–	–	–	–	100	–	–	–
Menéndez 2013	32/170	Clinician ICD-10	2	43.8	–	28.1	–	–	18.8	21.9	50	0	–	–
Verma 2013	126/698 18.1	Clinician ICD-10	2	–	–	–	–	–	–	–	19.3	–	–	–
Grover 2015	780	Clinician DSQ	2	78.2	67.9	56.4	47.8	49.1	50.8	51.3	51.3	20.5	20.5	22.6

Study	Sample	Assessment	Design										
Chadda 1995	50/50	Clinician IBQ DSM-III-R	1	–	–	–	–	–	–	–	–	20/42	2/16	12/8
Sukla 2000	40/40	Clinician	2	–	–	–	–	–	–	–	–	–	–	–
Perme 2005	25/32	Clinician SSI, CFS DSM-IV	1	***	–	–	–	–	–	***	–	–	–	–
Rajkumar 2014	19/27 F+/F–	Clinician Family history ICD-10	2	67.4	–	32.6	–	17.4	–	17.4	10.5/22.2	47.4/3.7	–	–
Bhatia 1989	31/48 64.6	Clinician ICD-9	2	70.8	–	–	–	–	62.4	68.7	–	39.5	20.8	–
Bhatia 1991	93/144	Clinician HAMD ICD-9	2	70.8	58.3¥	56.3	45.8	56.3	62.4	68.7	25.8	46.2	22.9	22.9
Grover 2015	264	Clinician SKAQ ICD-10	2	–	–	–	–	–	–	–	35.6	15.1	12.9	51.9

NOTE: Original studies published until July 2015 in PubMed database, using key words: "Dhat syndrome," "Dhat," and "semen-loss." *Inclusion criteria* (N = 18): Design: CS: cross-sectional; C: cohort; CC: case-control; RCT: randomized controlled clinical trials. Diagnostic criteria: ICD-9 or 10 (WHO criteria), DSM-III-R, IV, or V (APA criteria). *Exclusion criteria* (N = 37): Samples fewer than 30 cases; Reviews, case reports, and series of case-report articles. We collected *author*, year and country of the study data; *sociodemographic data* (age, age of onset, marital status, educational level, locality); *setting* (OPS: outpatient psychiatry units, sexual /marriage clinics; rural; tertiary care hospitals (TCH); community); *Dhat symptomatology* (1: semen loss upon urination, or 2: any other circumstance: night emission, masturbation, …); and other symptoms; *comorbidity* (sexual dysfunction, depression disorders, anxiety, stress-related or somatization disorders; and both sexual dysfunction and mental disorders); and *assessment tools*:

ADI: *Amritsar Depressive Inventory*: self-report instrument for depression symptomatology; HAMD: *Hamilton Depression Rating Scale*; GHQ: *Global Health Questionnaire*; DSQ: *Dhat Syndrome Questionnaire*; ICD-10: *International Classification of Diseases* (World Health Organization, 1992); SSI: *Somatization Screening Index*; SIBQ: *Screening Version of Illness Behaviour Questionnaire*; CFS: *Chalder Fatigue Scale*; SKAQ-II: *Sex Knowledge and Attitude Questionnaire*; IBQ: *Illness Behaviour Questionnaire*.

**Dhat syndrome showed two times and a half times greater risk (OR: 2.66; 95%CI: 1.51-4-68) of suffering from psychological distress (GHQ-12).

***Dhat syndrome patients showed a different pattern of illness beliefs and behavior compared with controls.

¥18.6% presented suicidal ideation

Dhat syndrome has a clear clinical description: a persistent preoccupation with semen loss and its consequences, together with moderate-to-severe distress or dysfunction, leading the patient to seek help (Prakash & Mandai, 2014; Prakash et al., 2012). Previous studies have shown that the syndrome is not due to another medical condition such a urinary tract infection or a sexually transmitted disease (Menéndez et al., 2013). We do not know yet whether there is a underlying familial or genetic vulnerability to dhat; the only study performed so far in this field (Rajkumar & Bharadwaj, 2014) suffered from several methodological limitations. From the cross-sectional information obtained, we know that dhat syndrome may present either alone, with comorbid sexual dysfunction, with comorbid psychiatry disorder (depression, anxiety, somatization), or with any of these conditions (Grover et al., 2015a; Deb & Balhara, 2013). Due to the lack of longitudinal studies, however, it is difficult to establish the causal direction of comorbidity. All of the information we have found comes from case reports, cross-sectional surveys, case-control studies, or some small cohort studies (see Grover et al., 2015a; Udina et al., 2013; Deb & Balhara, 2013, for reviews; also see Menéndez et al., 2013). Recently, data from a retrospective longitudinal study in 264 dhat syndrome patients (Grover et al., 2015c) suggested that comorbid sexual dysfunction and psychiatric disorders may occur subsequent to the onset of the condition. The study manifested several limitations, including its retrospective design, the risk of recall bias, and the absence of a control group.

Dhat syndrome may be common in patients with certain sociodemographic features (e.g., strong beliefs about semen and sexual taboos), personality traits, genetics, or life events who find themselves under levels of stress. Patients with dhat syndrome report fatigue, weakness, pain, insomnia, anxiety, anhedonia, and low levels of activity. This is a clinical profile that runs parallel to what is called "illness behavior," and acute self-limited condition (Ranjith & Mohan, 2006). In vulnerable subjects, the condition may become chronic, resulting in abnormal illness behavior and the development of anxiety, depression, or somatoform symptomatology. Future longitudinal studies are needed to identify the risk factors for dhat syndrome by observing the natural history of the syndrome and comorbidity.

ASSESSMENT OPTIONS

In recent years, efforts have been made to assess dhat syndrome with specific tools such as clinical interviews (Sharan et al., 2003). Methodological difficulties facing these studies include a high degree of variability in the reporting of its symptomatology and the emergence of misconceptions due to the absence of a specific instrument to assess its many dimensions.

Recently, Grover and colleagues (2014a) designed a comprehensive self-report questionnaire for the evaluation of dhat syndrome. The questionnaire contains dichotomous questions, (i.e., yes/no), multiple choice questions, open-ended questions, and various other reporting formats. The items are grouped into five main domains: characteristics of the syndrome, situations in which there is a passage of dhat, the reasons for it, psychological symptoms accompanying the syndrome (using the depression items of the Patient Health Questionnaire (PHQ-9) [Spitzer et al., 1999] and the somatic items of PHQ-15, [Kroenker et al., 2002]), and help-seeking and beliefs regarding treatment. The instrument demonstrated good content validity and has been translated into English and nine other languages. The Hindi and English versions evidenced good test-retest reliability (Grover et al., 2014a).

DIFFERENTIAL DIAGNOSIS

Differential diagnosis for dhat syndrome requires the consideration of several other disorders. First, urological problems such as urinary tract infections, sexually transmitted diseases, or genital abnormalities must first be ruled out through physical examination, urine sediment, and additional biological tests (Menéndez et al., 2013; Gautam et al., 2008; Bhatia, 1999). Most authors found no changes in the sediment or the presence of spermatozoids in urine (Menéndez et al., 2013; Kendurkar et al., 2008; Bhatia & Malik, 1991). The findings regarding oxaluria or phosphaturia are contradictory, with some authors reporting positive results (e.g., Chadda & Aluja, 1990), but not others (e.g., Menéndez et al., 2013).

Moreover, sexual dysfunction is the most prevalent medical comorbidity, present in 50%–60% of patients. Premature ejaculation and erectile difficulties are those most frequently described (Grover et al., 2015c; Grover et al., 2015a, Menéndez et al., 2013; Udina et al., 2013). It is important to note that, at least in some cases, sexual dysfunction was the reason for consulting a clinician, and dhat syndrome was detected through subsequent assessment (Grover et al., 2015c; Verma et al., 2013; Kendurkar et al., 2008; Gautham et al., 2008) (see Table 16.2).

Among psychiatric disorders, stress reactions, somatization, depression, and anxiety disorders are the most prevalent comorbidities. Finally, dhat syndrome only rarely presents in a psychotic form. There are some case reports of delusions related to dhat in the context of a formal psychotic disorder. For instance, "he described pain and weakness due to loss of a whitish substance from his penis with high degree of conviction" (Patra et al., 2014, p.171). This also can be found in major depression disorder with psychotic features. For example, Aneja et al. (2015) reported that, "he strongly believed that his illness was a result of gradual loss of semen in urine and excessive masturbation in childhood" (p. 83).

TREATMENT OPTIONS

Very few studies have focused on the treatment of dhat syndrome (Salam et al., 2012; Shukla & Sing, 2000; Bhatia & Malik, 1991; Chadda & Ahuja, 1990; Behere & Natraj, 1984). Data from Grover et al. (2015a) confirmed the previous reports of most other authors (e.g., Deb & Balhara, 2013; Khan, 2005). Specifically, patients with dhat syndrome consulted family doctors, Ayurvedic and homeopathic practitioners, and local sex-health specialists, in this order. Sometimes patients moved from one system of medicine to another (Kattimani et al., 2013; Mumford, 1996). Most patients acquired knowledge of the syndrome through peers, relatives, colleagues, or through the media and nonspecialist publications (Grover et al., 2015a; Mumford, 1996; Bhatia & Malik, 1991). As we will note later, the mean time to seek medical help averages four years—a period of time long enough to facilitate the development of secondary depression, anxiety disorders, or other psychosocial dysfunctions.

Some authors have recommended empathic listening, reassurance, the correction of erroneous beliefs (Wig, 1960), psychoeducation (Behere & Natraj, 1984), and cognitive behavioral therapy (CBT; Salam et al., 2012; Chadda & Ahuja, 1990). Psychoeducation should be one of the key therapeutic approaches to these patients. More generally, dhat syndrome patients are often badly misinformed about sexual matters, not only in relation to dhat/semen but in relation to almost all aspects of sexuality and anatomy (Grover et al., 2015b; Prakash & Rao, 2010). Psychosocial treatments also should focus on clarifying patients' misconceptions about the production and loss of semen through masturbation, excessive sexual activity, and nocturnal emissions (Salam et al., 2012). As Grover et al. (2015b, p. 5) noted, the Indian Psychiatric Society recommends that in patients with comorbid sexual dysfunctions, dhat syndrome should be treated first, because this may help to improve their overall sexual functioning.

Cultural adaptation of psychotherapy is a promising area for addressing the cultural concept of distress as well as psychiatric problems in general (e.g., Hinton, 2006). In dhat syndrome, supportive group psychotherapy focusing on psychoeducation and relaxation combined with Ayurvedic therapy lasting one month has proven more successful than Ayurvedic treatment alone for improving depressive symptomatology (Shukla & Singh, 2000). A specific CBT module for patients with dhat syndrome has been developed (Salam et al., 2012), consisting of a baseline assessment of patients, a basic sex education program, cognitive restructuring, and behavioral strategies. Application of the module to six cases of dhat syndrome obtained good outcomes; however, these results must be confirmed in controlled studies using larger samples.

Psychopharmacological therapies also have been used to treat dhat syndrome. A third of patients received at least one medication: antidepressants, benzodiazepines, or multivitamins (Grover et al., 2015a; Menéndez et al., 2013; Udina et al., 2013). Less information is available regarding the therapeutic response. Antidepressant therapy, mainly selective serotonin reuptake inhibitors, has been proposed in some studies as a monotherapy, or in conjunction with counseling (Bhatia & Malik, 1991; Dhikav et al., 2008). Others have suggested psychoeducation and use of minor tranquilizers (Behere & Natraj, 1984). Few studies have used a controlled and double-blind design, and the majority were not randomized and evidenced a high dropout rate (Bhatia & Malik, 1991). Bhatia and Malik (1991) found a 17% response to counseling alone versus 54% to imipramine or lorazepam in a randomized, controlled study. In a noncontrolled study, Dhikav et al. (2008) evidenced a better response with antidepressants plus counseling

(66%) than with counseling alone (34%). Behere and Natraj (1984) observed a 66% response with the combination of psychoeducation and minor tranquilizers.

Due to the heterogeneity of dhat patients with or without sexual dysfunction or psychiatric comorbidity, the clinical and therapeutic management of these patients should be individualized. Those without comorbidity may respond primarily to a psychoeducation approach; while those with comorbidity might benefit from cognitive behavioral therapy and psychopharmacological treatment.

RECOMMENDATIONS FOR FUTURE WORK

Dhat syndrome appears to be a heterogeneous syndrome that predominantly affects men who are originally from the Indian subcontinent and southeast Asia (Prakash et al., 2014). Due to processes of globalization and population migration, however, dhat syndrome now can be detected, diagnosed, and treated worldwide. Clinical psychiatry has to take account of culture (Kohrt et al., 2014), and a comprehensive medical and psychological approach for these patients must acknowledge the cultural background of the syndrome.

Although studies of this syndrome have increased in recent years, there is still a great need for epidemiological studies that can better establish its prevalence in the general population (including statistical control for confounding factors and bias). With regard to comorbidity, we cannot rule out the possibility of Berkson's bias, given that, not surprisingly, all the studies have been performed in clinical settings (mostly tertiary care hospitals). Epidemiological studies in the community also would improve the field's ability to detect risk factors, including personality traits, family history, life events, and beliefs.

The use of specific validated tools to assess the syndrome also could expand our knowledge of the characteristics of dhat. In this connection the *Comprehensive Questionnaire for Assessment of Dhat Syndrome* (Grover et al., 2014a) appears to be a good option, showing good psychometric properties and with versions available in several languages. Similarly, screening for depression, anxiety, and somatization syndromes using validated measures such as the PHQ-9 (Spitzer et al., 1999) and the PHQ-11 (Kroenke et al., 2002) or using structured interviews such as the *Mini International Neuropsychiatry Interview* (MINI) (Sheehan et al., 1998) would also aid in the diagnosis of comorbid conditions. This will assist in the clinical management and treatment of these patients.

Longitudinal studies also would be useful for collecting data on the naturalistic follow-up and outcomes of dhat syndrome (with and without comorbidity) as well as on treatment response. Controlled studies assessing the sexual knowledge and attitudes of dhat syndrome patients in the community are also needed to improve psychoeducation and sexual dysfunction therapies. Controlled randomized clinical trials comparing psychopharmacological treatments or assessing culturally adapted CBT among the various groups of dhat syndrome patients will also help the development of new therapeutic approaches.

ACKNOWLEDGMENTS

This study was carried out in part with the support of the Agency of University and Research Funding Management of the Catalan Government (SGR2014/ 1411) (R. Martín-Santos) and the Mental Health CIBER (Centro de Investigación Biomédica en Red de Salud Mental, CIBERSAM, Spain).

REFERENCES

American Psychiatric Association. (APA). (2000). *Diagnostic and statistical manual of mental disorders: DSM-IV-R.* Washington, DC: American Psychiatric Publishing.

American Psychiatric Association. (2013). *Diagnostic and statistical manual of mental disorders: DSM-5.* Washington, DC: American Psychiatric Association.

Aneja, J., Grover, S., Avasthi, A., Mahajan, S., Pokhrel, P., & Triveni, D. (2015). Can masturbatory guilt lead to severe psychopathology? A case series. *Indian Journal of Psychological Medicine, 37,* 81–86.

Balhara, Y.P. (2011). Culture-bound syndrome: Has it found its right niche? *Indian Journal of Psychological Medicine, 33,* 210–215.

Behere, P.B., & Natraj, G.S. (1984). Dhat syndrome: the phenomenology of a culture bound sex neurosis of the orient. *Indian Journal of Psychiatry, 26,* 76–78.

Bhatia, M.S., Bohra, N., & Malik, S.C. (1989). "Dhat" syndrome—a useful clinical entity. *Indian Journal of Dermatology, 34,* 32–41.

Bhatia, M.S., & Malik, S.C. (1991). Dhat syndrome: a useful diagnostic entity in Indian culture. *British Journal of Psychiatry, 159,* 691–695.

Bhatia, M.S. (1999). An analysis of 60 cases of culture bound syndromes. *Indian Journal of Medicine and Science, 53,* 149–152.

Cheng, T.A. (1989). Symptomatology of minor psychiatric morbidity: a cross-cultural comparison. *Psychological Medicine, 19,* 697–708.

Chaturvedi, S.K., Chandra, P.S., lssac, M.K., & Sodarashan, C.Y. (1993). Somatization misattributed to non-pathological vaginal discharge. *Journal of Psychosomatic Research, 37,* 575–579.

Chaturvedi, S. (1988). Psychasthenic syndrome related to leucorrhea in Indian women. *Journal of Psychosomatic Obstetrics and Gynecology, 8,* 67–72.

Chadda, R.K., & Ahuja, N. (1990). Dhat syndrome. A sex neurosis of the Indian subcontinent. *British Journal of Psychiatry,156,* 577–579.

Chadda, R.K. (1995). Dhat syndrome: Is it a distinct clinical entity? A study of illness behavior characteristics. *Acta Psychiatrica Scandinavica, 91,*136–139.

De Silva, P., & Dissanayake, S.A. (1989). The use of semen syndrome in Sri Lanka: A clinical study. *Sex and Marital Therapy, 4,* 195–204.

Deb, K.S., & Balhara, Y.P.S. (2013). Dhat syndrome: a review of the world literature. *Indian Journal of Psychological Medicine, 35,* 326–331.

Dewaraja, R., & Sasaki, Y. (1991). Semen-loss syndrome: a comparison between Sri Lanka and Japan. *American Journal of Psychotherapy, 45,* 14–20.

Dhikav, V., Aggarwal, N., & Anand, K.S. (2007). Is Dhat syndrome a culturally appropriate manifestation of depression? *Medical Hypotheses, 69,* 698.

Dhikav, V., Aggarwal, N., Gupta, S., Jadhavi, R., & Singh, K. (2008). Depression in Dhat syndrome. *Journal of Sexual Medicine, 5*, 841–844.

Gautham, M., Singh, R., Weiss, H., Brugha, R., Patel, V., Desai, N.G., Nandam, D., Kielmann, K., & Grosskurth, H. (2008). Socio-cultural, psychosexual, and biomedical factors associated with genital symptoms experienced by men in rural India. *Tropical Medicine and International Health, 13*, 384–395.

Grover, S., Gupta, S., Mehra, A., & Acasthi, A. (2015b). Comorbidity, knowledge and attitude towards sex among patients with Dhat syndrome: a retrospective study. *Asian Journal of Psychiatry*. Advance online publication. doi:10.1016/j.ajp.2015.07.002

Grover, S., Avasthi, A., Gupta, S., Dan, A., Neogi, R., Behere, B., Lakdawala, B., Tripathi, A., Chakborty, K., Sinha, V., Bhatia, M.S., Patjoshi, A., Rao, T.S.S., & Rozatkar, A. (2015c). Phenomenology and beliefs of patients with Dhat syndrome: a nationwide multicentric study. *International Journal of Social Psychiatry*. Advance online publication. doi:10.1177/002076401559187

Grover, S., Avasthi, A., Gupta, S., Dan, A., Neogu, R., Behere, P.B., ... Rozatkar, A. (2015a). Comorbidity in patients with Dhat Syndrome: a nationwide multicentric study. *Journal of Sexual Medicine, 12*, 1398–1401.

Grover, S., Avasthi, A., Aneja, J., Shankar, G., Mohan, R., Nehra, R., & Padhy, S.K. (2014a). *Comprehensive Questionnaire for Assessment of Dhat Syndrome*: Development and use in patient population. *Journal of Sexual Medicine, 11*, 2485–2495.

Grover, S., Kate, N., Avasthi, A., Rajpal, N., & Umamaheswari, V. (2014b). Females too suffer from Dhat syndrome: A case series and revisit of the concept. *Indian Journal of Psychiatry, 56*, 388–392.

Hamilton, M. (1960). A rating scale for depression. *Journal of Neurology, Neurosurgery, and Psychiatry, 23*(1), 56–62.

Hinton, D.E. (2006). Special issue—Culturally sensitive CBT. *Cognitive and Behavioral Practice, 13*, 246–248.

Jadhav, S. (2007). Dhis and Dhat: Evidence of semen retention syndrome amongst white Britons. *Anthropological Medicine, 14*, 229–239.

Kattimani, S., Menon, V., & Shrivastava, M.K. (2013). Is semen loss syndrome a psychological or physical illness? A case for conflict of interest. *Indian Journal of Psychological Medicine, 35*, 420–422.

Kendurkar, A., Kaur, B., Agarwal, A.K., Singh, H., & Agarwal, V. (2008). Profile of adult patients attending a marriage and sex clinic in India. *International Journal of Social Psychiatry, 54*, 486–493.

Keshavan, M.S. (2014). Culture bound syndromes: diseases entities or simple concepts of distress? *Asian Journal of Psychiatry, 12*, 1–2.

Khan, N. (2005). Dhat syndrome in relation to demographic characteristics. *Indian Journal of Psychiatry, 47*, 54–57.

Kohrt, B.A., Rasmussen, A., Kaiser, B.N., Hariz, E.E., Maharjan, S.M., Mutamba, B.B., ... Hinton, D.E. (2014). Cultural concepts of distress and psychiatric disorders: literature review and research recommendations for global mental health epidemiology. *International Journal of Epidemiology, 43*, 365–406.

Kroenke, K., Spitzer, R.L., & Williams, J.B. (2002). The PHQ-15: validity of a new measure for evaluating the severity of somatic symptoms. *Psychosomatic Medicine, 64*, 258–266.

Malhotra, H.K., & Wig, N.N. (1975). Dhat syndrome: a culture-bound sex neurosis of the orient. *Archives of Sexual Behavior, 4*, 519–528.

Mehta, V., De, A., & Balachandran, C. (2009). Dhat syndrome: a reappraisal. *Indian Journal of Dermatology, 54*, 89–90.

Menéndez, V., Fernandez, A., Placer, J., García-Linares, M., Tarragon, S., & Liso, E. (2013). Dhat syndrome, an emergent condition within urology in Spain. *World Journal of Urology, 31*, 941–945.

Mumford, D.B. (1996). The "Dhat syndrome": a culturally determined symptom of depression? *Acta Psychiatrica Scandinavica, 94*, 163–167.

Patra, S., Sidana, A., & Gupta, N. (2014). Delusion of dhat: The quandary of the form-content dichotomy! *Indian Psychiatry Journal, 23*, 171–172.

Perme, B., Ranjith, G., Mohan, R., & Chandrasekaran, R. (2005). Dhat: (Semen loss) syndrome: a functional somatic syndrome of the Indian subcontinent? *General Hospital Psychiatry, 27*, 215–217.

Prakash, O., Kar, S.K., & Sathyanarayana Rao, T.S. (2014). Indian story on semen loss and related Dhat syndrome. *Indian Journal of Psychiatry, 56*, 377–382.

Prakash, O., & Rao, T.S.S. (2010). Sexuality research in India: An update. *Indian Journal of Psychiatry, 52*, 260–263.

Prakash, S., & Mandai, P. (2014). Is the DSM-5 position on dhat syndrome justified? *Asian Journal of Psychiatry, 12*, 155–157.

Prakash, S., & Mandai, P. (2015). Is Dhat syndrome indeed a culturally determined form of depression? *Indian Journal of Psychological Medicine, 37*, 107–109.

Raguram, R., Jadhav, S., & Weiss, M. (1994). Historical perspectives on Dhat syndrome. *Nimhans Journal, 12*, 117–124.

Rajkumar, E.P., & Bharadwaj, B. (2014). Dhat syndrome: evidence for a depressive subtype. *Asian Journal of Psychiatry, 9*, 57–60.

Ranjith, G., & Mohan, R. (2006). Dhat syndrome as a functional somatic syndrome: Developing a sociosomatic model. *Psychiatry, 69*, 142–150.

Salam, K.P.A., Sharma, M.P., & Prakash, O. (2012). Development of cognitive-behavioral therapy intervention for patients with Dhat syndrome. *Indian Journal of Psychiatry, 54*, 367–374.

Sharan, P., Avasthi, A., Gupta, N., Mohanty, M., Gill, S., & Jain, A. (2003). Development of Dhat syndrome interview schedule. *Indian Journal of Psychiatry, 45*(suppl), 88.

Sheehan, D.V., Lecubrier, Y., Harnett-Sheehan, K., Amorim, P., Janavs, J., Weiller, E., ... Dunbar., G. (1998). The M.I.N.I. International neuropsychiatric Interview (MINI). The development and validation of a structured diagnostic psychiatric interview. *Journal of Clinical Psychiatry, 59* (20 suppl): 22–33.

Shukla, P.R., & Singh, R.H. (2000). Supportive psychotherapy in Dhat syndrome patients. *Journal of Personality Clinical Studies, 16*, 49–52.

Singh, G. (1985). Dhat syndrome revisited. *Indian Journal of Psychiatry, 27*, 119–122.

Spitzer, R.L., Kroenke, K., & Williams, J.B. (1999). Validation and utility of a self-report version of PRIME-MD: The PHQ primary care study. Primary Care Evaluation of Mental Disorders. Patient Health Questionnaire. *JAMA, 10*, 1737–1744.

Sumathipala, A., Siribaddana, S.H., & Bhugra, D. Culture-bound syndromes: the story of Dhat syndrome. *British Journal of Psychiatry, 184*, 200–209.

Trollope-Kumar, K. (2001). Cultural and biomedical meanings of the complaint of leukorrhea in South Asian women. *Tropical Medicine and International Health, 6,* 260–266.

Udina, M., Foulon, H., Corcoles, D., & Martín-Santos, R. (2012). Dhat syndrome: report of six cases. .*Medicina Clinica (Barc), 138,* 320.

Udina, M., Foulon, H., Bhatacharyya, S., Valdés, M., & Martín-Santos, R. (2013). Dhat syndrome: a systematic review. *Psychosomatics, 54,* 212–218.

Verma, R., Mina, S., Ul-Hassan, S., & Balhara, Y.P.S. (2013). A descriptive analysis of patients presenting to psychosexual clinic at a tertiary care center. *Indian Journal of Psychological Medicine, 35,* 241–247.

Wig, N.N. (1960). Problems of mental health in India. *Journal of Clinical and Social Psychiatry, 17,* 48–53.

World Health Organization (WHO). (1992). *The ICD-10 classification of mental and behavioral disorders: diagnostic criteria for research.* Geneva, Switzerland: WHO.

17

Ataques de Nervios

ROBERTO LEWIS-FERNÁNDEZ AND IRENE LÓPEZ ■

CLINICAL VIGNETTES

A 33-year-old Puerto Rican woman born in the United States is brought to an emergency room following a suicide attempt. She found out that day that her fiancé was murdered in a drug-related incident in Puerto Rico. Upon hearing the news, she brooded for several hours. Then, suddenly, she cried out and attempted to drink a bottle of bleach. When her brother knocked the bottle away, she fell to the ground, shaking, screaming, and crying. She recalled nothing that happened after she first cried out. Prior to the incident she had no previous psychiatric history (Lewis-Fernández, 2014).

A 35-year-old divorced Dominican woman was evaluated for facial pain. A week before, she learned that her ex-husband had remarried in the Dominican Republic. During the next few days, she became increasingly agitated and developed insomnia and anorexia. During her evaluation, she started screaming and alternated between being mute and mumbling unintelligibly in both Spanish and English. She was admitted to the inpatient psychiatric unit where, at one point, she ate plastic flowers from a vase and reported hearing her daughter's voice telling her to kill herself (Oquendo, Horwath, & Martínez, 1992).

What do these cases have in common? In each instance an ataque de nervios, *or "attack of nerves," had occurred following intense familial stress. Each episode, however, was precipitated by a distinct type of stressor. Further, their association with psychopathology also differs. In this chapter, we discuss this cultural concept of distress common among Latinos and show how, depending on the context, its relationship with psychopathology can vary, ranging from a normative response to stress to a marker of severe psychopathology. First, we provide an overview of the historical and cultural context in which ataque has been described, review its role in current diagnostic systems, and discuss its symptomatology and epidemiology. We end by reviewing the various means available to assess and treat ataque and by providing recommendations for future research.*

HISTORICAL AND CULTURAL CONTEXT

Studied for over half a century, *ataque de nervios* is one of the best-assessed cultural concepts of distress. It first appeared in the U.S. mental health literature in the 1950s, reported by U.S. military psychiatrists stationed in Puerto Rico. Initially identified by the problematic label of "Puerto Rican Syndrome," episodes of ataques were described as "spectacular" and "bizarre" "seizures" that occurred among recently inducted male recruits in response to the stressors associated with weapons training and combat courses (Fernández-Marina, 1961; Mehlman, 1961; Rothenberg, 1964; Rubio, Urdaneta, & Doyle, 1955). A gamut of reactions was associated with the "Puerto Rican Syndrome" label, including a partial loss of consciousness, convulsions, sudden verbal and physical outbursts, crying, and "pseudo-suicidal" attempts (see Table 17.1). In keeping with the psychoanalytic theory of the time, these investigators attributed ataques to specific indigenous child-rearing practices that allegedly predisposed sufferers to the hysterical discharge of aggressive drives. The power relationships embodied in the military, and the colonial situation represented by the presence of the U.S. armed forces in Puerto Rico, usually were left unanalyzed in these discussions.

Work since the 1970s by Latino mental health professionals and medical anthropologists working in Latino communities began to apply a sociocultural (in addition to a clinical) perspective to understanding ataques (Abad & Boyce, 1979; De La Cancela, Guarnaccia, & Carrillo, 1986; Guarnaccia, De La Cancela, & Carrillo, 1989; Lewis-Fernández, 1998; Lewis-Fernández & Aggarwal, 2015). Latino mental health professionals argued that ataque was a culturally recognized and sanctioned expression of strong emotion that should be understood as a form of communication about family relationships. Women's manifestations of ataques, in particular, were seen as a means of protesting the effects of economic disenfranchisement and male domination on their own and their relatives' lives. This indirect and relatively accepted form of resistance substituted for more direct and challenging types of protest.

Recent research has examined the relationship of ataque to psychiatric disorders and the epidemiology of ataque in Puerto Rico and the United States (Guarnaccia, 1993; Guarnaccia et al., 2009; Interian et al., 2005; Lewis-Fernández, Guarnaccia et al., 2002; López, Ramírez, Guarnaccia, Canino, & Bird, 2011; López et al., 2009). It also has situated ataque in relation to other cultural concepts of distress common among Latinos, such as *nervios* (Guarnaccia, Lewis-Fernández, & Rivera Marano, 2003; Guarnaccia, Rivera, Franco, & Neighbors, 1996; Lewis-Fernández et al., 2010) and described the relationship among ataque, traumatic exposure, dissociative capacity, and anxiety sensitivity (Cintrón, Carter, & Sbrocco, 2005; Hinton, Chong, Pollack, Barlow, & McNally, 2008; Lewis-Fernández, Garrido-Castillo et al., 2002; Lewis-Fernández et al., 2010). Ataque is now understood as a form of communication—an *idiom of distress*—regarding a person's reaction to adversity. It relies on dissociative and somatic expressions that are patterned by cultural understandings of what constitutes appropriate or transgressive emotions

Table 17.1. Attempts at Categorizing the Symptoms of Ataque de Nervios

Reference	Symptoms
Rubio et al. (1955)	**Presentation Occurs in One of Five Reactions:** 1. **Reaction #1:** (15.3%): Partial loss of consciousness, convulsions, hyperventilation, moaning, profuse salivation, aggression to self or others (e.g., biting, scratching) 2. **Reaction #2:** (24.8%): Sudden outbursts of verbal and physical hostility, with destructiveness and assaultiveness, expression of persecutory trends, hyperactivity 3. **Reaction #3:** (11.4%): Infantile emotionality and behavior. Sobbing and crying, dependency on others 4. **Reaction #4:** (9.4%): Pseudosuicidal attempts (superficial scratches on wrists, forearm, and chest by razor blades, pens, and pins; ingestion of rat poison or disinfectants; attempted hangings) 5. **Reaction #5:** (39.1%) Mild dissociation, inability to concentrate, forgetfulness, loss of interest in personal appearance, preoccupation, flat affect.
Mehlman (1961)	Extreme fright, agitation, violence, mutism, pseudoepilepsy, bizarre detached uncommunicative violent attitudes, self-mutilation, psychotic behaviors (including coprophagia and catatonic posturing), foaming at the mouth, with subsequent amnesia and confusion.
Guarnaccia, Rubio-Stipec, & Canino (1989)	Chest pain, temporary blindness, paralysis, fainting, unconsciousness, unusual spells, shortness of breath, rapid and pronounced heart beat, dizziness, weakness, sickly for most of life, crying spells, shouting uncontrollably, trembling, becoming physically and verbally aggressive
Guarnaccia et al. (1996)	**Affective dimension:** Screaming, crying, anxiety, depression, fear, anguish, anger **Bodily sensations:** Trembling, palpitations, dyspnea, chest pain, chills, headache, aphonia, upset stomach, fatigue, weakness, hypoesthesia in parts of the body, sweaty hands, convulsions, seizures **Action dimension:** Aggression toward self, wanting to die, suicide attempts, suicidal ideation; aggression toward others or things; inability to eat or sleep **Alterations in consciousness:** fainting, loss of consciousness, dizziness, sense of going crazy, amnesia, hallucinations, many thoughts or memories

Febo San Miguel et al. (2006)	**Externalizing:** Feeling angry, crying, screaming, falls/convulsions, aggression, breaking things, suicidal thoughts, fainting, losing consciousness, amnesia **Internalizing:** Nervous, frightened, trembling, pronounced and rapid heart beat, headache, suffocation, dyspnea, afraid of going crazy, dizziness

Lewis-Fernández, Guarnaccia, & Ruiz (2009)	1. Exposure to a frequently sudden, stressful stimulus, typically eliciting feelings of fear, grief, or anger, and involving a person close to the subject, such as a spouse, child, family member, or friend. Severity of the trigger ranges from mild–moderate (i.e., marital argument, disclosure of migration plans) to extreme (i.e., physical or sexual abuse, acute bereavement).
	
	2. Initiation of the episode immediately upon exposure to the stimulus, or after a period of brooding or emotional "shock."
	
	3. Once the acute attack begins, rapid evolution of an intense affective storm characterized by a primary affect usually congruent with the stimulus (such as anger, fear, grief) and a sense of loss of control (*emotional expressions*).
	
	4. These are accompanied by all, or some, of the following:
	
	  a. bodily sensations: trembling, chest tightness, headache, difficulty breathing, heart palpitations, heat in the chest, paresthesias of diverse location, difficulty moving limbs, fainting, blurred vision, or dizziness (*mareos*).
	
	  b. behaviors (action dimension): shouting, crying, swearing, moaning, breaking objects, striking out at others or at self, attempting to harm self with nearest implement, falling to the ground, shaking with convulsive movements, or lying "as if dead."
	
	5. Cessation may be abrupt or gradual, but it is usually rapid, and often results from the ministration of others, involving expressions of concern, prayers, or use of rubbing alcohol (*alcoholado*). There is return of ordinary consciousness and reported exhaustion.
	
	6. The attack is frequently followed by partial or total amnesia for the events of the acute attack: loss of consciousness, depersonalization, mind going blank, and/or general unawareness of surroundings (*alterations in consciousness*). Some ataques, however, exhibit no alterations in consciousness.

DSM-IV (APA, 1994) and DSM-5 (APA, 2013)	Symptoms of intense emotional upset, including acute anxiety, anger or grief, screaming and shouting uncontrollably; attacks of crying, trembling, heat in the chest rising into the head; and becoming verbally and physically aggressive. Dissociative experiences (e.g., depersonalization, derealization, amnesia), seizure–like or fainting episodes, and suicidal gestures are prominent in some *ataques* but absent in others.

and behaviors in Latino communities (Guarnaccia et al., 1996; Lewis-Fernández, 1998; Lewis-Fernández & Aggarwal, 2015).

ROLE IN CURRENT DIAGNOSTIC SYSTEMS

Ataque was first included in the mental health nosology in the *Diagnostic and Statistical Manual of Mental Disorders – Fourth edition* (DSM-IV) Glossary of Culture-Bound Syndromes (American Psychiatric Association [APA], 1994). *Culture-bound syndromes* were defined at the time as recurring patterns of distressing behaviors that were thought to be prevalent in and "bound" to particular localities, and which were not necessarily equivalent to any single diagnostic entity. Ataque was described as a cluster of symptoms centered on a sense of loss of control that was common among Caribbean Latinos (APA, 1994). In DSM-5, the concept of *culture-bound syndrome* was substituted by that of *cultural concept of distress*, which highlights the fact that different types of cultural concepts exist—not only syndromes, but also idioms of distress and explanations—and which emphasizes the cultural patterning of *all* expressions of distress, including the DSM categories (APA, 2013).

Although DSM-IV noted the potential association of ataque with several diagnoses, including anxiety, mood, dissociative, and somatoform disorders, it did not clarify how the cultural concept and the diagnoses were related or how the cultural concepts could be used in clinical practice. Moreover, listing the "culture-bound syndromes" in a separate appendix at the back of the book hindered their clinical use (Lewis-Fernández, Guarnaccia, & Ruíz, 2009; López & Ho, 2013). DSM-5 clarified some of these points, noting that cultural concepts represent ways of expressing distress that do not have a one-to-one correspondence with any diagnostic entity; the correspondence is more likely to be one-to-many in either direction:

> [S]ymptoms or behaviors that might be sorted by DSM-5 into several disorders may be included in a single folk concept, and diverse presentations that might be classified by DSM-5 as variants of a single disorder may be sorted into distinct concepts by an indigenous diagnostic system (APA, 2013, p.758).

The folk label (e.g., ataque) contributes important information over and above the psychiatric diagnosis, by clarifying symptoms and etiological attributions that could otherwise be confusing and that may, in fact, guide a patient's treatment expectations. Therefore, these cultural expressions should be included in case formulations. Moreover, cultural concepts sometimes apply to a wider range of experiences than diagnoses in terms of severity. This includes presentations that do not meet DSM criteria for any mental disorder. For example, some ataques constitute normative expression of nonpathological distress (e.g., when they occur at funerals), whereas others may be associated with one or more diagnoses.

The DSM-5 entry for ataque lists psychiatric disorders that share phenomenological similarities with this cultural concept of distress (APA, 2013). These include anxiety (e.g., panic, other specified), somatic symptom (e.g., conversion), stressor and trauma-related (other specified) dissociative (other specified), and/ or disruptive and impulse control disorders (e.g., intermittent explosive disorder). This list does not include conditions with which ataque is often comorbid, such as major depression and generalized anxiety disorder, but which do not share its paroxysmal character.

Presently, ataque is not included in the 10th edition of the *International Classification of Diseases and Related Health Problems* (ICD-10; World Health Organization [WHO], 1992), nor is it recommended for inclusion in ICD-11. This is primarily due to concerns about its diagnostic criteria. Ataque is, however, a very common syndrome in Latin America and the Caribbean (Razzouk, Nogueira, & de Jesus Mari, 2011).

Ataques are mentioned in the third edition of the *Glosario Cubano de Psiquiatría* (*Cuban Glossary of Psychiatry*; GC-3), which is an adaptation of the ICD-10 (Otero Ojeda et al., 2008; WHO, 1992). In GC-3, ataque is listed (without a specific code) under the dissociative and conversion disorders. It also is mentioned in a section titled, *Syndromes of Difficult Location* under the broader category of *nervios*, another cultural concept of distress. In GC-3, the clinician is cautioned that in certain contexts ataques are culturally normative, although there is passing reference to their association with mood, neurotic, and personality disorders.

In contrast, ataque is included more extensively in the *Guía Latinoamericana de Diagnóstico Psiquiátrico-Versión Revisada* (*Latin American Guide to Psychiatric Diagnosis – Revised Version*; GLADP-VR), the Latin American regional adaption of ICD-10 (APAL, 2012; Saavedra, Mezzich, Otero, & Salloum, 2012). As in GC-3, in GLADP-VR ataque is coded under the dissociative and conversion disorders, but it is also listed separately under a section titled, *Cultural Syndromes Specifically for Latin Americans*. There, ataque is described in some detail and receives its own classification code (F48.8 *Ataques de Nervios*: Puerto Rico). Thus, although ataque is included in DSM-5, GC-3, and GLADP-VR, the manuals vary as to how much the clinician is informed that ataque may represent a nonpathological expression of distress and about the range of disorders with which it shares phenomenological similarities.

SYMPTOMATOLOGY

An *ataque de nervios* is an emotional and behavioral paroxysm that is typically understood to arise directly from the impact on the person's nervous system (*nervios*) as a result of an overwhelming experience—often but not always of traumatic proportions—that causes the person to lose control over his/her emotions and behaviors. The exact symptoms of the emotional fit (Trautman, 1961) may differ from person to person and the primary emotion may be loss, grief, anger, or fear (Lewis-Fernández et al., 2009). In a representative community sample in Puerto Rico, the most common symptoms of a person's first ataque ($N = 77$) were: nervousness (90%), crying (88%), trembling (77%), palpitations (75%), chest tightness (75%), headache (70%), becoming "hysterical" (69%), fear (65%), losing control (64%), and shortness of breath (61%) (Guarnaccia et al., 1996). More infrequent symptoms, such as suicidal ideation, may indicate greater severity: About 7%–14% of ataques result in suicide attempts during the acute stage of an episode (Guarnaccia et al., 1996; 2009). Although some ataques are similar to panic attacks, careful phenomenological dissection indicated that only 36% fulfilled DSM-IV-TR criteria for panic attack and 17% for panic disorder (Lewis-Fernández, Guarnaccia et al., 2002).

Attempts to categorize the symptoms of ataque are listed in Table 17.1. Qualitative research in Puerto Rico organized ataque along four dimensions—emotional symptoms, bodily symptoms, aggressive symptoms, and alterations in consciousness—all centered on the overarching feeling of losing control (Guarnaccia et al., 1996). Later research grouped ataque symptoms into two nonorthogonal factors that were believed to overlap with internalizing and externalizing disorders (Febo San Miguel et al., 2006). In a clinical sample, two main subtypes of ataque were proposed which were associated with specific symptom profiles. Patients whose ataques were characterized by intense fearfulness, asphyxia, and chest tightness were more likely to receive diagnoses of panic disorder, whereas patients whose ataques were dominated by anger and aggressive behaviors (e.g., breaking things) were more likely to meet criteria for co-occurring mood disorders (Salmán et al., 1998). Ataques, however, should only be considered pathological if symptoms produce long-lasting distress or functional impairment.

PREVALENCE AND ASSOCIATED FEATURES

Ataques occur throughout the lifespan, from early childhood (López et al., 2009), to adolescence (Zayas & Gulbas, 2012), to middle age and beyond (Weingartner, Robison, Fogel, & Gruman, 2002). Demographically, both adults and children have risk factors typically associated with psychopathology. Among adults, ataque was found to be more common in women over the age of 45, with less than a high school education, who were formerly married (i.e., divorced, widowed, or separated) and were out of the labor force (Guarnaccia, Canino, Stipec, & Bravo, 1993; Guarnaccia et al., 2009). Among children, ataque is generally more common in girls, older youth (Guarnaccia, Martinez, Ramírez, & Canino, 2005; López et al., 2009), and children who perceive themselves to be poor (Guarnaccia et al., 2005).

The prevalence of ataque varies depending on the characteristics of the sample and the time frame assessed (Table 17.2). In a representative community sample in Puerto Rico, 16% of respondents reported at least one ataque during their lifetime, making it one of the most frequently reported syndromes on the Island (Guarnaccia et al., 1993). Epidemiological research in the United States indicates a lifetime prevalence of 5%–11% among adult Latinos, with the highest rate among Puerto Ricans (Guarnaccia et al., 2009). Prevalence is substantially higher in clinical samples, with lifetime estimates of 26%–55% (Alcántara, Abelson, & Gone, 2011; Lewis-Fernández, Guarnaccia, Patel, Lizardi, & Díaz, 2005; Weingartner et al., 2002). Among respondents in a clinic with a high proportion of anxiety disorder patients, 66% of Puerto Ricans and Dominicans reported at least one ataque in the last month (Hinton, Lewis-Fernández, & Pollack, 2009).

In children, prevalence in clinical samples is likewise higher than in representative community samples. Over 25% of children in a representative mental health sample in Puerto Rico reported at least one ataque during their lifetime compared with 9% of a representative community sample (Guarnaccia et al., 2005). Representative samples of Puerto Rican children in San Juan and the South Bronx revealed lower lifetime prevalence rates (5.4% and 4.3%, respectively), although ataque remained one of the most-reported mental health syndromes in the study (López et al., 2009).

The frequency of ataque in community samples ranges considerably. In one study, 28% of adult sufferers had only one ataque in their lifetime, while 13% had two, 21% had three to five, and 23% had six or more; meanwhile 15% were unsure (Lewis-Fernández et al., 2005). The frequency of ataque in clinical samples has also varied greatly (Hinton et al., 2008; Lewis-Fernández, Garrido-Castillo et al., 2002). Among Puerto Rican children with ataque in San Juan and the South Bronx, 61% and 57%, respectively, had one to three episodes in the last year (López et al., 2009). Ataque frequency can be considered a marker of ataque severity and is correlated with anxiety sensitivity and the capacity to dissociate (Hinton et al., 2008; Lewis-Fernández, Garrido-Castillo et al., 2002).

In terms of onset, ataques typically occur immediately after, or within a day of, a stressor: 65%–90% of individuals report having an ataque following a stressful event (Cintrón et al., 2005; Lewis-Fernández, Guarnaccia et al., 2002; Rubens, Felix, Vernberg, & Canino, 2014). Ataques are usually brief; about 33%–67% last less than an hour (Cintrón et al., 2005; Lewis-Fernández, Guarnaccia et al., 2002).

Cessation of an *ataque* can be gradual or abrupt, with sufferers typically reporting amnesia and exhaustion following the experience (Guarnaccia et al., 1996). However, 54%–58% indicated that they felt better and relieved after an episode (Lewis-Fernández, Guarnaccia et al., 2002), in part because they were able to express how they felt (e.g., saying, "*me desahogué*" or "I let it out"). Individuals who reported feeling better following an episode were also less likely to endorse panic disorder symptoms than those who expressed fear after the ataque (Lewis-Fernández, Guarnaccia et al., 2002). Sufferers tended to return to their premorbid level of functioning fairly quickly, usually within moments or days after the attack (Guarnaccia et al., 1996; 2003).

Despite being brief, ataque often is associated with certain long-term consequences. Compared with individuals without ataque, sufferers had higher odds of reporting multiple unexplained neurological symptoms (Interian et al., 2005), of describing their health as only fair or poor (Dienfach, Robison, Tolin, & Blank, 2003; Guarnaccia et al., 1993), and of reporting mental health-related disability and the use of outpatient mental health care (Lewis-Fernández et al., 2009). Similarly, children with ataque were more limited in their activities and reported

Table 17.2. PREVALENCE OF *ATAQUE DE NERVIOS*

Reference	Sample	N	Site	Age	Ethnicity	Prevalence
Guarnaccia, Rubio-Stipec, & Canino (1989)	Representative Community	1,513	Puerto Rico	Over 17 years	Puerto Rican	23%
Guarnaccia et al. (1993)	Representative Community	912	Puerto Rico	Over 17 years	Puerto Rican	16%
Weingartner et al. (2002)	Clinical	303	Northeastern United States	Over 17 years	Puerto Rican	26%
Lewis-Fernández, Garrido-Castillo et al. (2002)	Clinical	37	Northeastern United States	Over 17 years	Puerto Rican	43.2%
Lewis-Fernández et al. (2005)	Consecutive Clinical	186	Puerto Rico & Northeastern United States	Over 17 years	89 Island Puerto Rican 97 Mainland Puerto Rican	55.1% Island 51.5% Mainland
Guarnaccia et al. (2005)	Representative Community & Clinical	2,653	Puerto Rico	4–17 years	1,897 Community: Puerto Rican 767 Clinical: Puerto Rican	9% community 26% clinical
Hinton et al. (2008)	Clinical	70	Lowell, MA	Over 17 years	Puerto Rican	66% had 1 + *ataque* in last month
Hinton et al. (2009)	Clinical	140	Lowell, MA	Over 17 years	119 Puerto Rican 21 Dominican	66% had 1 + *ataque* in last month

López et al. (2009)	Representative Community	2,491	San Juan, Puerto Rico & the South Bronx, NY	5–13 years	1,353 Island Puerto Rican 1,138 Mainland Puerto Rican	5.4% in San Juan 4.3% in South Bronx
Guarnaccia et al. (2009)	Representative Community	2,554	Coterminous United States	Over 17 years	868 Mexican 577 Cuban 495 Puerto Rican 614 Other Latino	10.9% Puerto Rican 6.2% Cuban 6.0% Mexican 5.4% Other Latino
Alcántara et al. (2011)	Community	82	Midwestern United States	Over 17 years	Mexican American	41.5%

NOTE: All prevalence rates are lifetime unless otherwise noted. Presence of *ataque* was assessed differently across studies. Methods ranged from asking participants whether they had ever had an ataque to meeting a pre-established cutoff out of a list of symptoms.

more somatic concerns than those without ataque. In particular, they were more likely to report asthma, headaches, or epilepsy/seizures, and had more stomach-aches than their peers (López et al., 2011).

THEORIES OF ETIOLOGY

What causes ataque? Early psychoanalytic explanations postulated that ataques were due to an overpowering id and overwhelmed ego (Mehlman, 1961). The explosive nature of the episode was thought to result from excessive physical contact—either because of cramped quarters or because of excessive handling and fondling during childhood. This was believed to have led to libidinal over-arousal (Fernández-Marina, 1961; Rothenberg, 1964). In this view, delayed wean-ing through extended bottle-feeding and use of pacifiers further reduced a child's ability to tolerate frustration (Rothenberg, 1964). The low frustration tolerance, along with heightened sensitivity, eventually led to an ataque.

During the 1970s and 1980s, ataque was examined as a culturally acceptable form of expressing distress (Guarnaccia, De La Cancela, & Carrillo, 1989). Given the centrality of family to many Latinos, disruptions in familial bonds—such as separation, divorce, an argument, or witnessing an accident involving a family member—were identified as precipitants of ataque (Guarnaccia et al., 1993; López & Ho, 2013). In fact, among Puerto Rican children in New York City, ataque was associated with a higher number of stressful life events, including incidents related to family conflict (López et al., 2009).

Other precipitants have been investigated. Natural disasters, such as hurri-canes and mudslides, are reliable correlates of ataque (Guarnaccia et al., 1993). Research indicated, however, that exposure to these events, in the context of ele-vated exposure to other stressors, such as peer violence, did *not* add a statistically significant additional risk for ataque in community samples (Rubens et al., 2014). Violence, particularly in childhood, may thus play a key role in the occurrence of ataque. This is further substantiated by research indicating that children with ataque reported a greater exposure to violence than those without ataque (López et al., 2009).

It is still unclear, however, what role childhood trauma, in particular, may have in predisposing one to ataque. Whereas one study in a clinical sample noted an association between childhood trauma and ataque (Schecter et al., 2000), another did not find this association, in part because of the high level of exposure to trauma across cohorts with and without ataque (Lewis-Fernández, Garrido-Castillo et al., 2002). Trauma may be a necessary but not a sufficient precondition for the occur-rence of ataque. Trauma, in turn, may increase anxiety sensitivity and/or dissocia-tive capacity, which are associated with ataque occurrence and severity (Hinton et al., 2008; Lewis-Fernández, Garrido-Castillo et al., 2002).

Although stressors such as these have been implicated in precipitating ataques, other studies have shown that many sufferers do not, or cannot always, identify a precipitating event, suggesting that ataque also may be the result of accumulated suffering rather than one specific event (Cintrón et al., 2005; Lewis-Fernández, Guarnaccia et al., 2002). A multifactorial model is, therefore, needed to explain the occurrence and frequency of ataques and to contextualize the suffering that is associated with them (De La Cancela et al., 1986).

ASSESSMENT

Ataque has been assessed in various ways. To identify ataque sufferers, scales have been developed by combining items from earlier questionnaires, such as the somatization section of the *Diagnostic Interview Schedule* (Guarnaccia, Rubio-Stipec, & Canino, 1989) and the somatoform section of the *Composite International Diagnostic Interview* (CIDI; Interian et al., 2005). These proxy measures usually were developed for secondary analyses of existing datasets and relied on phenomenological similarities between the items and ethnographic descriptions of ataque. Respondents were scored as positive if they met a symptom cutoff score and had some degree of impairment.

A second wave of epidemiological research incorporated queries about ataque into new data collection efforts, often based on a single question that asked respondents whether they had "ever had an *ataque de nervios*" (Guarnaccia et al., 1993) or on a full CIDI module based on a symptom list derived from epidemiological and clinical research (Guarnaccia et al., 2010). Despite inherent methodological limitations, the single-question approach— sometimes combined with a few additional questions such as "How many *ataques* have you had in your life?"—has been very fruitful (Alcántara et al., 2011; Guarnaccia et al., 1993; Hinton et al., 2008; 2009; Lewis-Fernández et al., 2010; López et al., 2009; Weingartner et al., 2002). Although recall bias is a concern, Latinos tend to know what ataque refers to when asked. For example, when Hispanic American immigrants living in Spain were presented with hypothetical vignettes of individuals experiencing distress based on the DSM-IV description of ataque, they were more likely to identify these cases correctly than were Spanish nationals (Durá-Vila & Hodes, 2012). Recent ataque scales collapsed symptoms into internalizing and externalizing clusters based on epidemiological research. (Febo San Miguel et al., 2006). These clusters were reliable (Cronbach's α = .83 and .77, respectively) and moderately correlated (r = .49). To date, however, these scales have not been used to screen for ataque, nor have cutoffs been established.

Clinical research in the mid-1990s prepared in-depth clinician-administered interviews based on the ethnographic research that led to the ataque description in DSM-IV. *The Explanatory Model Interview Catalogue* gathered information about the first and a subsequent episode of ataque, apparent precipitants, and family history of the cultural concept (Guarnaccia et al., 1996; Lewis-Fernández, Garrido-Castillo et al., 2002; Lewis-Fernández, Guarnaccia et al., 2002). These interviews were used to characterize the ataque episodes in substantial detail, including comparing them to psychiatric disorders.

DIFFERENTIAL DIAGNOSIS

Not all episodes of ataque are associated with psychopathology (Guarnaccia et al., 1993). Ataque is comorbid, however, with a range of psychological disorders among youth and adults, including mood, anxiety, dissociative, somatoform, stressor and trauma-related, and disruptive disorders (Guarnaccia et al., 1993; 2005; Lewis-Fernández, Garrido-Castillo et al., 2002; Liebowitz et al., 1994; López et al., 2009). But what distinguishes ataque from these disorders?

First, it is important to note that ataque does not correlate exclusively with one particular psychiatric diagnosis and cannot be treated as simply a culturally shaped version of a specific psychiatric disorder. Instead, ataque is a marker of being overwhelmed by adversity, which can be associated with a range of disorders. Second, it is important to distinguish between syndromes that share phenomenological features with ataque—such as transient, ego-dystonic, emotional paroxysms (e.g., panic attacks)—and disorders that are comorbid with ataque. The latter are longer lasting conditions that co-occur with ataque (e.g., mood disorders). Their comorbidity may be due to shared risk factors, or to one condition predisposing to the other—the temporal sequence of their onsets remains to be elucidated (Lewis-Fernández, Guarnaccia et al., 2002). In fact, the comorbidity of ataque is extensive. Among adults in Puerto Rico, ataque sufferers had 4.35 times the odds of meeting criteria for a psychiatric diagnosis compared with those without the cultural syndrome (Guarnaccia et al., 1993). Likewise, Island children with ataques had 4.3 times the odds of any psychiatric disorder when assessed in community settings and 2.3 times the odds in a clinical setting (Guarnaccia et al., 2005).

In terms of paroxysmal conditions resembling ataque, a given ataque episode may meet criteria for one or more of these conditions because of their phenomenological similarities. For example, an ataque may fulfill criteria for panic attack or for acute dissociative reaction (a subtype of other specified dissociative disorder) depending on its symptoms. Both the folk and professional labels should be used in diagnosis and treatment planning, because each contributes useful information. The similarities and differences among ataque and panic attacks and panic disorder have been extensively studied (Lewis-Fernández, Guarnaccia et al., 2002). In epidemiological studies in Puerto Rico, adults and children with ataque had 25–30 times the odds of meeting criteria for panic disorder compared with respondents without ataque (Guarnaccia et al., 1993; 2005). These elevated odds ratios are due to the very low prevalence of panic disorder among respondents who did not report ataque (e.g., 0.4% of adults). This finding indicates that it is rare to find panic disorder in Puerto Rico among community residents who do not identify as suffering from ataque (Lewis-Fernández et al., 2005).

However, the converse is not true; in Puerto Rico only 9% of community-based adults with ataque met criteria for panic disorder (Guarnaccia et al., 1993). Likewise, in clinical samples, most ataque sufferers did not meet criteria for panic disorder (Salmán et al., 1998; Lewis-Fernández, Guarnaccia et al., 2002). Among

66 ataque sufferers attending an anxiety disorders clinic in New York, only 44% reported that their best-remembered ataques met the 10-minute crescendo required by DSM-IV for panic attacks, and only 26% of these ataques were uncued by precipitants; for 65% of respondents, all of their ataques over their lifetime had been cued. Unlike most panic attacks, after an ataque individuals report feeling relief, and may only experience limited avoidance or anticipatory dread (Cintrón et al., 2005). One study, however, found that 80% of best-remembered ataques met DSM-IV criteria for at least one post-episode sequela, such as behavior change related to the attacks (Lewis-Fernández, Guarnaccia et al., 2002). Ataques are also more likely during the day, as opposed to nocturnal panic attacks, and to occur in the company of others.

Two other kinds of paroxysmal conditions share phenomenological simi-larities with ataque: acute dissociative experiences—such as those receiving a DSM-5 diagnosis of other specified dissociative disorder (APA, 2013)—and sudden suicidal episodes (Trautman, 1961). Severity of ataques, assessed as lifetime number of episodes, is positively and independently related to self-reported dissociative symptoms as measured with the *Dissociative Experiences Scale*, and to clinician-diagnosed dissociative disorders as assessed with the *Structured Clinical Interview for DSM-IV* (Hinton et al., 2008; Lewis-Fernández, Garrido-Castillo et al., 2002; Lewis-Fernández et al., 2010). Regarding suicide, in a nationally representative community sample of diverse U.S. Latino sub-ethnicities (N = 2,554), lifetime history of ataque was independently associ-ated with suicidal ideation (OR = 2.4) after adjusting for multiple covariates. This suggested that the cultural syndrome conveys additional risk beyond recognized risk factors such as psychiatric diagnosis and traumatic exposure (Lewis-Fernández et al., 2009). During ataque episodes, sufferers may make goal-directed or ill-formed attempts at self-harm, increasing the morbidity (and occasional mortality) of the syndrome.

TREATMENT

There is no systematic research on the treatment of ataque. Several case studies have focused on reducing the patient's general level of distress and on establishing trust and rapport rather than on treating the ataque per se (Lewis-Fernández, 1996; Lizardi, Oquendo, & Graves, 2009; Schechter, Kaminer, Grienenberger, & Amat, 2003). One study detailed the assessment and treatment of a parent-child dyad in which the mother was positive for ataque (Schechter et al., 2003). Information regarding the mother's ataque precipitants—and her illness attributions—was used to strengthen the parent-child bond via guided play therapy.

General treatment principles may be useful in caring for a person with ataques. Because intolerance of negative affect and arousal symptoms are associated with anxiety severity, clinicians may help sufferers to tolerate these experiences (Hinton et al., 2009). Practices that reduce arousal, such as meditation and breath-ing exercises (Hinton et al., 2009), may help prevent or reduce future episodes.

One study showed how progressive muscle relaxation, together with cognitive coping and grounding exercises, helped a client manage her ataques (Sánchez & Shellcross, 2012).

At a minimum, clinicians need to ensure the safety of the sufferer during an ataque. Providing support and acknowledging the overwhelming nature of the experience are both vital in helping someone who has experienced an ataque. Culturally sanctioned ways of doing so include the use of rubbing alcohol (Lewis-Fernández et al., 2009) or a tincture of alcohol and herb-infused distilled water known as *agua de florida* (floral water), which not only rallies community support but also likely responds to hidden etiological explanations related to hot-cold concepts of disease—the applied liquids cool the nervous system (Harwood, 1971). In addition, clinicians can support the person's own efforts to return to a state of *control* and *tranquilidad* (equanimity), helping him/her regain a sense of homeostasis after the episode (Lewis-Fernández, 2008; Lewis-Fernández & Aggarwal, 2015). If the ataques are associated with impairment, longer-term treatment could focus on helping clients learn to identify the triggers that precipitate an ataque and to express their emotions in a less explosive manner.

Key to all recommendations is the need for a collaborative treatment approach. It is important for clinicians to understand how the patient views the problem and to use this information to help guide the therapeutic approach (Hinton et al., 2008; Lewis-Fernández, Guarnaccia et al., 2002; Lizardi et al., 2009). The use of standardized cultural assessments, such as the *DSM-5 Cultural Formulation Interview*, could be useful in this regard (Lewis-Fernández et al., 2016). Obtaining a family history could be informative, given that 37.2% and 46.4% of children in community and clinical samples, respectively, have a family history of ataque (Guarnaccia et al., 2005). Integrating family genograms into treatment may help.

Finally, some clients may not view their ataque as a problem. Instead, they may focus primarily on the precipitating stressors rather than the episode itself. This is suggested by data showing that only about one third of community respondents seek help for the ataques themselves (Cintrón et al., 2005). Future work should investigate forms of healing that address the larger structural issues associated with the ataque (De La Cancela et al., 1986). Feminist therapy, for example, may be particularly useful because of its emphasis on social action and empowerment (Rivera-Arzola & Ramos-Grenier, 1997).

RECOMMENDATIONS FOR FUTURE WORK

Many questions remain regarding ataque de nervios. Although there is now substantial information on its prevalence and psychiatric and demographic correlates, we know much less about etiology, predictors, and developmental course. Although stressful life events, such as some forms of traumatic exposure, appear necessary to the emergence of ataques, these are not sufficient, given that a fair proportion of exposed individuals do not develop ataques. It remains unclear what factors lead to the emergence of the cultural syndrome once the person is exposed to trauma. A multifactorial model of ataque onset must include elements such as gender roles, poverty, anxiety sensitivity, dissociative capacity, family modeling of similar behaviors, and specific cultural understandings of the value of remaining in emotional control, to name a few, which combine to place sufferers at risk of ataque. For example, how do cultural understandings, such as gender roles, get translated into physical symptoms in culturally specific ways?

Further work is needed on potential mechanisms of action that would account for the impact of these predisposing elements. In particular, what distinguishes those who are exposed to stress, and develop ataques, as opposed to those who are exposed but do not develop ataques? If stress is key to the occurrence of an ataque, do the types of stressors differ for men and women? What is the impact of temperamental traits, such as impulsivity, on the risk of ataque and the specific phenomenology of the condition? Additionally, if early trauma can disrupt neural circuitry, what role does culture play in the expression of this dysregulation? How does an inborn or very early capacity for dissociation combine with other risk factors to give rise to highly dissociative episodes? Are there cultural understandings of the self and of how strong emotions should be managed that predispose persons to highly dissociative ataques?

What are the developmental stages of risk that individuals go through? Are there cohort effects—possibly related to evolving cultural characteristics of the society as a whole—that distribute risk unevenly across age cohorts? Are recent generations at a different level of risk than older ones? What social cues predispose to its emergence? For example, what would be the impact of migration into different cultural settings, such as Spain as compared to the United States, on the risk of ataque? Future research also should continue to assess the relation between ataque and other conditions, such as fit-like noninjurious suicidal behavior (Guarnaccia et al., 2009; Trautman, 1961; Zayas & Gulbas, 2010).

Finally, given the risk of recall bias with retrospective studies, it is vital to assess ataques prospectively. Longitudinal research would help clarify the role of specific risk factors and developmental stages. Such study designs would also provide information on how ataques may change over the course of one's life. Prospective designs also allow for systematic treatment studies, which are currently nonexistent. In sum, the study of ataque has progressed rapidly since the mid-20th century, but much remains to be known about this cultural concept of distress.

REFERENCES

Abad, V., & Boyce E. (1979). Issues in the psychiatric evaluations of Puerto Ricans: A socio-cultural perspective. *Journal of Operational Psychiatry, 10*(1), 28–39. doi: http://dx.doi.org/10.1177/136346158101800217

Alcántara, C., Abelson, J.L., & Gone, J.P. (2011). Beyond anxious predisposition: Do *padecer de nervios* and *ataque de nervios* add incremental validity to predictions of current distress among Mexican mothers? *Depression & Anxiety, 29*(1), 23–31. doi: 10.1002/da.20855

American Psychiatric Association. (1994). *Diagnostic and statistical manual of mental disorders* (4th ed.). Washington, DC: Author.

American Psychiatric Association. (2013). *Diagnostic and statistical manual of mental disorders* (5th ed.). Washington, DC: Author.

Asociación Psiquiátrica de América Latina. (2012*). Guía Latinoamericana de diagnóstico psiquiátrico, Versión revisada* (GLADP-VR) [Latin American guide to psychiatric diagnosis, (Rev. Version). Lima, Peru: Asociación Psiquiátrica de América Latina.

Cintrón, J.A., Carter, M.M., & Sbrocco, T. (2005). *Ataques de nervios* in relation to anxiety sensitivity among island Puerto Ricans. *Culture, Medicine & Psychiatry, 29*(4), 415–431. doi: 10.1007/s11013-006-9001-7

De La Cancela, V., Guarnaccia, P.J., & Carrillo E. (1986). Psychosocial distress among Latinos: A critical analysis of *ataques de nervios. Humanity and Society, 10,* 431–447.

Dienfach, G.J., Robison, J.T., Tolin, D.F., & Blank, K. (2003). Late-life anxiety disorders among Puerto Rican primary care patients: Impact on well-being, functioning, and service utilization. *Journal of Anxiety Disorders, 18,* 841–858. doi: 10.1016/janxdis.203.10.005

Durá-Vila, G., & Hodes, M. (2012).Cross-cultural study of idioms of distress among Spanish nationals and Hispanic American migrants: *susto, nervios* and *ataque de nervios. Social Psychiatry and Psychiatric Epidemiology, 47*(10), 1627–1637. doi: 10.1007/s00127-011-0468-3

Fernández-Marina, R. (1961). The Puerto Rican syndrome: Its dynamics and cultural determinants. *Psychiatry, 24*(1), 79–82. doi: 10.1521/00332747.1961.11023256

Febo San Miguel, V.E., Guarnaccia, P.J., Shrout, P., Lewis-Fernández, R., Canino, G., & Ramírez, R.R. (2006). A quantitative analysis of *ataque de nervios* in Puerto Rico: Further examination of a cultural syndrome. *Hispanic Journal of Behavioral Sciences, 28*(3), 313–330. doi: 10.1177/0739986306291441

Guarnaccia, P.J. (1993). *Ataques de nervios* in Puerto Rico: Culture-bound syndrome or popular illness. *Medical Anthropology, 15,* 157–170. doi: 10.1080/01459740.1993.9966087

Guarnaccia, P.J., De La Cancela, V., & Carrillo, E. (1989). The multiple meanings of *ataques de nervios* in the Latino community. *Medical Anthropology, 11,* 47–62. doi: 10.1080/01459740.1989.9965981

Guarnaccia, P.J., Canino, G., Stipec, M., & Bravo, M. (1993). The prevalence of *ataques de nervios* in the Puerto Rico Disaster Study: The role of culture in psychiatric epidemiology. *The Journal of Nervous and Mental Disease, 181*(3), 157–165. doi: 10.1097/00005053-199303000-00003

Guarnaccia, P.J., Lewis-Fernández, R., & Rivera Marano, M.R. (2003). Toward a Puerto Rican popular nosology: *Nervios* and *ataque de nervios. Culture, Medicine & Psychiatry, 27*(3), 339–366. doi: 10.1023/A:1025303315932

Guarnaccia, P.J., Lewis-Fernández, R., Martinez Pincay, I., Shrout, P., Guo, J., Torres, M., . . . Alegría, M. (2009). *Ataque de nervios* as a marker of social and psychiatric vulnerability: Results from the NLAAS. *International Journal of Social Psychiatry, 56*(3): 298–309. doi: 10.1177/0020764008101636.

Guarnaccia, P.J., Martinez, I., Ramírez, R., & Canino, G. (2005). Are *ataques de nervios* in Puerto Rican children associated with psychiatric disorder? *Journal of the American Academy of Child & Adolescent Psychiatry*, 44(11), 1184–1192. doi: 10.1097/01.chi.0000177059.34031.5d

Guarnaccia, P.J., Rivera, M., Franco, F., & Neighbors, C. (1996). The experiences of *ataques de nervios*: Towards an anthropology of emotions in Puerto Rico. *Culture, Medicine and Psychiatry*, 20(3), 343–367. doi: 10.1007/BF00113824

Guarnaccia, P.J., Rubio-Stipec, M., & Canino, G. (1989). *Ataques de nervios* in the Puerto Rican Diagnostic Interview Schedule: The impact of cultural categories on psychiatric epidemiology. *Culture, Medicine and Psychiatry*, 13, 275–295. doi: 10.1007/BF00054339

Harwood, A. (1971). The hot-cold theory of disease: Implications for treatment of Puerto Rican patients. *Journal of the American Medical Association*, 216(7), 1153–1158. doi: 10.1001/jama.1971.03180330029005.

Hinton, D.E., Chong, R., Pollack, M.H., Barlow, D.H., & McNally, R.J. (2008). *Ataque de nervios*: Relationship to anxiety sensitivity and dissociation predisposition. *Depression and Anxiety*, 25(6), 489–495. doi: 10.1002/da.20309.

Hinton, D.E., Lewis-Fernández, R., & Pollack, M.H. (2009). A model of the generation of *ataque de nervios*: The role of fear of negative affect and fear of arousal symptoms. *CNS Neuroscience & Therapeutics*, 15, 264–275. doi: 10.1111/j.1755-5949.2009.00101.

Interian, A., Guarnaccia, P.J., Vega, W.A., Gara, M.A., Like, R.C., Escobar, J.I., & Díaz-Martínez, A.M. (2005). The relationship between *ataque de nervios* and unexplained neurological symptoms: A preliminary analysis. *Journal of Nervous and Mental Disease*, 193(1), 32–39. doi: 10.1097/01.nmd.0000149216.29035.31

Lewis-Fernández, R. (1998). *Eso no estaba en mí ... no pude controlarme: El control, la identidad, y las emociones en comunidades puertorriqueñas*. [That was not in me ... I could not control myself: control, identity, and emotion in Puerto Rican communities.] *Revista de Ciencias Sociales*, 4, 268–299.

Lewis-Fernández, R. (2014). Dissociations. In J.W. Barnhill (Ed.), *DSM-5: clinical cases* (pp. 169–171). Washington, DC: American Psychiatric Publishing.

Lewis-Fernández, R., & Aggarwal, N.K. (2015). Psychiatric classification beyond the DSM: An interdisciplinary approach. In L.J. Kirmayer, R.B. Lemelson, & C.A. Cummings (Eds.), *Revisioning psychiatry: Cultural phenomenology, critical neuroscience, and global mental health*. New York: Cambridge University Press, pp. 434-468.

Lewis-Fernández, R., Aggarwal, N.K., Hinton, L., Hinton, D.E., & Kirmayer, L.K. (Eds.) (2016). *The DSM-5 handbook on the cultural formulation interview*. Washington, DC: American Psychiatric Publishing.

Lewis-Fernández, R., Garrido-Castillo, P., Bennasar, M.C., Parrilla, E.M., Laria, A.J., Ma, G., & Petkova, E. (2002). Dissociation, childhood trauma, and *ataque de nervios* among Puerto Rican psychiatric outpatients. *American Journal of Psychiatry*, 159(9), 1603–1605. doi: 10.1176/appi.ajp.159.9.1603.

Lewis-Fernández, R., Gorritz, M., Raggio, G.A., Peláez, C., Chen, H., & Guarnaccia, P.J. (2010). Association of trauma-related disorders and dissociation with four idioms of distress among Latino psychiatric outpatients. *Culture, Medicine and Psychiatry*, 34, 219–243. doi:10.1007/s11013-010-9177-8

Lewis-Fernández, R., Guarnaccia, P.J., Martínez, I.E., Salmán, E., Schmidt, A., & Liebowitz, M. (2002). Comparative phenomenology of ataques de nervios, panic attacks, and panic disorder. *Culture, Medicine & Psychiatry*, *26*(2), 199–223. doi:10.1023/A:1016349624867.

Lewis-Fernández, R., Guarnaccia, P.J., Patel, S., Lizardi, D., & Díaz, N. (2005). *Ataque de nervios*: Anthropological, epidemiological, and clinical dimensions of a cultural syndrome. In A.M. Georgiopoulos & J.F. Rosenbaum (Eds.), *Perspectives in cross-cultural psychiatry* (pp. 63–85). Philadelphia, PA: Lippincott Williams & Wilkins.

Lewis-Fernández, R., Guarnaccia, P.J., & Ruiz, P. (2009). Culture-bound syndromes. In B.J. Sadock, V.A. Sadock, & P. Ruiz (Eds.), *Kaplan and Sadock's comprehensive textbook of psychiatry* (9th ed.; pp. 2519–2538). Philadelphia, PA: Lippincott Williams & Wilkins.

Liebowitz, M.R., Salmán, E., Jusino, C.M., Garfinkel, R., Street, L., Cárdenas, D. L., . . . Klein, D.F. (1994). *Ataque de nervios* and panic disorder. *American Journal of Psychiatry*, *151*(6), 871–875. doi: 10.1176/ajp.151.6.871

Lizardi, D., Oquendo, M.A., & Graver, R. (2009). Clinical pitfalls in the diagnosis of *ataque de nervios*: A case study. *Transcultural Psychiatry*, *46*(3), 463–486. doi: 10.1177/1363461509343090

López, I., & Ho, A. (2013). Culture-bound (or culturally salient?): The role of culture in disorder. In K.D. Keith (Ed.), *The encyclopedia of cross-cultural psychology*. Hoboken, NJ: Wiley-Blackwell. doi: 10.1002/9781118339893

López, I., Ramírez, R., Guarnaccia, P., Canino, G., & Bird, H. *Ataques de nervios* and somatic complaints among Island and Mainland Puerto Rican children. (2011). *CNS Neuroscience & Therapeutics*, *17*(3), 158–166. doi: 10.1111/j.1755-5949.2010.00137.x

López, I., Rivera, F., Ramírez, R., Guarnaccia, P., Canino, G., & Bird, H.R. (2009). *Ataques de nervios* and their psychiatric correlates in Puerto Rican children from two different contexts. *The Journal of Nervous and Mental Disease*, *3*(12), 923–929. doi: 10.1097/NMD.0b013e3181c2997d

Mehlman, R.D. (1961). The Puerto Rican syndrome. *The American Journal of Psychiatry*, *118*, 328–332. doi: 10.1176/ajp.118.4.328

Oquendo, M., Horwath, E., & Martínez, A. (1992). *Ataques de nervios*: Proposed diagnostic criteria for a culture specific syndrome. *Culture, Medicine & Psychiatry*, *16*, 367–376. doi: 10.1007/BF00052155

Otero Ojeda, A.A., Rabelo Pérez, V., Echazábal Campos, A., Calzadilla Fierro, L., Duarte Castañeda, F., Magriñat Fernández, J.M., & Acosta Nodal. C. (2008). *Tercer Glosario Cubano de Psiquiatría* [The third Cuban glossary of psychiatry]. La Habana, Cuba: Hospital Psiquiátrico de la Habana.

Razzouk, D., Nogueira, B, de Jesus Mari, J. (2011). The contribution of Latin American and Caribbean studies on culture-bound syndromes for the revision of the ICD-10: Key findings from a work in progress. *Revista Brasileira de Psiquiatria*, *33*(1), 513–520.

Rivera-Arzola, M., & Ramos-Grenier, J. (1997). Anger, *ataques de nervios*, and *la mujer Puertorriqueña*: Sociocultural considerations and treatment implications. In J.G. García & M.C. Zea (Eds.), *Psychological interventions and research with Latino populations* (pp. 125–141). Boston: MA: Allyn & Bacon.

Rothenberg, A. (1964). Puerto Rico and aggression. *American Journal of Psychiatry*, *120*(10), 962–970. doi: 10.1176/ajp.120.10.962

Rubens, S.L., Felix, E.D., Vernberg, E.M., & Canino, G. (2014). The role of peers in the relation between hurricane exposure and *ataques de nervios* among Puerto Rican adolescents. *Psychological Trauma: Theory, Research, Practice, and Policy, 6*(6), 716–723. doi: 10.1037/a0036701

Rubio, M., Urdaneta, M., & Doyle, J.L. (1955). Psychopathologic reaction patterns in the Antilles command. *U.S. Armed Forces Medical Journal, 6*(12), 1767–1772.

Saavedra, J.E., Mezzich, J.E., Otero, A., & Salloum, I.M. (2012). The revision of the Latin American guide for psychiatric diagnosis (GLADP) and an initial survey on its utility and prospects. *The International Journal of Person-Centered Medicine, 2*(2), 214–221. doi: 10.5759/ijpcm.v212.219

Salmán, E., Liebowitz, M.R., Guarnaccia, P.J., Jusino, C.M., Garfinkel, R., Street, L., ... Klein, D.F. (1998). Subtypes of *ataques de nervios*: The influence of coexisting psychiatric diagnosis. *Culture, Medicine & Psychiatry, 22*(2), 231–244. doi: 10.1023/A:1005326426885

Sánchez, A., & Shallcross, R. (2012). Integrative psychodynamic treatment of *ataque de nervios. Clinical Case Studies, 11*(1), 5–23. doi: 10.1177/1534650111436210

Schechter, D.S., Kaminer, T., Grienenberger, J.F., & Amat, J. (2003). Fits and starts: A mother-infant case-study involving intergenerational violent trauma and pseudoseizures across three generations. *Infant Mental Health Journal, 24*(5), 510–528. doi: 10.1002/imhj.10070

Schechter, D.S., Marshall, R., Salmán, E., Goetz, D., Davies, S., & Liebowitz, M.R. (2000). *Ataque de nervios* and history of childhood trauma. *Journal of Traumatic Stress 13*(3), 529–534. doi: 10.1023/A:1007797611148

Trautman, E.C. (1961). The suicidal fit: A psychobiologic study on Puerto Rican immigrants. *Archives of General Psychiatry, 5*(1), 76-83. doi:10.1001/archpsyc.1961.01710130078009.

Weingartner, K., Robison, J., Fogel, D., & Gruman, C. (2002). Depression and substance use in a middle aged and older Puerto Rican population. *Journal of Cross-Cultural Gerontology, 17*(2), 173–193. doi: 10.1023/A:1015861002809

World Health Organization. (1992). International statistical classification of diseases and related health problems (10th Rev.; ICD-10). Geneva: WHO.

Zayas, L.H., & Gulbas, L.E. (2012). Are suicide attempts by young Latinas a cultural idiom of distress? *Transcultural Psychiatry, 49*(5), 718–734. doi: 10.1177/1363461512463262

Miscellaneous Disorders

18

Alice in Wonderland Syndrome

JAN DIRK BLOM ■

VIGNETTE

A five-year-old boy is traveling back home with his family after a well-spent summer vacation in France. He falls asleep in the back of the car and wakes up to find that everything looks tilted. His parents think that maybe he slept too deeply, or that he is suffering from a stiff neck. But at home the complaint persists, and the boy stumbles and falls quite often. He is taken to the family physician, who examines him and orders an X-ray of his neck to check for structural abnormalities, only to find that nothing is wrong with it. He then refers the child to a neurologist and then to a psychiatrist. More diagnostic tests are run, including an electroencephalogram (EEG), magnetic resonance imaging (MRI) of the brain, and serological testing for viral encephalitis. Nothing out of the ordinary is found, even though the apparent obliquity of things—called plagiopsia, as the specialists explain—remains present for most of the day. The boy is offered a low dose of valproic acid for symptomatic treatment, but his mother declines after she has been told that spontaneous recovery is possible in such cases, especially in children. She is happy that after a year of uncertainty and worry her son's curious symptom now has a name, and that comparable cases have been described in the literature. So she decides for him to go on without any medical or psychological interventions. Over the course of another year, to everyone's relief, the boy does indeed find that the orientation of vertical lines has returned to normal.

The boy's story reminds me of a symptom I experienced myself, and in my mind I am transported back to a remote tropical beach on the island of Ko Pha Ngan, Thailand, where I see myself lying under a mosquito net after I contracted a viral infection due to food poisoning. Because of the fever, I am confined to a little bamboo hut by the seashore. Lying there in the damp darkness, I have the peculiar sensation that my hands are growing to the size of boxing gloves. When I look at them they seem perfectly normal, even though the impression persists that they might be a little swollen. But as soon as I look away or close my eyes, they once again feel as if they were the size of balloons. It is not an unpleasant sensation, merely curious, but nevertheless I am glad that it lasts only as long as the height of the fever. Before my temperature has fully stabilized, it subsides and never recurs.

A 14-year-old boy is less fortunate. While smoking cannabis, he has the anxious sensation that his head is shrinking and his tongue is growing to enormous proportions. After the effects of the joint wear off, he is relieved to find that his head and tongue regain their normal size. However, from then on he finds himself suffering from daily recurring episodes of derealization and depersonalization during which he has the sensation that stationary objects are moving away from him, his legs are growing shorter, and his hands are shrinking to the size of tiny stumps, especially in his pockets. The symptoms persist for over 35 years, during which time the boy grows into a man, finishes his education at a much lower level than anticipated, gets married, has children, and despite his incapacitating complaints succeeds in obtaining a minor in Spanish at the university, and in generating a steady income while working as a science reporter. Full diagnostic testing throughout the years never reveals anything out of the ordinary, and after having tried out various medicines from the groups of antipsychotics, antidepressants, antiepileptics, and benzodiazepines, it is finally a combination of lamotrigine and citalopram that helps him to reduce the frequency and intensity of the symptoms some 50%—even though at times they return at full force and go on to interfere with his daily functioning.

HISTORICAL AND CULTURAL CONTEXT

The term Alice in Wonderland syndrome (AIWS) was coined in 1955 by the British psychiatrist John Todd (1914–1987) as an umbrella term for symptoms such as those described here. As Todd asserted, he meant for the term "to draw attention to a singular group of symptoms intimately associated with migraine and epilepsy, although not confined to these disorders" (p. 701). The group comprised hyperschematia, hyposchematia, derealization, depersonalization, and somatopsychic duality, as well as illusory changes in the size, distance, or position of stationary objects in the visual field, illusory feelings of levitation, and illusory alterations in the sense of the passage of time (Todd, 1955).

Todd was well aware that he was not the first to describe these symptoms or to associate them with the fictional experiences of *Alice in Wonderland*. In 1954 he himself had preluded on the subject matter of his 1955 paper by describing a patient with micropsia (i.e., seeing things as smaller than they are) and Lilliputian hallucinations (visual hallucinations of objects with miniature proportions; Todd, 1954). However, perceptual distortions such as these had been described long before his time (Charcot, 1889; Veraguth, 1903; Bonnier, 1905; Wilson, 1916; Gelb & Goldstein, 1918; Pötzl, 1943; Seitelberger, 1952), and both Coleman (1933) and Lippman (1952) had drawn comparisons with the phenomena described in *Alice's Adventures in Wonderland*, the children's book written by Charles Lutwidge Dodgson (1832–1898), aka Lewis Carroll.

As originally suggested by Lippman (1952), the somaesthetic distortions described in Dodgson's book (Figure 18.1, Figure 18.2, and Figure 18.3) may well have been inspired by the author's own experiences. In Todd's own words, "The revelation that Lewis Carroll (Charles Lutwidge Dodgson) suffered from migraine arouses the suspicion that Alice trod the paths and byways of a Wonderland well known to her creator" (Anonymous, 1956). In a similar vein, it has been suggested that the split body image of the character Sylvie in another book by Dodgson, *Sylvie and Bruno*, may have been inspired by a migraine-associated illusion of the author himself (Podoll & Robinson, 1999; 2002). An alternative explanation for these surreal elements in Dodgson's stories is that he had either read about the hallucinogenic effects of *Amanita muscaria*, or perhaps experimented with this mushroom himself (Carmichael, 1996).

Whatever the historical course of events may have been, with Alice, Dodgson succeeded in creating a character who appealed as much to physicians as she did to the book's intended audience. Thus, by adopting the name, Alice in Wonderland syndrome, Todd chose a memorable phrase for a group of symptoms hitherto unknown to many.

Over the past 60 years this group of symptoms has gradually expanded (Lanska & Lanska, 2013). It now includes some 40 different visual phenomena characterized by distortions of the form, size, orientation, color, and/or speed of perceived objects (Table 18.1), and more than 15 somaesthetic and other non-visual distortions (Table 18.2). What these widely varying symptoms would seem to have in common is that they constitute distorted rather than hallucinatory or illusory percepts. Hallucinations are percepts experienced in the absence of an appropriate stimulus from the external world; illusions are percepts based on stimuli from the external world that are either misperceived or misinterpreted, in such a way that the object

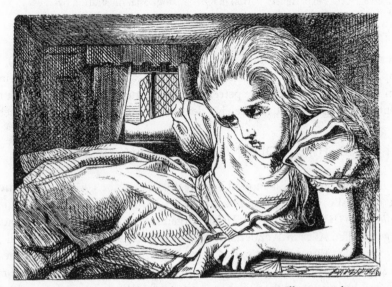

Figure 18.1 Alice experiences total body macrosomatognosia. Illustration by John Tenniel (1865).

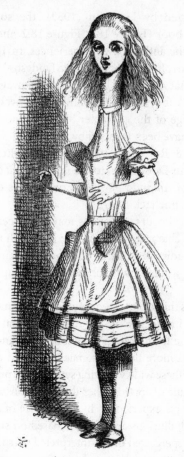

Figure 18.2 Alice experiences partial macrosomatognosia. Illustration by John Tenniel (1865).

appears to constitute something different from what it really is (Blom, 2010). The symptoms considered characteristic of AIWS, however, are percepts based on stimuli from the external world that are perceived in a distorted manner. They do not represent something different, but merely a deformed version of the objects themselves.

ROLE IN CURRENT DIAGNOSTIC SYSTEMS

The literature on AIWS is modest (Figure 18.4), as is the concept's role in current diagnostic systems. The *International Classification of Diseases, Clinical Modification* (ICD-9-CM, World Health Organization, 2008) features a diagnostic category called Alice in Wonderland syndrome (ICD-9-CM 293.89), as well as a category called Visual Distortions of Shape and Size (ICD-9-CM 368.14). The latter category falls under the heading, "Disorders of the Eye and Adnexa," and may, therefore, be considered the peripheral variant of AIWS. It lists metamorphopsia, micropsia, macropsia, and megalopsia as its clinical subtypes.

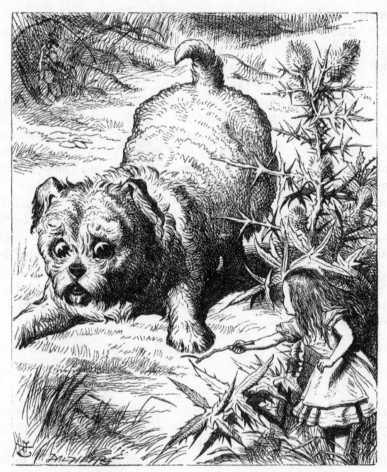

Figure 18.3 Alice experiences total body microsomatognosia. Illustration by John Tenniel (1865).

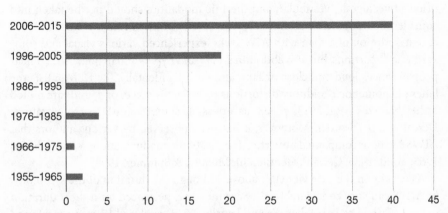

Figure 18.4 Number of scientific publications on AIWS per decennium in the international literature (N = 72).

Although the ICD-9-CM would seem to place more emphasis on visual rather than somaesthetic distortions, various authors have suggested that it is the latter group of distortions that deserve the status of obligatory symptoms of AIWS (Podoll, Ebel, Robinson, & Nicola, 2002; Lanska & Lanska, 2013; Liu, Liu, Liu, & Liu, 2014). This has led Lanska and Lanska (2013) to propose a typology wherein cases characterized by somaesthetic distortions are designated as "type A" or "true" AIWS, and cases with only visual distortions ("type B") or those with both visual and somaesthetic distortions ("type C") as "Alice in Wonderland-like syndromes."

The *Diagnostic and Statistical Manual of Mental Disorders – Fifth Edition* (DSM-5; APA, 2013) mentions the symptoms "two-dimensionality or flatness, exaggerated three-dimensionality, or altered size or distance of objects (i.e., macropsia or micropsia)," but does so only in the context of Depersonalization/Derealization Disorder (300.6). It does not mention AIWS or any of its other individual symptoms, even though Todd (1955) already had asserted that "complete or partial forms of the syndrome appear in the course of a wide variety of disorders" (p. 703), some of which (including schizophrenia) figure prominently in the DSM-5 and its predecessors. It is unclear why AIWS failed to be included in the DSMs, but this may well have contributed to the unfamiliarity of mental health professionals with the syndrome.

SYMPTOMATOLOGY

The symptoms considered characteristic of AIWS are diverse, even though they would seem to have in common, as we saw, that they constitute distortions of regular sense perception (i.e., distortions of visual, somaesthetic, temporal, and self-perception). Table 18.1 provides an overview of known visual distortions, and Table 18.2 describes somaesthetic and other nonvisual distortions. Although Todd's original paper does not hint at any distortions experienced in other sensory modalities, these overviews beg the question of whether parageusia, parosmia, and equivalent distortions in the auditory, sexual, coenesthetic, kinesthetic, proprioceptive, algesic, vestibular, and thermic modalities should not be taken into consideration as possible additional symptoms. A point in case is Hamed's (2010) case description of a man with AIWS who experienced various visual and somaesthetic distortions, but also abdominal pain and hyper- and hypoacusis. ("I hear people's voices loud and close or faint and far.") Incidentally, the DSM-5 lists the latter phenomenon ("auditory distortions . . . whereby voices or sounds are muted or heightened"; APA, 2013, p. 303) as a possible symptom of Depersonalization/Derealization Disorder. Moreover, it has been observed by various authors that AIWS can be accompanied by vertigo (i.e., vestibular hallucination; see Mayrhofer, 1963; Todd, 1955; Ceriani, Gentileschi, Muggia, & Spinnler, 1998).

As we saw in the case vignettes above, although the duration of the symptoms of AIWS can vary considerably, they are mostly experienced for a short duration of time (Critchley, 1953). Lanska and Lanska (2013) analyzed 17 cases, and found nine of them to have lasted fewer than five minutes, seven lasting for five to 30

Table 18.1. VISUAL DISTORTIONS (METAMORPHOPSIAS) THAT MAY OCCUR IN THE CONTEXT OF ALICE IN WONDERLAND SYNDROME

Type of Metamorphopsia	Characterization	Key Reference
Achromatopsia	The inability or strongly diminished ability to perceive color	Zeki (1990)
Akinetopsia	The inability to perceive motion	Zeki (1991)
Chloropsia	Green vision	Pinckers, Cruysberg, & Liem (1989)
Chromatopsia	Seeing things in a single hue (as in chloropsia, cyanopsia, erythropsia, ianothinopsia, and xanthopsia)	Pinckers, Cruysberg, & Liem (1989)
Complicated metamorphopsia	A metamorphopsia that alters the affective assessment of the extracorporeal environment, rendering it either beautiful, ugly, or frightening	Critchley (1953)
Corona phenomenon	An extra contour around objects	Klee & Willanger (1966)
Cyanopsia	Blue vision	Pinckers, Cruysberg, & Liem (1989)
Dyschromatopsia	Color confusion	Zeki (1990)
Dysmegalopsia	A diminished ability to appreciate the size of objects	Wilson (1916)
Dysmetropsia	A change in the apparent size and distance of objects	Wilson (1916)
Dysmorphopsia	Lines and contours appearing to be wavy	Lunn (1948)
Dysplatopsia	Objects appearing flattened and elongated	Wieser (2000)
Enhanced stereoscopic vision	An exaggeration of the depth and detail of visually perceived objects	Critchley (1949)
Entomopia	Seeing multiple images, as if perceived through an insect's eye	Lopez, Adornato, & Hoyt (1993)
Erythropsia	Red vision	Pinckers, Cruysberg, & Liem (1989)

(continued)

Table 18.1. CONTINUED

Type of Metamorphopsia	Characterization	Key Reference
Gyropsia	Seeing an illusory, circular movement	Ey (1973)
Hemimetamorphopsia	A visual distortion of only one half of an object	Nijboer, Ruis, van der Worp, & de Haan (2008)
Hyperchromatopsia	Colors seen as exceptionally bright	ffytche & Howard (1999)
Ianothinopsia	Purple vision	Pinckers, Cruysberg, & Liem (1989)
Illusory splitting	A vertical splitting of objects	Podoll & Robinson (2002)
Illusory visual spread	A perceived extension, expansion, or prolongation of objects	Critchley (1949)
Inverted vision	Objects appearing rotated (usually in the coronal plane, over 90° or 180°)	Winslow (1868)
Kinetopsia	Illusory movement	Ey (1973)
Loss of stereoscopic vision	Objects appearing two-dimensional or "flat"	Critchley (1949)
Macroproxiopia	Objects appearing larger and closer than they are	Critchley (1953)
Macropsia	Seeing things larger than they are	Critchley (1949)
Micropsia	Seeing things smaller than they are	Critchley (1949)
Microtelepsia	Objects appearing smaller and farther away than they are	Taylor, Scheffer, & Berkovic (2003)
Monocular metamorphopsia	Metamorphopsia for one eye	Willanger & Klee (1966)
Mosaic vision	A fragmentation of perceived objects into irregular, crystalline, polygonal facets, interlaced as in a mosaic	Sacks (1970)
Palinopsia	Illusory reoccurrence of visual percepts (as in polyopia, illusory visual spread, and the trailing phenomenon)	Critchley (1949)

Table 18.1. CONTINUED

Type of Metamorphopsia	Characterization	Key Reference
Pelopsia	Objects appearing closer than they are	Ey (1973)
Plagiopsia	Objects appearing as if tilted	Critchley & Ferguson (1933)
Polyopia	Seeing multiple identical copies of a single image	Klüver (1966)
Porropsia	Stationary objects appearing to move away	Vujić & Ristić (1939)
Prosopometamorphopsia	Apparent distortion of faces	Bodamer (1947)
Simple metamorphopsia	A metamorphopsia that does not alter the affective assessment of the extracorporeal environment	Critchley (1953)
Teleopsia	Objects appearing to be farther away than they are	Wilson (1916)
Trailing phenomenon	A series of discontinuous stationary images trailing behind a moving object	Asher (1971)
Visual allachaesthesia	Objects appearing dislocated into the opposite visual field	Beyer (1885)
Visual perseveration	An illusory reoccurrence of visual percepts after an object has moved out of focus	Critchley (1949)
Xanthopsia	Yellow vision	Pinckers, Cruysberg, & Liem (1989)
Zoom vision	Vision fluctuating between micropsia and macropsia, or between microtelepsia and macroproxiopia	Sacks (1970)

NOTE: Adapted from Blom, 2010.

minutes, and a single one lasting for two days. Most episodes would seem to be self-limiting, even though they may sporadically recur from time to time across decades (Dooley, Augustine, Gordon, Brna, & Westby, 2014), whereas in other cases they may be experienced for years or even decades on end, virtually without interruption (Willanger & Klee, 1966; Blom, Looijestijn, Goekoop, Diederen, Rijkaart, Slotema, & Sommer, 2011; Blom, Sommer, Koops, & Sacks, 2014).

A salient detail is that patients sometimes report that, after visual fixation on an object, metamorphopsias arise only after an interval of several seconds (Willanger &

Table 18.2. Somaesthetic Distortions and Other Nonvisual Distortions that May Occur in the Context of Alice in Wonderland Syndrome

Type of Distortion	Characterization	Key Reference
Aschematia	Inadequate representation of the space occupied by some part of the body	Bonnier (1905)
Derealization	Experiencing the world as unreal	Mayer-Gross (1935)
Depersonalization	Experiencing oneself as unreal	Dugas (1898)
Hyperschematia	Overrepresentation of the space occupied by some part of the body	Bonnier (1905)
Hyposchematia	Underrepresentation of the space occupied by some part of the body	Bonnier (1905)
Illusory feeling of levitation	Sensation of floating in the air	Todd (1955)
Palisomaesthesia	Illusory reoccurrence of somaesthetic percepts	Feldman & Bender (1970)
Paraschematia	Inappropriate representation of the space occupied by some part of the body	Bonnier (1905)
Partial macrosomatognosia	Experiencing a part of the body as larger	Frederiks (1963)
Partial microsomatognosia	Experiencing a part of the body as smaller	Frederiks (1963)
Protracted duration	Deceleration of psychological time	Hoff & Pötzl (1934)
Quick-motion phenomenon	Acceleration of psychological time	Hoff & Pötzl (1934)
Splitting of the body image	Sensation of one's own body being split in two, usually down the middle	Podoll & Robinson (2002)
Time distortion	Altered experience of psychological time	Hoff & Pötzl (1934)
Total body macrosomatognosia	Experiencing the whole body as larger	Frederiks (1963)
Total body microsomatognosia	Experiencing the whole body as smaller	Frederiks (1963)

NOTE: Adapted from Blom, 2010.

Klee, 1966; Blom et al., 2014). After this temporal delay they begin to see faces and/or objects in a distorted manner, but during the first few seconds their perception is unaltered. In the historical literature this is considered a sign of cerebral asthenopia (Pötzl, 1928; Willanger & Klee, 1966), a phenomenon that will be explained further in the section on theories of etiology.

PREVALENCE RATE AND ASSOCIATED FEATURES

Epidemiological surveys and clinical prevalence studies of AIWS are lacking, but the syndrome is generally considered rare. Studies among clinical populations, however, indicate that its prevalence may well be underestimated (Smith, Wright, & Bennett, 2015). This suspicion would seem to be confirmed by three studies of individual types of metamorphopsia in the general population.

The first study involved a cross-sectional survey of macropsia and micropsia among 1,480 adolescents aged 13–18 years, which yielded lifetime prevalence rates of 5.6% for boys and 6.2% for girls for either of these symptoms (Abe & Suzuki, 1986a; 1986b). The second one was a cross-sectional study of macropsia, micropsia, and time distortions, carried out among 3,224 high school students, also aged 13–18 years (Abe, Oda, Araki, & Igata, 1989). This study yielded six-month prevalence rates of 3.8% for micropsia, 3.9% for macropsia, 2.5% for slow-motion illusions (i.e., protracted duration), and 1.3% for fast-motion illusions (i.e., the quick-motion phenomenon). The third study in the general population, by Lipsanen, Lauerma, Peltola, and Kallio (1999), among 297 individuals with a median age of 25.7 years, yielded lifetime prevalence rates of 30.3% for teleopsia, 18.5% for metamorphopsia (i.e., dysmorphopsia), 15.1% for macropsia, and 14.1% for micropsia. Moreover, the latter study indicated that within the group of people with visual distortions, 38.9% had experienced a single symptom, 33.6% two, 10.6% three, and 16.8% had experienced four symptoms. This might either hint at a common underlying pathological process for all four types of distortion, or at a stochastic process by means of which the presence of a single type of distortion significantly lowers the threshold for other types of distortion to join in.

The remaining literature consists chiefly of case reports and modest case series, the largest of which comprised 48 patients from a pediatric cohort (Liu et al., 2014).

Associated features of AIWS may range from hallucinations, illusions, and other perceptual symptoms to derealization, depersonalization, headaches, epileptic seizures, and clinical signs of encephalitis, depending on the context in which the symptoms occur.

THEORIES OF ETIOLOGY

The symptoms characteristic of AIWS traditionally are considered organic in nature, in the sense that they are attributed to physical pathologies of the

perceptual system. Most of them are attributed to central (as opposed to peripheral) nervous mechanisms. Dysmorphopsia (i.e., seeing straight lines as wavy) is
a type of metamorphopsia that can at once be of central and of peripheral origin. In the latter case, it is attributed to intraocular pathology (notably retinal
detachment). Another example is plagiopsia (i.e., seeing things as tilted, as in the
five-year old boy described earlier), which is sometimes attributed to labyrinthine
disease (Mayrhofer, 1942; Deecke, Mergner, & Plester, 1981).

Central metamorphopsias, on the other hand, are attributed to functional or
structural pathologies of the central nervous system. The vast network that comprises the visual network contains extremely selective neuron populations and
even single-cell columns in "low-level" regions of the visual network (notably
cortical areas V1–V5) that encode for specific aspects of visual perception (as
opposed to "higher-order," integrative regions, which have a function in object
perception, object recognition, and other more "cognitive" processes). The
empirical basis for the specialized function of these neuron populations stems
in large part from the work of Hubel and Wiesel (1962; 2005) on the receptive
fields in the cat's striate cortex. In humans, specific neurobiological correlates
have been described for several types of metamorphopsia; for others, educated
guesses have been made (for overviews, see ffytche & Howard, 1999; ffytche,
Blom, & Catani, 2010). Some of them are attributed purely to aberrant activity
of certain circumscript areas (such as bilateral ventrolateral occipital lesions in
V5 in cases of akinetopsia, i.e., the inability to perceive motion; see Zeki, 1991);
others to pathologies of the optic tract or to higher-order mismatches between
individual components of the visual network, which can vary interindividually.

Likewise, some somaesthetic distortions are attributed to functional or structural
pathologies of the somatosensory cortex, notably those affecting the temporoparietal
junction (Ceriani et al., 1998), whereas others would seem to involve mismatches
between regions that have varying functions in representing the body schema.

Structural pathologies may include any type of brain lesion, ranging from isch-
emic and hemorrhagic to neoplastic, while functional ones may include blood
flow alterations (notably hypoperfusion), electrophysiological aberrations (notably focal epileptic activity in temporoparietal or occipital regions), and cortical
spreading depression (as in migraine). Incidentally, structural pathologies also
may give rise to symptoms of AIWS via functional aberrations, as described in a
case of epilepsy caused by a cavernous angioma (Philip, Kornitzer, Marks, Lee, &
Souayah, 2015).

The phenomenon of cerebral asthenopia mentioned earlier is historically
attributed to a heightened fatigability of otherwise normally functioning, "lower-
level" neuron populations in the visual cortex (Willanger & Klee, 1966), due to
which those neuron populations cease to exert their normal function (Bay, 1953).
If a neuron population specialized for horizontal lines, for example, fails to exert
its proper function while a test subject is looking at a white rectangle, the image
perceived is bound to have a distorted shape.

The etiological agents responsible for mediating the symptoms of AIWS are
very diverse (Table 18.3), but in clinical practice the majority of pathological

Table 18.3. CONDITIONS IN THE CONTEXT OF WHICH SYMPTOMS OF AIWS
HAVE BEEN DESCRIBED

Conditions	Key References
Infectious diseases	
Acute disseminated encephalomyelitis	Coven, Horasanlı, Sönmez, Coban, & Dener (2013)
Coxsackie B1 virus encephalitis	Wang, Liu, Chen, Chang, & Huang (1996)
Cytomegalovirus	Losada-Del Pozo, Cantarín-Extremera, García-Peñas, Duat-Rodríguez, López-Marín, Gutiérrez-Solana, & Ruiz-Falcó (2011)
Epstein-Barr virus encephalitis (infectious mononucleosis)	Piessens, Indesteege, & Lemkens (2011)
H1N1 influenza virus encephalitis	Augarten & Aderka (2011)
Influenza A virus encephalitis	Kuo, Yeh, Chen, Weng, & Tzeng (2012)
Lyme neuroborreliosis	Binalsheikh, Griesemer, Wang, & Alvarez-Altalef (2012)
Meningococcal meningitis	Trolle (1951)
Neurosyphilis	Wilson (1916)
Scarlet fever	Brumm, Walenski, Haist, Robbins, Granet, & Love (2010)
Typhoid encephalopathy	Kitchener (2004)
Varicella zoster encephalitis	Soriani, Figgioli, Scarpa, & Borgna-Pignatti (1998)
Central nervous system lesions	
Brain tumor	Geyer (1963)
Cavernous angioma	Philip, Kornitzer, Marks, Lee, & Souayah (2015)
Cerebral arteriosclerosis	Veraguth (1903)
Cerebral thrombosis	Critchley (1949)
Hemorrhagic stroke	Camacho Velasquez, Rivero Sanz, Tejero Juste, & Suller Marti (2015)
Ischemic stroke	Camacho Velasquez, Rivero Sanz, Tejero Juste, & Suller Marti (2015)
Microembolization following open heart surgery	Meyendorf (1982)
Robin Hood syndrome	Morland, Wolff, Dietemann, Marescaux, & Namer (2013)
Traumatic encephalopathy	Willanger & Klee (1966)
Wallenberg's syndrome	Bjerver & Silfverskiöld (1968)

(continued)

Table 18.3. CONTINUED

Conditions	Key References
Peripheral nervous system lesions	
Eye disease	Bay (1953)
Labyrinthine disease	Deecke, Mergner, & Plester (1981)
Paroxysmal neurological disorders	
Epilepsy	Heo, Cho, Lee, Park, Kim, & Lee (2004)
Headache with neurological deficits and cerebrospinal fluid (CSF) lymphocytosis	Zeiner, Steinmetz, & Foerch (2015)
Migraine	Ilik & Ilik (2014)
Psychiatric disorders	
Delusional misidentification syndrome	Takaoka Norikatsu Ikawa Nobuya Niwa (2001)
Depressive disorder	Bui, Chatagner, & Schmitt (2010)
Derealization/depersonalization disorder	Wiesse (1979)
Dissociative disorder	Lipsanen, Lauerma, Peltola, & Kallio (1999)
Schizoaffective disorder	Blom, Looijestijn, Goekoop, Diederen, Rijkaart, Slotema, & Sommer (2011)
Schizophrenia	Coleman (1933)
Medications	
5-HT$_2$ agonists	Dubois & Vanrullen (2011)
Cough medicine (containing dihydrocodeine and *dl*-methylephedrine)	Takaoka & Takata (1999)
Dextromethorphan	Losada-Del Pozo, Cantarín-Extremera, García-Peñas, Duat-Rodríguez, López-Marín, Gutiérrez-Solana, & Ruiz-Falcó (2011)
Montelukast	Bernal Vañó & López Andrés (2013)
Oseltamivir	Jefferson, Jones, Doshi, & Del Mar (2009)
Topiramate	Evans (2006)
Illicit substances	
Amanita muscaria	Brvar, Možina, & Bunc (2006)
Amphetamines	Curran, Byrappa, & McBride (2004)
Ayahuasca	Critchley (1929)
Cannabis	Losada-Del Pozo, Cantarín-Extremera, García-Peñas, Duat-Rodríguez, López-Marín, Gutiérrez-Solana, & Ruiz-Falcó (2011)

(continued)

Table 18.3. CONTINUED

Conditions	Key References
Cocaine	Unnithan & Cutting (1992)
LSD	Lerner & Lev Ran (2015)
MDMA	Litjens, Brunt, Alderliefste, & Westerink (2014)
Mescaline	Klüver (1966)
Toluene-based solvent	Takaoka, Ikawa, & Niwa (2001)
Trichlorethylene	Todd (1954)
Miscellaneous	
Hyperpyrexia	Eshel, Eyov, Lahat, & Brauman (1987)
Hypnagogic state	Jürgens, Ihle, Stork, & May (2011)
Hypnopompic state	Schneck (1971)
Hypnotherapy	Schneck (1969)
Sensory deprivation	Heron (1961)

cases are attributed either to migraine, epilepsy, or infection. In the medical literature, infection is by far the most common cause of AIWS in children, even though in more than half of the cases no cause can be found (Liu et al., 2014). As a consequence, perhaps, hyperpyrexia also is accepted as a possible etiological agent (Eshel, Eyov, Lahat, & Brauman, 1987; Lahat, Eshel, & Arlazoroff, 1991).

Last but not least, various psychodynamic interpretations of the symptoms of AIWS have been published, characterizing them in designated cases as "hysterical," "transcortical," or "psychogenic" in nature (Wilson, 1916; Schneck, 1961; Meyers, 1977; Wiesse, 1979; Schneck, 1984). Some caution in adopting these terms may be warranted, however, because none of the papers involved indicated that adjuvant investigations were undertaken to rule out the possibility of underlying organic pathology. The influence of "mental" factors may be apparent in some cases, as, for example, in Wilson's (1916) claim that he himself was able to terminate episodes of micropsia at will when he was a child, but even this remarkable feat does not rule out the possibility that the symptom itself may well have had an organic etiology.

That said, it is worthwhile remembering that prevalence studies in the general population indicate that the majority of metamorphopsias would seem to be experienced in the absence of any overt (psycho)pathology. This is in line with observations made by Critchley (1953), who wrote, "Metamorphopsia is by no means confined to patients with organic focal disease of the brain. Indeed, most cases occur in quite different circumstances. Some of them are met with in normal, though sensitive, aesthetic and introspective individuals."

ASSESSMENT OPTIONS

People experiencing metamorphopsias and other symptoms of AIWS often have a hard time describing them, even to themselves. Therefore, the assessment of AIWS and its individual symptoms stands and falls with proper history taking, based on a thorough knowledge of the various types of distortion that can be encountered. It may be helpful to show patients illustrations of these distortions to aid them in recognizing and describing them. History taking also should focus on the various possible conditions associated with AIWS (see the section on differential diagnosis). Depending on the outcome, a general physical examination, neurological examination, psychiatric assessment, blood tests, an EEG, and an MRI scan of the brain may be useful, even though the latter two do not tend to yield many positive findings (Liu et al., 2014). This may well be due to the fact that focal epileptic activity—if present—does not always show on scalp recordings, and that the spatial resolution of MRI scans is not always sufficient to visualize relatively small lesions. A promising technique is functional MRI, with the aid of which cerebral activation patterns concomitant with perceptual distortions can be visualized (Brumm, Walenski, Haist, Robbins, Granet, & Love, 2010; Blom et al., 2011).

DIFFERENTIAL DIAGNOSIS

The differential diagnosis of AIWS is complex, because it involves at least three levels of conceptualization. At the symptomatological level, its individual symptoms must be differentiated from perceptual symptoms that fall under different headings, notably illusions and (simple and geometrical) hallucinations. At the nosological level, a long list of associated disorders should be taken into account. Todd (1955) already noted that AIWS can appear in the context of "migraine, epilepsy, cerebral lesion, intoxication with phantastica drugs, the deliria of fevers, hypnagogic states, and schizophrenia," but even he was aware that this list was not complete, while "discounting descriptions of the artificial and perverted experience of subjects under the influence of phantastica [i.e., hallucinogenic] drugs (mescaline, etc.)" (p. 703). Table 18.3 provides a list of disorders in the context of which AIWS and its individual symptoms have been described. It should be noted, however, that associated disorders such as these are not necessarily etiologies. So in the final analysis, differential diagnosis also involves addressing the etiological level, that is, assessing the factors that can be considered responsible for sparking the process that mediated the symptoms of AIWS in a particular case. In cases of (prior) substance abuse, notably the possibility of hallucinogen-induced persistent perception disorder (HPPD) should be taken into account (Litjens, Brunt, Alderliefste, & Westerink, 2014). Because the latter syndrome also has been described in the context of cannabis use, the third patient from our case vignette fulfills the diagnostic criteria of HPPD, even though his perceptual symptoms, per se, fully comply with the criteria of AIWS.

TREATMENT OPTIONS

Most cases of AIWS are considered benign, especially in children, in the sense that the symptoms tend to have a short duration and that they are self-limiting (Weidenfeld & Borusiak, 2011; Liu et al., 2014). An important exception would seem to be AIWS in the context of encephalitides such as Epstein-Barr virus encephalitis (Kuo, Chiu, Shen, Ho, & Wu, 1998). In other cases, however, the need for treatment should be carefully assessed, especially when the symptoms are present only fleetingly, when there is little or no burden of disease, and when there is no demonstrable pathology (as in our first case vignette).

When treatment is considered necessary, there are various additional issues to be taken into account. Due to the overwhelmingly large number of possible etiological factors and associated disorders, the treatment of AIWS and its individual symptoms should primarily be directed at alleviating the underlying pathology. For the purpose of symptomatic treatment, evidence-based protocols are lacking. In clinical practice, however, most patients are treated with medications from the groups of antiepileptics, migraine prophylaxes, antibiotics, or antiviral agents. Contrary to clinical intuition, perhaps, there would seem to be little room for the use of antipsychotics. One of the very few papers mentioning their use is one by Losada-Del Pozo, Cantarín-Extremera, García-Peñas, Duat-Rodríguez, López-Marín, Gutiérrez-Solana, and Ruiz-Falcó (2011).

As Table 18.3 indicates, topiramate, 5-HT_2 antagonists, and various other types of medication may need to be avoided. This also may hold true for the antipsychotic agent risperidone, which makes sense because of its potential to lower the threshold for epileptic activity (Morehead, 1997). However, given that the evidence for the reputed harmful effects of these types of medication stems from case reports, it is unclear whether these substances might not still be effective in cases with a different underlying etiology.

RECOMMENDATIONS FOR FUTURE WORK

Sixty years after Todd's seminal contribution, a lot of work has been done to further our understanding of AIWS. And yet more work is waiting to be done.

First of all, the operational definition of AIWS and its diagnostic criteria are in need of further development. A historical reconstruction of Todd's considerations might be helpful, as it is currently unclear why he chose to include distortions in some sensory modalities and not in others. More specifically, the question remains whether distortions in the olfactory, gustatory, auditory, sexual, coenesthetic, kinesthetic, proprioceptive, algesic, vestibular, and thermic modalities should not be added to the list of possible symptoms of AIWS. More importantly, however, the validity of AIWS as an independent nosological construct needs to be assessed, as well as its overlap with related syndromes such as HPPD (also referred to as "LSD-induced Alice in Wonderland syndrome," see Lerner & Lev Ran, 2015).

Secondly, patient sample sizes are in need of drastic expansion to allow for sufficient statistical power of empirical studies of AIWS. In conformity with recent initiatives to create international databases for rare diseases, one might consider creating a database for cases of AIWS, with special attention for phenomenological characteristics, diagnostic findings (including substance abuse), natural course, and treatment results. For such a database to be effective, all new cases of AIWS should be subjected to a systematic assessment, including proper history taking, EEG, and MRI of the brain. In addition, functional imaging techniques such as fMRI during active phases of AIWS may be helpful in establishing specific neurobiological correlates of individual symptoms.

Thirdly, it may be worthwhile to conduct epidemiological surveys for AIWS in the general population. Considering the results of the above-mentioned surveys of individual symptoms among adolescents, the symptoms may well be more common than hitherto assumed. Symptoms of AIWS tend to be transient in nature, and because the individuals experiencing them may fear being labeled as "mentally ill" they may well refrain from consulting a health professional, causing the symptoms to go undetected in the eyes of clinicians and scientists.

In the fourth place, AIWS is in need of proper representation in international diagnostic classifications such as the ICD (which might benefit from expanding its diagnostic criteria) and the DSM (which might benefit from including the syndrome and its individual symptoms).

Last but not least, our insight into the nature of AIWS might be enhanced by network analyses of the mutual relationships of individual symptoms, as well as their relationships with the perceptual networks underlying them.

REFERENCES

Abe, K., Oda, N., Araki, R., & Igata, M. (1989). Macropsia, micropsia, and episodic illusions in Japanese adolescents. *Journal of the American Academy of Child and Adolescent Psychiatry, 28*, 493–496.

Abe, K., & Suzuki, T. (1986a). Prevalence of some symptoms in adolescence and maturity: Social phobias, anxiety symptoms, episodic illusions and idea of reference. *Psychopathology, 19*, 200–205.

Abe, K., & Suzuki, T. (1986b). Age trends of social phobias, anxiety symptoms, morning dysphoria, early awakening and episodic illusions in 9–60 years of age. In C. Shagass (Ed.), *Biological psychiatry (Development in psychiatry)* (pp. 607–609). New York: Elsevier.

American Psychiatric Association. (2013). *Diagnostic and statistical manual of mental disorders. Fifth edition.* Washington, DC: American Psychiatric Association.

[Anonymous] (1956). The "Alice in Wonderland" syndrome: Relation to migraine. Based on an article by J. Todd, *Canadian Medical Association Journal,* 73: 701, November 1, 1955. In Abbott Laboratories. *What's New. Special Christmas Edition 1956* (pp. 22–24). North Chicago, IL: Abbott Laboratories.

Asher, H. (1971). "Trailing" phenomena—A long-lasting LSD side effect. *American Journal of Psychiatry, 127,* 1233–1234.

Augarten, A., & Aderka, D. (2011). Alice in Wonderland syndrome in H1N1 influenza. *Pediatric Emergency Care, 27,* 120.

Bay, E. (1953). Disturbances of visual perception and their examination. *Brain, 76,* 515–550.

Bernal Vañó, E., & López Andrés, N. (2013). Un caso de síndrome de Alicia en el país de las maravillas en probable relación con el uso de montelukast. *Annales de Pediatría, 78,* 127–128.

Beyer, E. (1895). Über Verlagerungen im Gesichtsfeld bei Flimmerskotom. *Neurologische Zentrallblatt, 14,* 10–15.

Binalsheikh, I.M., Griesemer, D., Wang, S., & Alvarez-Altalef, R. (2012). Lyme neuroborreliosis presenting as Alice in Wonderland syndrome. *Pediatric Neurology, 46,* 185–186.

Bjerver, K., & Silfverskiöld, B.P. (1968). Lateropulsion and imbalance in Wallenberg's syndrome. *Acta Neurologica Scandinavica, 44,* 91–100.

Blom, J.D. (2010). *A dictionary of hallucinations.* New York: Springer.

Blom, J.D., Looijestijn, J., Goekoop, R., Diederen, K.M.J., Rijkaart, A.-M., Slotema, C.W., & Sommer, I.E.C. (2011). Treatment of Alice in Wonderland syndrome and verbal auditory hallucinations using repetitive transcranial magnetic stimulation. A case report with fMRI findings. *Psychopathology, 44,* 337–344.

Blom, J.D., Sommer, I.E.C., Koops, S., & Sacks, O.W. (2014). Prosopometamorphopsia and facial hallucinations. *Lancet, 384,* 1998.

Bodamer, J. (1947). Die Prosopagnosie. *Archiv für Psychiatrie und Nervenkrankheiten, 179,* 6–53.

Bonnier, P. (1905). L'aschématie. *Revue Neurologique, 13,* 605–609.

Brumm, K., Walenski, M., Haist, F., Robbins, S.L., Granet, D.B., & Love, T. (2010). Functional magnetic resonance imaging of a child with Alice in Wonderland syndrome during an episode of micropsia. *Journal of the American Association for Pediatric Ophthalmology and Strabismus, 14,* 317–322.

Brvar, M., Možina, M., & Bunc, M. (2006). Prolonged psychosis after Amanita muscaria ingestion. *Wiener Klinische Wochenschrift, 118,* 294–297.

Bui, E., Chatagner, A., & Schmitt, L. (2010). Alice in Wonderland syndrome in major depressive disorder. *Journal of Neuropsychiatry and Clinical Neuroscience, 22,* 352.

Camacho Velasquez, J.L., Rivero Sanz, E., Tejero Juste, C., & Suller Marti, A. (2015). Síndrome de Alicia en el país de las maravillas en patología cerebrovascular. *Neurología.* Advance online publication JDB: DOI: 10.1016/j.nrl.2014.09.009 .

Carmichael, C. (1996). Wonderland revisited. *London Miscellany, 28,* 19–28.

Ceriani, F., Gentileschi, V., Muggia, S., & Spinnler, H. (1998). Seeing objects smaller than they are: Micropsia following right temporo-parietal infarction. *Cortex, 34,* 131–138.

Charcot, J.-M. (1889). *Leçons du Mardi à La Salpêtrière. Policlinique* 1888–1889. Paris: E. Lecrosnier & Babé.

Coleman, S.M. (1933). Misidentification and non-recognition. *Journal of Mental Science, 79,* 42–51.

Coven, I., Horasanlı, B., Sönmez, E., Coban, G., & Dener, S. (2013). The Alice in Wonderland syndrome: An unusual in acute disseminated encephalomyelitis. *American Journal of Emergency Medicine, 31,* 638.e1–638.e3.

Critchley, M. (1929). The ayahuasca and jagé cults. *British Journal of Inebriety, 26,* 218–222.

Critchley, M. (1949). Metamorphopsia of central origin. *Transactions of the Ophthalmologic Society of the UK, 69,* 111–121.

Critchley, M. (1953). *The parietal lobes.* London: Edward Arnold & Co.

Critchley, M., & Ferguson, F.R. (1933). Migraine. *Lancet, 221,* 123–126.

Curran, C., Byrappa, N., & McBride, A. (2004). Stimulant psychosis: Systematic review. *British Journal of Psychiatry, 185,* 196–204.

Deecke, L., Mergner, T., & Plester, D. (1981). Tullio phenomenon with torsion of the eyes and subjective tilt of the visual surround. *Annals of the New York Academy of Sciences, 374,* 650–655.

Dooley, J.M., Augustine, H.F., Gordon, K.E., Brna, P.M., & Westby, E. (2014). Alice in Wonderland and other migraine associated phenomena—Evolution over 30 years after headache diagnosis. *Pediatric Neurology, 51,* 321–323.

Dubois, J., & Vanrullen, R. (2011). Visual trails: Do the doors of perception open periodically? *PLoS Biology, 9,* e1001056.

Dugas, L. (1898). Un cas de dépersonnalisation. *Revue Philosophique de la France et de L'Étranger, 45,* 500–507.

Eshel, G.M., Eyov, A., Lahat, E., & Brauman, A. (1987). Alice in Wonderland syndrome, a manifestation of acute Epstein-Barr virus infection. *Pediatric Infectious Disease Journal, 6,* 68.

Evans, R.W. (2006). Reversible palinopsia and the Alice in Wonderland syndrome associated with topiramate use in migraineurs. *Headache, 46,* 815–818.

Ey, H. (1973). *Traité des Hallucinations.* Paris: Masson et Cie., Éditeurs.

Feldman, M., & Bender, M.B. (1970). Visual illusions and hallucinations in parieto-occipital lesions of the brain. In E. Keup (Ed.), *Origin and mechanisms of hallucinations. Proceedings of the 14th Annual Meeting of the Eastern Psychiatric Research Association held in New York City, November 14–15, 1969* (pp. 23–35). New York: Plenum Press.

ffytche, D.H., Blom, J.D., & Catani, M. (2010). Disorders of visual perception. *Journal of Neurology, Neurosurgery, and Psychiatry, 81,* 1280–1287.

ffytche, D.H., & Howard, R.J. (1999). The perceptual consequences of visual loss: "Positive" pathologies of vision. *Brain, 122,* 1247–1260.

Frederiks, J.A.M. (1963). Macrosomatognosia and microsomatognosia. *Psychiatry, Neurology and Neurosurgery, 66,* 531–536.

Gelb, A., & Goldstein, K. (1918). Zur Psychologie des optischen Wahrnehmungs- und Erkennungsvorganges. *Zeitschrift für die gesamte Neurologie und Psychiatrie, 41,* 1–141.

Geyer, K.-H. (1963). Zentrale Störungen des Formensehens. Zur Pathogenese der Metamorphopsie. *Deutsche Zeitschrift für Nervenheilkunde, 184,* 378–387.

Hamed, S.A. (2010). A migraine variant with abdominal colic and Alice in Wonderland syndrome: A case report and review. *BMC Neurology, 10,* 2.

Heo, K., Cho, Y.J., Lee, S.-K., Park, S.A., Kim, K.-S., & Lee, B.I. (2004). Single-photon emission computed tomography in a patient with ictal metamorphopsia. *Seizure, 13,* 250–253.

Heron, W. (1961). Cognitive and physiological effects of perceptual isolation. In P. Solomon, P.E. Kubzansky, P.H. Leiderman Jr., J.H. Mendelson, R.Trumbull, & D.Wexler (Eds.), *Sensory deprivation. An investigation of phenomena suggesting a revised concept of the individual's response to his environment* (pp. 6–33). Cambridge, MA: Harvard University Press.

Hoff, H., & Pötzl, O. (1934). Über eine Zeitrafferwirkung bei homonymer linksseitiger Hemianopsie. *Zeitschrift für die gesamte Neurologie und Psychiatrie*, *151*, 599–641.

Hubel, D.H., & Wiesel, T.N. (1962). Receptive fields, binocular interaction and functional architecture in the cat's visual cortex. *Journal of Physiology*, *160*, 106–154.

Hubel, D.H., & Wiesel, T.N. (2005). *Brain and visual perception*. Oxford: Oxford University Press.

Ilik, F., & Ilik, K. (2014). Alice in Wonderland syndrome as aura of migraine. *Neurocase*, *20*, 474–475.

Jefferson, T., Jones, M., Doshi, P., & Del Mar, C. (2009). Possible harms of oseltamivir— A call for urgent action. *Lancet*, *374*, 1312–1313.

Jürgens, T.P., Ihle, K., Stork, J.H., & May, A. (2011). "Alice in Wonderland syndrome" associated with topiramate for migraine prevention. *Journal of Neurology, Neurosurgery & Psychiatry*, *82*, 228–229.

Kitchener, N. (2004). Alice in Wonderland syndrome. *International Journal of Child Neuropsychiatry*, *1*, 107–112.

Klee, A., & Willanger, R. (1966). Disturbances of visual perception in migraine. *Acta Neurologica Scandinavica*, *42*, 400–414.

Klüver, H. (1966). *Mescal and mechanisms of hallucinations*. Chicago, IL: University of Chicago Press.

Kuo, S.C., Yeh, Y.W., Chen, C.Y., Weng, J.P., & Tzeng, N.S. (2012). Possible association between Alice in Wonderland syndrome and influenza A infection. *Journal of Neuropsychiatry and Clinical Neurosciences*, *24*, E7–E8.

Kuo, Y.T., Chiu, N.C., Shen, E.Y., Ho, C.S., Wu, M.C. (1998). Cerebral perfusion in children with Alice in Wonderland syndrome. *Pediatric Neurology*, *19*, 105–108.

Lahat, E., Eshel, G., & Arlazoroff, A. (1991). "Alice in Wonderland" syndrome: A manifestation of infectious mononucleosis in children. *Behavioural Neurology*, *4*, 163–166.

Lanska, J.R., & Lanska, D.J. (2013). Alice in Wonderland Syndrome: Somesthetic vs visual perceptual disturbance. *Neurology*, *80*, 1262–1264.

Lerner, A.G., & Lev Ran, S. (2015). LSD-associated "Alice in Wonderland syndrome" (AIWS): A hallucinogen persisting perception disorder (HPPD) case report. *Israel Journal of Psychiatry and Related Sciences*, *52*, 67–69.

Lippman, C.W. (1952). Certain hallucinations peculiar to migraine. *Journal of Nervous and Mental Diseases*, *116*, 346–351.

Lipsanen, T., Lauerma, H., Peltola, P., & Kallio, S. (1999). Visual distortions and dissociation. *Journal of Nervous and Mental Disease*, *187*, 109–112.

Litjens, R.P., Brunt, T.M., Alderliefste, G.J., & Westerink, R.H. (2014). Hallucinogen persisting perception disorder and the serotonergic system: A comprehensive review including new MDMA-related clinical cases. *European Neuropsychopharmacology*, *24*, 1309–1323.

Liu, A.M., Liu, J.G., Liu, G.W., & Liu, G.T. (2014). "Alice in Wonderland" syndrome: Presenting and follow-up characteristics. *Pediatric Neurology*, *51*, 317–320.

Lopez, J.R., Adornato, B.T., & Hoyt, W.F. (1993). "Entomopia": A remarkable case of cerebral polyopia. *Neurology*, *43*, 2145–2146.

Losada-Del Pozo, R., Cantarín-Extremera, V., García-Peñas, J.J., Duat-Rodríguez, A., López-Marín, L., Gutiérrez-Solana, L.G., & Ruiz-Falcó, M.L. (2011). Características y evolución de los pacientes con síndrome de Alicia en el País de las Maravillas. *Revista de Neurología, 53,* 641–648.

Lunn, V. (1948). *Om Legemsbevidstheden.* Copenhagen: Ejnar Munksgaard.

Mayer-Gross, W. (1935). On depersonalization. *British Journal of Medical Psychology, 15,* 103–122.

Mayrhofer, J. (1942). Über kombinierte labyrinthäre und occipitale Symptome nach Hinterhaupts-Schuß. *Zeitschrift für die gesamte Neurologie und Psychiatrie, 174,* 613–625.

Meyendorf, R. (1982). Psychopatho-ophthalmology, gnostic disorders, and psychosis in cardiac surgery. *Archives of Psychiatry and Neurological Sciences, 232,* 119–135.

Meyers, W.A. (1977). Micropsia and testicular retractions. *Psychoanalytic Quarterly, 46,* 580–604.

Morehead, D.B. (1997). Exacerbation of hallucinogen-persisting perception disorder with risperidone. *Journal of Clinical Psychopharmacology, 17,* 327–328.

Morland, D., Wolff, V., Dietemann, J.L., Marescaux, C., & Namer, I.J. (2013). Robin Hood caught in Wonderland: Brain SPECT findings. *Clinical Nuclear Medicine, 38,* 979–981.

Nijboer, T.C.W., Ruis, C., van der Worp, H.B., & de Haan, E.H.F. (2008). The role of Funktionswandel in metamorphopsia. *Journal of Neuropsychology, 2,* 287–300.

Philip, M., Kornitzer, J., Marks, D., Lee, H.J., & Souayah, N. (2015). Alice in Wonderland Syndrome associated with a temporo-parietal cavernoma. *Brain Imaging and Behavior, 9,* 910–912. Advance online publication.

Piessens, P., Indesteege, F., & Lemkens, P. (2011). Alice in Wonderland syndrome and upper airway obstruction in infectious mononucleosis. *B-ENT, 7,* 51–54.

Pinckers, A., Cruysberg, J.R.M., & Liem, T.A. (1989). Chromatopsia. *Documenta Ophthalmologica, 72,* 385–390.

Podoll, K., & Robinson, D. (1999). Lewis Carroll's migraine experiences. *Lancet, 353,* 1366.

Podoll, K., & Robinson, D. (2002). Splitting of the body image as somesthetic aura symptom in migraine. *Cephalalgia, 22,* 62–65.

Podoll, K., Ebel, H., Robinson, D., & Nicola, U. (2002). Sintomi essenziali ed accessori nella sindrome di Alice nel paese delle meraviglie. *Minerva Medica, 93,* 287–293.

Pötzl, O. (1928). *Die Optisch-Agnostische Störungen.* Leipzig: F. Deuticke.

Pötzl, O. (1943). Über Anfälle vom Thalamustypus. *Zeitschrift für die gesamte Neurologie und Psychiatrie, 176,* 793–800.

Sacks, O. (1970). *Migraine.* New York: Vintage Books.

Schneck, J.M. (1961). Micropsia. *American Journal of Psychiatry, 118,* 232–234.

Schneck, J.M. (1969). Micropsia. *Psychosomatics, 10,* 249–251.

Schneck, J.M. (1971). Micropsia. *Psychiatric Quarterly, 45,* 542–544.

Schneck, J.M. (1984). Psychogenic micropsia in fact and fiction. *Journal of the American Medical Association, 251,* 2350.

Seitelberger, F. (1952). Über Phantomerscheinungen bei Thalamuserkrankungen. *Wiener Zeitschrift für Nervenheilkunde und deren Grenzgebiete, 4,* 259–265.

Smith, R.A, Wright, B., & Bennett, S. (2015). Hallucinations and illusions in migraine in children and the Alice in Wonderland syndrome. *Archives of Disease in Childhood, 100,* 296–298.

Soriani, S., Figgioli, R., Scarpa, P., & Borgna-Pignatti, C. (1998). "Alice in Wonderland" syndrome and varicella. *Pediatric Infectious Disease Journal, 17,* 935–936.

Takaoka, K., Ikawa, N., & Niwa, N. (2001). "Alice in Wonderland" syndrome as a precursor of delusional misidentification syndromes. *International Journal of Psychiatry in Clinical Practice*, 5, 149–151.

Takaoka, K., & Takata, T. (1999). "Alice in Wonderland" syndrome and Lilliputian hallucinations in a patient with a substance-related disorder. *Psychopathology*, 32, 47–49.

Taylor, I., Scheffer, I.E., & Berkovic, S.F. (2003). Occipital epilepsies: Identification of specific and newly recognized syndromes. *Brain*, 126, 753–769.

Todd, J. (1954). Trichlorethylene poisoning with paranoid psychosis and Lilliputian hallucination. *British Medical Journal*, 1, 439–440.

Todd, J. (1955). The syndrome of Alice in Wonderland. *Canadian Medical Association Journal*, 73, 701–704.

Trolle, E. (1951). *Late prognosis in meningococcal meningitis.* Copenhagen: Danish Science Press.

Unnithan, S.B., & Cutting, J.C. (1992). The cocaine experience: Refuting the concept of a model psychosis? *Psychopathology*, 25, 71–78.

Veraguth, O. (1903). Ueber Mikropsie und Makropsie. *Deutsche Zeitschrift für Nervenheilkunde*, 24, 453–464.

Vujić, V., & Ristić, J. (1939). Ein Fall von Porropsie mit gestörter palpatorischer Größenschätzung. *Deutsche Zeitschrift für Nervenheilkunde*, 150, 30–38.

Wang, S.M., Liu, C.C., Chen, Y.J., Chang, Y.C., & Huang, C.C. (1996). Alice in Wonderland syndrome caused by coxsackievirus B1. *Pediatric Infectious Disease Journal*, 15, 470–471.

Weidenfeld, A., & Borusiak, P. (2011). Alice-in-Wonderland syndrome—a case-based update and long-term outcome in nine children. *Child's Nervous System*, 27, 893–896.

Wieser, H.G. (2000). Temporal lobe epilepsies. In P.J. Vinken & G.W. Bruyn (Eds.), *Handbook of Clinical Neurology, Vol. 73. The Epilepsies, Part II.* Amsterdam: Verlag Hans Huber.

Wiesse, J. (1979). Derealisationsphänomene: Psychophysiologische Untersuchung und psychodynamische Interpretation bei einem 9-jahrigen Jungen mit Mikropsien. *Praxis der Kinderpsychologie und Kinderpsychiatrie*, 28, 133–136.

Willanger, R., & Klee, A. (1966). Metamorphopsia and other visual disturbances with latency occurring in patients with diffuse cerebral lesions. *Acta Neurologica Scandinavica*, 42, 1–18.

Wilson, S.A.K. (1916). Dysmetropsia and its pathogenesis. *Transactions of the Ophthalmological Society UK*, 36, 412–444.

Winslow, F. (1868). *On obscure diseases of the brain and disorders of the mind. Fourth edition.* London: Churchill.

World Health Organization. (2008). *The international classification of diseases, 9th revision, clinical modification. sixth edition.* Geneva, Switzerland: World Health Organization.

Zeiner, P.S., Steinmetz, H., & Foerch, C. (2015). Pseudomigräne mit Liquorpleozytose. "Alice-im-Wunderland"-Syndrom. *Nervenarzt.* Advance online publication.

Zeki, S. (1990). A century of cerebral achromatopsia. *Brain*, 113, 1721–1777.

Zeki, S. (1991). Cerebral akinetopsia (visual motion blindness). A review. *Brain*, 114, 811–824.

19

Factitious Disorders

BRENDA BURSCH AND ROBERT HASKELL ■

VIGNETTE

By the time Anita Hansen, as we shall call her, arrived in the office of a pediatric neurologist at a prominent academic hospital, both her mother and her new pediatrician were in search of a miracle. Anita, age 10 years, had been suffering from multiple illnesses, including medication-resistant epilepsy, with grand mal, absence, partial complex, and myoclonic seizures; right-sided hemiparesis, ataxia and memory deficits, all understood to be expressions of a stroke-like syndrome; and sensoneuronal hearing loss mitigated only somewhat by hearing aids. She had urinary retention and multiple urinary tract infections, which led to the placement of bilateral ureteral stents, as well as gastroesophageal reflux disease (GERD), multiple food allergies, and intermittent bloody diarrhea. She also had been diagnosed with central hypoventilation syndrome, which at one point caused such frequent and frightening episodes of apnea—described as "near Sudden Infant Death Syndrome (SIDS) episodes" by her physicians at the time—that Anita received a tracheostomy at age three years, later closed when she no longer required the support of a ventilator.

Mrs. Hansen, as Anita's pediatrician had explained to the neurologist, was a single mother and a respiratory therapist by training who, in a remarkable coincidence, had written a master's thesis on "Near SIDS Events" four years before her daughter's birth. She struck the neurologist as a compassionate and well-informed advocate for Anita, strikingly articulate and detailed in her account of her daughter's long illness, and very well prepared, having arrived at the office with a thick folio of records from a gamut of pediatric subspecialists, including pulmonologists, endocrinologists, urologists, cardiologists, gastroenterologists, orthopedic surgeons, and other neurologists. Anita's care, she explained, became her life's work on the day she resuscitated her two-week-old daughter after she stopped breathing in her arms.

That one little girl should suffer from so many illnesses and have received so little in the way of effective treatment was tragic, as the neurologist pointed out straightaway to Mrs. Hansen, but also strange—a thought that he kept to himself. "I grew up in a family where almost everyone had serious medical problems," Mrs. Hansen told him, "so this stuff doesn't faze me as it might other mothers."

Anita was a cheerful, placid girl, a smiler, and a giggler. She made her way around the office with the use of a walker, and her speech, though rudimentary for someone her age (a fact not surprising given how much school she had missed), was fluent and appropriate. Her mother had taught her basic sign language, and she was able to understand the neurologist's questions by looking directly at him when he spoke, then turning to her mother, who translated with her hands. She explained that she had "problems with balance" and "problems with memory." But she was a sometimes diffident historian who would laugh, shake her head, or say, "Ask my mom," when the neurologist probed further.

The neurologist arranged for a scheduled hospital admission the following week, explaining to Mrs. Hansen that Anita needed to be placed on 24-hour video-EEG so that her brainwaves and seizure activity could be closely monitored. He also hoped that careful observation would allow him to test his vague but creeping hypothesis that Anita, her mother, or both were manufacturing her symptoms.

Mrs. Hansen brought Anita to the hospital on the assigned date and told the admitting nurse that she would "need to handle all aspects of care," including blood draws (since Anita had small, friable veins) and meals (on account of Anita's numerous food allergies). Though the nurse bristled slightly at Mrs. Hansen's controlling style, she told Anita's neurologist that Anita was fortunate to have such a tireless crusader for a mother. But the neurologist demurred, sharing his concerns with the team and urging that, wherever possible, Anita be assessed and treated under conditions that prevented any tampering by her mother.

Though her anticonvulsant medications were discontinued, Anita had no seizures throughout her six-day hospitalization. Her hearing aids were removed at the time of admission, and when Anita was asked about the fact that she appeared to be hearing with no difficulty, she explained that she was "lip-reading," even though she responded appropriately when her interlocutors' backs were turned. A physical therapist gently insisted that Anita walk the hallways unaided, and although her gait and balance problems disappeared almost immediately, Anita continued to say—and, indeed, appeared to believe—that she was too unsteady to walk on her own, regularly touching a wall or a floor even though this contact clearly did not aid her ambulation. Anita also underwent a thorough psychological evaluation, which indicated that, while clearly not psychotic, she seemed to have difficulty picking reality and fantasy apart. The psychologist's findings were also consistent with a history of severe medical trauma resulting from years of tests, procedures, hospitalizations, and treatments.

Concerned that Anita was the victim of Factitious Disorder Imposed on Another (FDIA)—also known as Munchausen Syndrome by Proxy—the neurologist decided to contact an expert on the topic at another prominent medical center in the area for consultation. The Hansens, it turned out, were a powerful, if distant, memory at this other hospital. Seven years earlier, the child psychiatrist on the inpatient Pediatric service had been consulted after Anita's seizures, apnea, and intermittent hypoglycemia were systematically challenged and disproven by another suspicious doctor.

The psychiatrist vividly recalled meeting with Mrs. Hansen for the first time. She told him about her extended family's myriad medical troubles, explained that she was not surprised by the medical team's impression of illness falsification since her daughter had occasional "good periods," and—something he told the neurologist he would never forget—shared her belief that Anita would die young.

The child psychiatrist also described an interview at the time with Anita's maternal grandfather, who acknowledged that her grandmother had suffered from severe multiple sclerosis, but was not sure what Mrs. Hansen had meant when she referred to the family's many health problems. He said that his wife's illness had been difficult for his daughter, an only child who received little attention, with her mother confined to her bed and her father absorbed in his wife's care from the moment he came home from work. The psychiatrist inquired about Mrs. Hansen's health during her childhood, and her father recalled that, when she was 11 years old, she fell from a tree and broke both of her arms. Recovery took much longer than expected, and her father had to hire a temporary night nurse for his wife so that he could attend to his daughter during her convalescence. After that, he remembered, Anita's mother "always had something—headaches, stomach problems, fainting spells," though he'd heard little about these in recent years.

The psychiatrist had previously diagnosed Mrs. Hansen with FDIA and reported her to the city's child protective services agency. Anita was placed in foster care, and her mother was ordered to participate in counseling. But at her attorney's urging, the court prohibited Mrs. Hansen's therapist from speaking with Anita's clinicians, and because of this, the psychiatrist explained, he lost track of the Hansens. He was sorry to learn that Anita was back in her mother's care, where she not only remained a victim of Mrs. Hansen's mental illness but now also appeared to believe her symptoms to be real.

After speaking with the expert and learning of the previous diagnosis of FDIA, the neurologist confronted Mrs. Hansen. She conceded that Anita had been briefly removed from her home years earlier because she had been, as she put it, "a bit overprotective." The neurologist asked her why she had omitted this chapter in an otherwise painstaking summary of her daughter's medical ordeal, and why her daughter's outsized medical chart excluded the psychiatric notes or any mention of FDIA. Mrs. Hansen smiled and calmly explained that her religious beliefs prevented her from "perpetuating a lie."

HISTORICAL/CULTURAL CONTEXT

In Factitious Disorders, the patient exaggerates, fabricates, simulates, and/or induces symptoms of medical and/or psychiatric illnesses—in himself or in another person—with no concrete incentive beyond the pleasure, consolation, or status conferred by being a patient (or by being closely identified with a patient). Many stories of illness unfold like the one above: one unsuspecting doctor after another accepts in good faith an accounting of symptoms, and one doctor after another is pressed into the service not of treatment and recovery, but of the illness itself. FDIS/FDIA is one of few disorders in which we may think of the patient as a perpetrator, and in which we may feel compelled to resort to subterfuge to confirm a diagnosis. This aspect of the disorder carries unavoidable ethical and counter-transferential implications that make its treatment especially complicated.

Though malingering, in which symptoms are fabricated in order to win something good or avoid something bad, appeared in the Old Testament and was the subject of a treatise by the famous second-century Roman physician Galen of Pergamon (Feldman, 2004), who was the first of many to enumerate the ruses of terrified soldiers, factitious disorder as we now define it only came into focus in the last century. In a 1934 paper titled "Polysurgery and Polysurgical Addiction," Karl Menninger identified a category of patients for whom surgery was its own reward. In a 1951 article in the *Lancet*, Richard Asher coined the term Munchausen Syndrome to describe an illness "which most doctors have seen, but about which little has been written." He named it for the title character in Rudolf Raspe's *The Surprising Adventures of Baron Munchausen*, who boasted of riding on a cannon-ball, among other fabulous exploits. In 1977, Sir Roy Meadow described what he called Munchausen Syndrome by Proxy. Displaying a moral outrage not always at home in medicine; he called it "the hinterland of child abuse." Factitious Disorder first appeared in the DSM-III in 1980. (The term Munchausen Syndrome never appeared in the DSM, and although it initially described a more severe or chronic form of FD, the two terms are now used interchangeably.)

Factitious Disorder came to prominence in the 20th century, at a time when physicians had attained a social status unknown to them in earlier eras. The illness appears to be tethered to the prevailing values of a particular time and place, which is why the predominant symptoms of Factitious Disorder have shifted according to broader cultural shifts (Brown & Scheflin, 1999). In the United States, an over-abundance of medical care (for which managed care was designed as a corrective) has provided a fertile terrain for the disorder, as has the overabundance of all manner of media. In the last 50 years, as the media has focused variously on Vietnam veterans, victims of child abuse or rape, AIDS sufferers, escapees from cults, and those who have endured grievous iatrogenic injuries, new contexts and new constellations of symptoms have invited and incited the FD patient. Because these patients often intensify their symptoms when they know that they are being observed (Szoke & Boillet, 1999), and because attention is a key patient aim in the disorder, our clinical suspicion should rise wherever there is significant attention to be gained and whenever the symptoms themselves seem "fashionable."

In 2000, Marc Feldman pointed to the shaping power of the zeitgeist when he wrote about "virtual factitious disorder," otherwise known as Munchausen by Internet. Feldman observed that online medical chat rooms, support groups, and websites about medicine for laypeople made it easy not only to find sympathy but also to fictionalize the symptoms that are likely to beget it, all from behind the curtain of a computer screen. The doctor shopping that has always been regarded as a red flag in Factitious Disorder enables the patient to make himself unknown over and over again, but where better to do this than in the acentric and anonymous corridors of the Web?

ROLE IN CURRENT DIAGNOSTIC SYSTEM
AND SYMPTOMATOLOGY

Factitious Disorder diagnostic criteria published in the *Diagnostic and Statistical Manual of Mental Disorders, 5th Edition* (DSM-5; American Psychiatric Association, 2013) represents the most up-to-date formal conceptualization of this phenomenon. The diagnosis of Factitious Disorder Imposed on Self requires that the individual deceptively falsified physical or psychological signs or symptoms, or induced injury or disease; that the individual represents himself or herself to others as genuinely ill, impaired, or injured; and that the behavior is internally motivated. Such individuals are diagnosed with Factitious Disorder Imposed on Self when neither external rewards nor other forms of psychopathology better account for the deceptive illness falsification. The course of illness is further defined by adding a specifier in order to reflect a single episode or recurrent episodes. If the afflicted individual deceptively falsifies physical or psychological signs or symptoms, or induces injury or disease in another, then the diagnosis of Factitious Disorder Imposed on Another is applied. Although the diagnostic criteria in the World Health Organization's *International Classification of Diseases, 10th Revision* (ICD-10) overlap with the DSM-5 criteria, ICD-10 includes "motivation to adopt the sick role" as a criterion, which is based upon inference rather than objective findings.

Methods of illness falsification can include exaggeration, fabrication, simulation, symptom coaching, and induction. Although a genuine medical condition may be present, the deceptive behavior causes others to view such individuals (or their victims) as excessively ill or impaired, which can lead to unnecessary clinical assessments and treatments.

PREVALENCE RATE AND ASSOCIATED FEATURES

Due to the secretive, and sometimes criminal, nature of this behavior, there are numerous barriers to prevalence research. An Italian community study using interviews and rating scales to assess lifetime prevalence rates and estimated risks of DSM-IV psychiatric disorders determined the lifetime prevalence of factitious disorders in the general population was 0.1% (Faravelli et al., 2004). Because the study was based on self-report, one might consider this a low estimate.

Using the National Hospital Discharge Survey data for the years 1997–2006 to examine point prevalence among hospitalized patients, Hamilton et al. (2013) found that factitious disorder was an assigned diagnosis in 9.3 per 100,000 patients (<0.0001%). In high-risk samples, the point prevalence estimates are expectedly higher. For example, a prospective study of patients with fevers of unknown origin suggested the presence of a factitious disorder in 9.0% (Aduan, Fauci, Dale, Herzberg, & Wolff, 1979), and a study of psychiatric inpatients suggested the presence of a factitious disorder in 8.0% (Catalina, Gómez Macias, & de Cos, 2008). Not surprisingly, there is some evidence that clinicians believe that a factitious disorder is present more frequently than it is diagnosed (Swanson, Hamilton, & Feldman, 2010).

In an examination of factitious disorders impacting children, an expert team carefully reviewed medical records and collateral information for 751 child patients (ranging in age from 11 months to 16 years, mean age 6.9 years) referred to the Pediatric Unit of Agostino Gemelli Hospital in Rome between November 2007 and March 2010 (Ferrara et al., 2013). They found that FDIS was present in 14/751 patients, resulting in a point prevalence of 1.8%. An additional four patients were the victims of FDIA for a point prevalence of 0.53%. Factitious fever was present in 12.5% of patients admitted for hyperpyrexia.

Individuals with FDIS or FDIA are at risk for experiencing great psychological distress or functional impairment by causing harm to themselves and others. Family, friends, and healthcare professionals also are often adversely affected by their behavior. Factitious disorders are similar to substance use disorders, eating disorders, impulse-control disorders, and pedophilic disorder in both the persistence of the behavior and the effort to conceal the disordered behavior through deception.

Many afflicted individuals report highly dysfunctional families of origin and the experience of severe abuse and/or neglect as children, suggesting that these biographical features may be risk factors. They may come from families that, while appearing quite conventional on the surface, failed to protect children from significant abuse or conflict. Sometimes they are identified as caregivers in their families of origin. They frequently report childhood traumas such as serious illness, abandonment, intense family conflict, or death of a person close to them.

The disorder may begin in childhood or adulthood after a rewarding medical care contact or hospitalization that caused the individual to feel protected, gave him or her a sense of affection or attention, or was otherwise emotionally satisfying. With time, the emotionally rewarded sick role behavior becomes habitual and difficult to stop. Cognitive compartmentalization can contribute to denial in the sufferer. For example, a parent may think to herself that it is safe to briefly induce illness in her child since she is in control of the situation. Some sufferers have an aggressive, confrontational style, while others are more passive. Most consider themselves victims and have a tendency to externalize blame. Comorbidity among personality disorders, somatic symptom disorders, and factious disorders is common (Bass & Jones, 2011). Substance misuse, self-destructive behavior, post-traumatic stress disorder, and learning disorders are regularly noted, and variation in intelligence, socioeconomic status, education, and ethnicity has been identified (Bools, Neale, & Meadow, 1994; Sheridan, 2003). Limited data suggest that factitious-disordered men, who are most often seen in severe cases of FDIS, are often less overtly cooperative and endearing than the women.

THEORIES OF ETIOLOGY

Although the causes of Factitious Disorder are poorly understood, most theorists believe that a childhood history of abuse, neglect, loss, or deprivation lies at the root of the illness and accounts for the patient's focus on a degree and quality of attention that early life experience denied. It has, in other words, been viewed as a disorder of reenactment, in which the fabrication of symptoms allows for the regression into or attempted correction of early attachment patterns. As R. J. Carlson wrote in 1984, "The fabrication of symptoms may serve as a mechanism whereby these individuals can temporarily relate to others, overcome their isolation, obtain caring, have certainty of their needs being met, and possibly act out previous family dynamics."

Not surprisingly, Factitious Disorder shares many of the putative causes of personality disorders (particularly borderline, histrionic, and narcissistic personality disorders) and can be understood as a severe form of character pathology in its own right. In both FD and personality disorders, the long-term sequelae of traumatic childhood experiences may include an unstable or fragmented sense of self, deficits in affect development and regulation, impaired reality testing, self-injury motivated by a need (conscious or not) for attention or punishment, and the use of primitive defenses such as denial.

The history of Factitious Disorder patients also frequently reveals early health problems, hospitalizations, or experiences with the illnesses and treatment of family members. Menninger (1934) understood the factitious production of symptoms as an aggressive act against a physician who stood in for a "perceived sadistic parent," and certainly, FDIS/FDIA patients demonstrate a high degree of unconscious aggression toward healthcare providers and express frequent disappointment in them. Other psychodynamic interpretations of the illness have understood symptoms as a fulfillment of pathologic dependency needs, unconscious masochistic urges, or revenge fantasies.

Scholars of various theoretical orientations have viewed the illness as motivated by the fantasy of physicians as a uniquely potent source of nurturing. Through the care provided by doctors and nurses, these patients learned that the health professions offered a promise of attention, consolation, and nurturing not present elsewhere in their lives (Cramer, Gershberg, & Stern, 1971). Inevitably, some of these Factitious Disorder patients were drawn to the health professions themselves; for many, like the mother in our earlier vignette, a high degree of medical knowledge can lead to a more prolonged and destructive course of illness.

To date, there is no conclusive evidence of the involvement of particular brain structures, neurotransmitters, or other biomarkers in Factitious Disorder. But what makes the origins of this illness so difficult to uncover is the barrier to the truth posed by the patients themselves, whose frequent refusal to accept their diagnosis or to provide factually accurate histories makes FDIS/FDIA among psychiatry's most perplexing illnesses.

ASSESSMENT OPTIONS

No diagnostic tests or paper and pencil measures exist to diagnose this disorder reliably. Medical, psychiatric, and/or developmental disorders can be falsified in numerous ways, including exaggeration (embellishment of a legitimate symptom or problem), fabrication (false accounting of symptoms or medical history), simulation (creating the appearance of illness by methods such as putting blood in a urine sample, altering medical records, or tampering with medical tests), and induction (directly causing or exacerbating a problem, such as by medical neglect, poisoning, or suffocation). See Box 19.1 for a list of potential assessment approaches.

The medical record is a crucial data source because the information provided in clinical documentation is usually entered at the time of the healthcare

---

Box 19.1

Potential Assessment Procedures

- Chronological medical record analysis of symptom reporting and illness behavior compared to objective observations/findings.
- Interviews of individuals with significant contact with the individual suspected of Factitious Disorder (e.g., school personnel, other clinicians, or extended family members) and, in cases of FDIA, interview of the suspected victim(s).
- Closely clinically monitored observation of individual (or victim), using the following approach:
    - First, observe symptoms and behaviors without changing treatments.
    - Second, observe while sequentially withdrawing treatments thought to be unneeded.
    - Third, observe during sequential challenging of suspected false claims (for example, feeding a suspected infant victim reported to be unable to eat).
- Analysis of objective data that is carefully collected to prevent tampering (including laboratory results, medical imaging, pathology reports, physical examination findings, work or school achievement, etc.) to determine whether it supports the individual's (or victim's) diagnosis. It is important to consider how symptoms could be induced, how data could have been altered, and if there is missing or incongruent data.
- Mental health assessment to evaluate for comorbidities and to determine whether suspicious behavior could be better explained by another problem or disorder.
- Testing of the suspected individual's ability to correct or revise his or her illness story and behavior when provided with feedback, education, support, and guidance.

---

visit, making it less susceptible to clinician recall bias or defensiveness that may arise within the context of a legal inquiry. To assess for FDIS/FDIA using a complete set of records, we suggest the creation of a chronological table of every telephone call, office appointment, emergency room visit, and hospitalization. Missed appointments and hospital discharges against medical advice are also important to track. The chronological table is designed to reveal patterns of healthcare utilization, including the number of healthcare facilities and specialty services involved in the family's care (Sanders & Bursch, 2002). Unlike a simple review of records, it allows for pattern analysis of the suspected individual. A thorough, carefully organized table lends itself to easy review of the family's illness and medical treatment trajectories, in addition to the behavior of family members during medical care contacts. Importantly, it also enables the clinician to cross-check information presented by the patient regarding past healthcare contacts and medical problems against the objective data. See Table 19.1 for an example.

When conducting a records-based behavioral analysis, it is important to (a) identify or consider the source of the documented information; (b) examine primary data (test results, rather than just the interpretation of test results); (c) note whether healthcare provider diagnoses or conclusions match objective data; (d) consider whether objective findings could have been falsified or induced; and (e) look at the history broadly to determine whether it makes sense. Literature exists to assist the evaluator in differentiating sudden infant death syndrome from suffocation (Kahn et al., 1992; Meadow, 1990; Samuels & Southall, 1995; Truman & Ayoub, 2002) and in identifying chronic intestinal pseudo-obstruction due to FDIS/FDIA (Hyman, Bursch, Beck, DiLorenzo, & Zeltzer, 2002) and failure to thrive due to illness falsification (Mash, Frazier, Nowacki, Worley, & Goldfarb, 2011).

DIFFERENTIAL DIAGNOSIS

Although direct expressions of behavioral motivation can clarify the diagnosis of an individual engaged in high health care utilization, clinicians typically are required to examine behavioral patterns to infer motivation and to develop diagnostic hypotheses. As in other compulsive or high-denial disorders, it is often only with time in therapy that FDIS/FDIA patients' motivations become evident to clinicians and to the patients themselves (Ayoub, 2010; Sanders, 1996). Nevertheless, accurate diagnosis can inform prognosis and treatment recommendations. This section includes guidance for accurate differential diagnosis.

Somatic Symptom Disorder or Conversion Disorder
(Functional Neurological Symptom Disorder)

In Somatic Symptom Disorder, there may be excessive attention to and treatment seeking for perceived medical concerns, but there is no evidence that the individual is routinely providing false information or behaving deceptively (Feldman, Hamilton, & Deemer, 2001; Krahn, Bostwick, & Stonnington, 2008). Although desire for medical interventions and the risk of overmedicalization may be similar, education on the biopsychosocial model of illness and a rehabilitation approach to treatment tends to be more acceptable to this population.

Malingering

Malingering is intentional illness falsification solely for purposes of obtaining tangible external items (e.g., money, time off work, child custody, medications, the cover-up of a crime). By contrast, the diagnosis of Factitious Disorder requires intentional illness falsification above and beyond that required for self-protection or for desired tangible external items. For example, Factitious Disorder should remain on the differential in a mother who has constructed an enduring story and life centered around falsified illness in her child even if the family, as part of that larger story, receives a vacation or computer donated to them by a non-profit agency for children with life-limiting illnesses. It is important to remember that both Malingering by proxy and FDIA can be abusive if a victim is misled to believe incorrectly that they are ill and/or if the victim is exposed to unnecessary evaluations or treatments (Burton, Warren, Lapid, & Bostwick, 2015; Chafetz & Dufrene, 2014).

Borderline Personality Disorder

Borderline personality traits and other personality disorder traits are commonly comorbid in adults with Factitious Disorder. Although deliberate self-harm in the absence of suicidal intent can occur in borderline personality disorder, these individuals do not typically lie about why they hurt themselves. Self-injury in Factitious Disordered individuals is more likely to be deceptively presented as evidence of an underlying medical problem.

Psychotic Disorders

Although it is possible for a Factitious Disordered individual to have psychotic symptoms (for example, auditory hallucinations telling her that she is a bad person or that doctors are conspiring against her), medical overutilization based solely on delusional health beliefs rules out the diagnosis of Factitious Disorder. A delusional parent will sometimes report symptoms not observed by clinicians, but he or she will typically point to normal variation as evidence of the problem (such as normal variation in skin pigment as evidence of parasites) and accurately report the skepticism of previous physicians. Reports of gruesome symptoms, such as melting organs or parasitic infestations, are more likely to be psychotic in

Table 19.1. Example Table Excerpt

Date	Patient	Location/ Clinician	Subjective/ Reported Problems	Objective Observations	Diagnosis/ Plan/Treatment	Other
3/4/02	Anita	University Medical Center ER & Inpatient Admission/ Dr. Summers	Per mom, at 1:45am, mom found baby apneic (pale, dusky, unresponsive to gentle stimulation); gave CPR after she determined baby was breathless & pulseless, after 2 rounds of breaths & compressions baby began to breathe, brought to hospital. No sxs of illness. Other med hx: Per mom, curdy vomit after each feeding x 3 weeks. She would also turn red, get fussy & arch her back. Admission meds: Zantac 2x/ day started 2 weeks ago for GER.	Feeding well (bottle fed); NAD; no ALTEs; no fevers; O2 sats 98-100% RA; resp unlabored; no apnea alarms, normal tone. Spinal tap: negative. EKG: WNL. Head ultrasound: negative. CXR: negative. UGI: WNL. Slight delay in gastric emptying, no reflux, no hernia, and normal peristalsis. Blood cultures: negative. Urine cultures: negative. WBC: 18.6.	Dx: Resp sxs, Apnea, Likely GER Hosp Tx: Antibiotics (during r-o sepsis work-up) DC Tx: Reglan 0.8mg po TID 30 min before feeds; Zantac 15mg po BID; Home Apnea monitor. Follow-up with PCP in 3–4 days.	Baby lives at home with single mother; no contact with father. Per H&P, mom was adopted so family hx unknown. Reports of children on apnea monitors who are far removed on biological dad's side (2nd or 3rd cousins).
3/9/11	Anita	Midtown Fire Dept EMS	Per mom, two month old baby had an apneic episode and required CPR for 1½ minutes, 3 rounds.	WNL	Transport to hospital. A suspected child abuse report was made by EMS due to mom's report of performing CPR & no signs on baby that she had.	

Date	Name	Provider	Narrative	Findings	Dx/Plan	Notes
3/9/11	Anita	Regional Hospital ER	Per mom, baby had an apneic episode while off the monitor (asleep in car seat—was pale, dusky limp, no breathing, no pulse) and required CPR for 1.5 minutes, 3 rounds. Appeared normal by the time EMS arrived. No illness sxs. Mom stopped both Zantac & Reglan shortly after last discharge. Baby continues to spit up after feeds with curdy looking formula & is intermittently fussy. Sxs improved on Enfamil AR.	O2 sats 99-100%; vital signs WNL. RSV negative; CXR WNL. Happy, playful.	Dx: Report of Apnea; GER Discussed restarting Zantac and Reglan, or starting Prevacid, in order to prevent episodes, but mom declined at this time. Plan: DC Home	Mom reported hx of a second cousin on pt's dad's side who died as an infant of unknown causes.
4/9/11	Anita	Midtown Fire Department EMS	Per mom, monitor went off. Baby was pale and blue around lips, mom got pt to breathe quickly.	WNL	Transport to hospital.	
4/9/11	Anita	Regional Hospital ER	Per mom, baby was blue and apneic. Also, mom had blood-tinged matter on her shirt and said that baby had vomited blood on her.	NAD, alert, smiling, pink, good resp. Pulse ox: 94–97%.	Dx: Apnea episode Tx: Prilosec	

nature (Elmer, George, & Peterson, 2000; Meehan, Badreshia, & Mackley, 2006; Trabert, 1995).

Anxiety Disorders

An excessively anxious individual might unintentionally overreact to normal physical functioning. In the case of "vulnerable child syndrome," due to an early traumatic event, a mother may experience the fear that her baby will not survive (Green & Solnit, 1964). Consequently, she may see the child as vulnerable and become more concerned than necessary about the child's health. High anxiety may lead to an excessive use of healthcare services and may place the child at risk for iatrogenic harm, but this parent does not meet criteria for Factitious Disorder unless deception is identified.

It is important to note that some Factitious Disordered mothers have created medical problems during their pregnancies (Bates, 2001). Porter, Heitsch, and Miller (1994) published a case report about a woman who induced premature rupture of the fetal membranes, causing the birth of twin infants who died from infection. Goss and McDougall (1992) published a case report of a mother who admitted inducing her delivery with a knitting needle and later falsifying illness in her child. Jones, Delplanche, Davies, and Rose (2015) presented a case of a 30-year-old pregnant woman evaluated for severe fetal growth restriction who was discovered to have fabricated her medical history when attempts were made to obtain past medical records.

Autism Spectrum Disorders

Some parents with Autism Spectrum Disorder (ASD) have children at risk for either overmedicalization or medical neglect. "Theory of mind" deficits, such as difficulty determining the intentions of others, impaired understanding of how their behavior affects others, and struggles with social reciprocity may be observed in these parents. As a result, they may incorrectly conclude that a doctor is being malevolent and/or irrational, resulting in interpersonal conflicts and misunderstandings with the treatment team. With limited ability to determine the motivations and intentions of others, some may develop a protective, suspicious stance. Some have limited perception of and limited empathic response to distress cues, which may be dangerous when they are parenting an ill child. Some may have difficulty tolerating benign abnormalities and will, therefore, seek unneeded surgical or medical corrections. Finally, individuals with ASD may exhibit obsessive-compulsive and/or perseverative behavior within their areas of interest, which could include medicine. If deception becomes a feature of this behavior, a comorbid Factitious Disorder diagnosis becomes appropriate.

Eating and Feeding Disorders

Individuals may restrict food intake, falsify dietary history, and/or utilize emetics or laxatives, to support a false story of unintentional weight loss or gain. When there are clear distortions regarding beliefs about appropriate feeding require- ments or practices and/or distorted perceptions about weight, but no evidence that the primary goal of the individual is to induce weight loss in order to suggest an underlying medical condition, an eating disorder diagnosis should be consid- ered and may be more likely (Honjo, 1996; Katz, Mazer, & Litt, 1985; Moszkowicz & Bjornholm, 1998; Scourfield, 1995).

The presence of a genuine medical condition does not preclude the diagnosis of FDIS/FDIA, as comorbid illness often occurs in affected individuals. It is impor- tant to provide standard-of-care services regardless of the presence of a factitious disorder.

TREATMENT OPTIONS

Individuals with a Factitious Disorder are often considered untreatable due to the high rates of denial and the compulsive nature of the behavior. Such individu- als typically have great difficulty identifying their problematic behavior and even greater difficulty stopping it. It is, therefore, unrealistic, and can, in fact, be dan- gerous, to assume that identification of the problem and confrontation of the indi- vidual is sufficient to curb the behavior. Psychotherapy can be effective in select cases, particularly when the illness falsification is relatively mild (with recent onset or low level of acuity), when the individual has admitted to the deceptive behav- ior, and, in the case of FDIA, when the individual has demonstrated remorse and empathy for the victim(s). Severe illness falsification, such as nonaccidental poi- soning and suffocation, is associated with poor prognosis and mortality.

General predictors associated with poor outcome among parents seeking reunification after committing child abuse are applicable to those with Factitious Disorder. They include the presence of one or more of the following: parental history of severe childhood abuse, persistent denial of abusive behavior, refusal to accept help, severe personality disorder, intellectual disability, psychosis, and alcohol or drug abuse (Jones, 1987).

Psychotherapeutic approaches to FDIS/FDIA vary, but they all include efforts to increase awareness and to reduce the risk of relapse. Because the rare and high- denial nature of this disorder precludes the initiation of formal randomized trials to compare treatment approaches, interventions should be selected based on iden- tified behaviors, psychiatric symptoms, and comorbidities. Treatment options to consider include narrative therapy, dialectical behavioral therapy, trauma-focused therapy, parent-child interactive therapy, and intensive family therapy. Among those with skills deficits, cognitive deficits, or learning disorders, basic skills build- ing also may be needed (for example, parent training and/or problem-solving skills). It is important to provide education about normal symptoms, development, and behavior whenever afflicted individuals need help understanding what is abnormal. The development of support systems and a relapse prevention plan are recommended. Safety measures, expert consultation, and careful supervision are needed whenever therapy and reunification are attempted in cases of FDIA.

RECOMMENDATIONS FOR FUTURE WORK

Given the many barriers to conducting research on Factitious Disorder, opportunities for the publication of pooled data may be the best way to advance our understanding of effective intervention approaches. With the adoption of electronic medical records, it may become possible to develop algorithms that assist the clinician by flagging high-risk cases and allowing for easier construction of a medical record table. A preliminary screening measure for early detection of illness falsification imposed upon a child has been developed and requires further validation (Greiner, Palusci, Keeshin, Kearns, & Sinal, 2013). Finally, a closer examination of potential underlying neurological risk factors may inform prevention and intervention efforts.

REFERENCES

Aduan, R.P., Fauci, A.S., Dale, D.C., Herzberg, J.H., & Wolff, S.M. (1979). Factitious fever and self-induced infection: a report of 32 cases and review of the literature. *Annals of Internal Medicine, 90*(2), 230–242.

American Psychiatric Association. (2013). *Diagnostic and Statistical Manual of Mental Disorders, fifth edition.* Arlington, VA: American Psychiatric Association.

Asher, R. (1951). Munchausen's syndrome. *Lancet, 1*(6650):339–341.

Ayoub, C. (2010). Munchausen by proxy. In R. Shaw & D. DeMaso (Eds.), *Textbook of pediatric psychosomatic medicine: consultation on physically ill children* (pp. 185–198). Washington DC: American Psychiatric Publishing, Inc.

Bass, C., & Jones, D. (2011). Psychopathology of perpetrators of fabricated or induced illness in children: case series. *The British Journal of Psychiatry, 199*(2),113–118. doi: 10.1192/bjp.bp.109.074088.

Bates, B. (2001). Be on the lookout for factitious preterm labor. *OB/GYN News.* http://www.thefreelibrary.com/Be+on+the+Lookout+for+Factitious+Preterm+Labor.-a072801697

Bools, C., Neale, B., & Meadow, S.R. (1994). Munchausen syndrome by proxy: A study of psychopathology. Child Abuse & Neglect, 18(9),773–788.

Brown, D., & Scheflin, A. (1999). Factitious disorders and trauma-related diagnoses. *Journal of Psychiatry & Law, 27*, 373–422. Retrieved from http://digitalcommons.law.scu.edu/cgi/viewcontent.cgi?article=1069&context=facpubs

Burton, M.C., Warren, M.B., Lapid, M.I., & Bostwick J.M. (2015). Munchausen syndrome by adult proxy: a review of the literature. *Journal of Hospital Medicine*, *10*(1), 32–35. doi:10.1002/jhm.2268.

Carlson, R.J. (1984). Factitious psychiatric disorders: diagnostic and etiological considerations. *Psychiatric Medicine*, *2*(4):383–388.

Catalina, M.L., Gómez Macias, V., & de Cos, A. (2008). Prevalence of factitious disorder with psychological symptoms in hospitalized patients. *Actas Españolas de Psiquiatría*, *36*, 345–349.

Chafetz, M., & Dufrene, M. (2014). Malingering-by-proxy: need for child protection and guidance for reporting. *Child Abuse & Neglect*, *38*(11), 1755–1765. doi: 10.1016/ j.chiabu.2014.08.015.

Cramer, B., Gershberg, M.R., & Stern, M. (1971). Munchausen syndrome: its relationship to malingering, hysteria, and the physician-patient relationship. *Archives of General Psychiatry*, *24*,573–578.

Elmer, K.B., George, R.M., & Peterson, K. (2000). Therapeutic update: use of risperidone for the treatment of monosymptomatic hypochondriacal psychosis. *Journal of the American Academy of Dermatology*, *43*(4), 683–686.

Faravelli, C., Abrardi, L., Bartolozzi, D., Cecchi, C., Cosci, F., D'Adamo, D., . . . Rosi, S. (2004). The Sesto Fiorentino study: background, methods and preliminary results. Lifetime prevalence of psychiatric disorders in an Italian community sample using clinical interviewers. *Psychotherapy and Psychosomatics*, *73*, 216–225.

Feldman, M.D. (2000). Munchausen by Internet: detecting factitious illness and crisis on the Internet. *Southern Medical Journal*, *93* (7), 669–672.

Feldman, M.D., Hamilton, J.C., & Deemer, H.N. (2001). Factitious disorder, in Somatoform and Factitious Disorders. In K.A. Phillips (Editor), *Review of Psychiatry, Vol 20, No 3* (pp 129–166). Washington, DC: American Psychiatric Publishing.

Feldman, M.D. (2004). *Untangling the web of Munchausen syndrome, Munchausen by proxy, malingering, and factitious disorder.* New York: Brunner-Routledge.

Ferrara, P., Vitelli, O., Bottaro, G., Gatto, A., Liberatore, P., Binetti, P., & Stabile, A. (2013). Factitious disorders and Munchausen syndrome: the tip of the iceberg. *Journal of Child Health Care,17*(4), 366–374. doi: 10.1177/1367493512462262.

Goss, P.W., & McDougall, P.N. (1992). Munchausen syndrome by proxy—A cause of preterm delivery. *The Medical Journal of Australia*, *157*(11–12), 814–817.

Green, M., & Solnit, A.J. (1964). Reactions to the threatened loss of a child: A vulnerable child syndrome. *Pediatrics*, *34*, 58–66.

Greiner, M.V., Palusci, V.J., Keeshin, B.R., Kearns, S.C., & Sinal, S.H. (2013). A preliminary screening instrument for early detection of medical child abuse. *Hospital Pediatrics*, *3*(1), 39–44.

Hamilton, J.C., Eger, M., Razzak, S., Feldman, M.D., Hallmark, N., & Cheek, S. (2013). Somatoform, factitious, and related diagnoses in the National Hospital Discharge Survey: Addressing the proposed DSM-5 revision. *Psychosomatics*, *54*, 142–148. doi: 10.1016/j.psym.2012.08.013.

Honjo, S. (1996). A mother's complaints of overeating by her 25-month-old daughter: a proposal of anorexia nervosa by proxy. *International Journal of Eating Disorders*, *20*(4), 433–437.

Hyman, P.E., Bursch, B., Beck, D., DiLorenzo, C., & Zeltzer L.K. (2002). Discriminating Munchausen syndrome by proxy from chronic digestive disease in toddlers. *Child Maltreatment*, 7(2),132–137.

Jones, D.P.H. (1987). The untreatable family. *Child Abuse & Neglect*, 11, 409–420.

Jones, T.W., Delplanche, M.L., Davies, N.P., & Rose, C.H. (2015). Factitious disorder-by-proxy simulating fetal growth restriction. *Obstetrics & Gynecology*, 125(3), 732–734. doi: 10.1097/AOG.0000000000000506.

Kahn, A., Groswasser, J., Rebuffat, E., Sottiaux, M., Blum, D., Foerster, M., Franco, P., Bochner, A., Alexander, M., Bachy, A., Richard, P., Verghote. M., Le Polain. D., & Wayneberg, J.L. (1992). Sleep and cardiorespiratory characteristics of infant victims of sudden death: a prospective case-control study. *Sleep*, 15(4), 287–292.

Katz, R.L., Mazer, C., & Litt, I.F. (1985). Anorexia nervosa by proxy. *Journal of Pediatrics*, 107(2), 247–248.

Krahn, L.E., Bostwick, M.J., & Stonnington, C.M. (2008). Looking toward DSM-V: Should factitious disorder become a subtype of somatoform disorder? *Psychosomatics* 49(4), 277–282.

Mash, C., Frazier, T., Nowacki, A., Worley, S., & Goldfarb, J. (2011). Development of a risk-stratification tool for medical child abuse in failure to thrive. *Pediatrics,128*(6), e1467–e1473. doi: 10.1542/peds.2011-1080.

Meadow, R. (1990). Suffocation, recurrent apnea, and sudden infant death. *Journal of Pediatrics*, 117(3):351–357.

Meehan, W.J., Badreshia, S., & Mackley, C.L. (2006). Successful treatment of delusions of parasitosis with olanzapine. *Archives of Dermatology*, 142(3), 352–355.

Menninger, K.A. (1934). Polysurgery and polysurgical addiction. *Psychoanalytic Quarterly*, (3):173–199.

Moszkowicz, M., & Bjornholm, K.I. (1998). Factitious illness by proxy presenting as anorexia and polydipsia by proxy. *Acta Paediatrica*, 87(5), 601–602.

Porter, G.E., Heitsch, G.M., & Miller, M.D. (1994). Munchausen syndrome by proxy: unusual manifestations and disturbing sequelae. *Child Abuse & Neglect*, 18(9):789–794.

Samuels, M.P., & Southall, D.P. (1995). Child abuse and apparent life-threatening events. *Pediatrics*, 96, 167–168.

Sanders, M.J. (1996). Narrative family therapy with Munchausen by proxy: A successful treatment case. *Family Systems & Health*, 14(2), 315–329.

Sanders, M.J., & Bursch, B. (2002). Forensic assessment of illness falsification, Munchausen by proxy, and Factitious Disorder, NOS. *Child Maltreatment*, 7(2), 112–124.

Scourfield, J. (1995). Anorexia by proxy: Are the children of anorexic mothers an at-risk group? *International Journal of Eating Disorders*, 18(4), 371–374.

Sheridan, M.S. (2003). The deceit continues: an updated literature review of Munchausen Syndrome by Proxy. *Child Abuse & Neglect*, 27(4), 431–451.

Swanson, L.M., Hamilton, J.C., & Feldman M.D. (2010). Physician-based estimates of medically unexplained symptoms: a comparison of four case definitions. *Family Practice*, 27, 487–493. doi: 10.1093/fampra/cmq051.

Szoke, A., & Boillet, D. (1999). Factitious disorder with psychological signs and symptoms: case reports and proposals for improving diagnosis. *Psychiatry On-Line*.

Trabert, W. (1995). 100 years of delusional parasitosis. Meta-analysis of 1,223 case reports. *Psychopathology*, 28(5), 238–246.

Truman, T.L., & Ayoub C.C. (2002). Considering suffocatory abuse and Munchausen by proxy in the evaluation of children experiencing apparent life-threatening events and sudden infant death syndrome. *Child Maltreatment*, 7(2), 138–148.

World Health Organization. International statistical classification of diseases and related health problems, 10th revision. Version 2010. http://apps.who.int/classifications/icd10/browse/2010/en Accessed July 13, 2015.

20

Diogenes Syndrome

BRIAN O'SHEA ■

VIGNETTE

A socially isolated female in her twenties who lived with her divorced mother in Ireland presented to her local mental health clinic with auditory hallucinations that commented on her actions, delusions of being spied on, poor personal hygiene, and vitamin B1 and iron deficiency. Her mother, based on a difficult lengthy interview and the contorted "magical" thinking and critical tone during her numerous telephone calls, appeared to have schizotypal personality disorder. Despite initial agreement to her daughter's voluntary admission to hospital she engaged in persistent entreaties to have her "only offspring" returned to her. Mother appeared to be totally unaware of own ambivalence: she wanted her daughter helped in an undefined way but could not tolerate the exposure, even to professionals, that this involved. After clinicians developed a tenuous rapport with the young patient, and after significant amelioration of her symptoms with antipsychotic medication, she had begun to entertain the possibility of residing in a supervised hostel. She demonstrated considerable subservience to her mother's instructions throughout her stay in hospital. At times this "obedience" intensified to fear of her mother's inordinate power to influence her regarding her acceptance or refusal of professional assistance.

In a dramatic gesture, her mother appeared on the ward one night and took her daughter, dressed in pyjamas, out of hospital. Attempts by staff to gain access to the patient's home proved fruitless. The door was not opened to them, the house and garden were in a dilapidated state, and the inside of the house appeared to be cluttered with heaps of rubbish and excrement. One could see that the toilet had been disconnected and there was no electricity going into the residence. Attempts to have the patient made a Ward of Court (placed under High Court protection) were unsuccessful because the "second opinion" psychiatrist was unable to contact her. Eventually it was discovered that mother and daughter had left for an unknown destination.

In this particular case, mother and daughter both appeared to be suffering from Diogenes syndrome as a specific manifestation of folie à deux. Folie à deux is a delusion transmitted from one person to another, the couple being emotionally very close. The recipient of the false belief is usually the passive partner and often recovers over a period of months if the two are separated. Diagnostic criteria include evidence that the people involved have been intimately associated; identical or near identical delusional themes; and acceptance, support, and sharing of each other's delusions. If one person develops the delusion first and "infects" another it is called folie communiquée. If both develop it at the same time it is called folie simultanée. We can only suggest that the mother forced her daughter to live in squalor and neglect as she did (folie communiquée), but we cannot say that the daughter would not have become ill if she had never lived with her mother (a variant of folie simultanée). Unfortunately, we were unable to thoroughly categorize their situation within this framework because the mother evaded a more thorough assessment.

HISTORICAL/CULTURAL CONTEXT

Diogenes syndrome (senile squalor syndrome) is named for Diogenes of Sinope or Διογένης ὁ Σινωπεύς (Wrigley & Cooney, 1992; O'Shea & Falvey, 1997; Cooney, 1997). Diogenes (c. 412 or 404–323 BCE), a Greek Cynic philosopher (Navia, 1996), was a native of Sinope (modern Sinop or Σινώπη on Cape Ince in Turkey). A beggar who admired poverty and decried human achievements, he lived in an Athenian tub and ate onions. Notably, he did not hoard and he enjoyed the company of other humans (Marcos & Gomez-Pellin, 2008). The Cynics advocated self-sufficiency and contentment and eschewed material possessions. Other names for the contemporary conception of the syndrome include *Augean stables syndrome* and *social breakdown of the elderly syndrome*. The stables in Greek myth belonged to Augeas (Augeias) who was king of Elis. The stables, unclean and housing many cattle, were cleaned by Heracles (Hercules) who achieved his task in a single day by rerouting rivers. Post (1982) called the phenomenon *senile recluse* and MacMillan and Shaw (1966) used the term *senile breakdown*.

Another historical precursor of Diogenes syndrome was Plyushkin, a character in Gogol's novel, *Dead Souls* (Gogol, 1961). He may have more closely fitted the concept of Diogenes syndrome than did Diogenes himself (Cybulska, 1998). The landowner Plyushkin saved everything he found, including food that went moldy.

Clark et al. (1975) coined the term Diogenes syndrome in 1975 specifically to describe gross self-neglect in old age.

Although symptoms of Diogenes are not currently a strong focus of scientific interest, the syndrome has received considerable coverage in the media. The play *The Dazzle* was based on the highly educated Collyer brothers, Homer and Langley, who lived in a filthy and dilapidated house in Harlem. The house was crammed with hoarded material. Homer starved to death. After two weeks of searching and the removal of 130 tons of rubbish Langley's body was discovered. He appears to have been smothered by a mountain of debris. When they died in

1947 Homer was 65 years old and Langley was 61 years old. They had set booby traps around the premises to trap intruders but one of these devices may have contributed to Langley's demise.

The actress Drew Barrymore won the best actress award for the 2009 TV movie *Grey Gardens* that tells the story of Edie Bouvier Beale (1917–2002), first cousin to Jackie Kennedy Onassis and sufferer from alopecia totalis. Edie was discovered in a squalid mansion in Bal Harbour, Florida, surrounded by flea infested cats and raccoons and a mountain of filthy cans.

In 2010 the Las Vegas police spent a month searching for the 67-year-old Billie Jean James, but it was her husband who unearthed her remains at home under a pile of garbage.

ROLE IN CURRENT DIAGNOSTIC SYSTEMS

Diogenes syndrome is found in neither the *Diagnostic and Statistical Manual of Mental Disorders* (DSM-5) nor in the *International Classification of Diseases* (ICD-10). It should be noted, however, that Diogenes syndrome is likely to represent a heterogeneous group of conditions (Clark et al., 1975; Drummond et al., 1997; Reyes-Ortiz, 2001; Amanullah et al., 2009). There are no universally accepted criteria (inclusionary or exclusionary) for this syndrome (Hanon et al., 2004).

Hoarding disorder, a separate but overlapping concept will be discussed briefly here. DSM-5 hoarding disorder (300.3), placed in the chapter on "obsessive-compulsive and related disorders," refers to persistent difficulty getting rid of possessions, regardless of their real value (American Psychiatric Association, 2013, p. 247). This, as is often found in Diogenes, leads to congestion of living areas. Decongestion only occurs when a third party intervenes. The practice leads to significant impairment in some aspect of living.

The most common psychiatric diagnoses in cases of abnormal hoarding appear to be Alzheimer's disease (AD), chronic paranoid schizophrenia, chronic alcoholism, and bipolar affective disorder (Irvine & Nwachukwu, 2014). A reaction to stress in later life has been postulated for Diogenes syndrome (e.g., the death of a close relative may be a precipitating factor in those with no psychiatric illness). Clark et al. (1975) suggested that such stress interacted with personality vulnerability, including schizotypy.

Regarding other correlates, cases of Diogenes have come from diverse social backgrounds, from the poverty-stricken to the upper echelons of society. Range of intelligence varies from high to low (Williams et al., 1998). Some cases may have frontal lobe dysfunction (Orrell & Sahakian, 1991; Lebert, 2005) as reflected in poor decision-making and hoarding. It is not uncommon, however, to find that the people store hoarded material in a logical manner, such as sorting jumpers and newspapers separately. Insight in OCD (obsessive-compulsive disorder) with hoarding may be associated with less insight than in OCD without hoarding (Murphy et al., 2010). OCD-related hoarding may be mediated by reduced activity in the cingulate cortex (Saxena et al., 2004).

Reported underlying disorders of abnormal hoarding include OCD, neurological insults, stimulant abuse, autism, anorexia nervosa (uneaten food), Prader-Willi syndrome (Barocka et al., 2004), Tourette syndrome (multiple motor and vocal tics), schizophrenia, schizotypal personality disorder, and obsessive-compulsive disorder. There may be a role for frontal lobe dysfunction in the etiology of both the wider concept of excessive hoarding and the narrower one of Diogenes syndrome.

Compulsive hoarding is common and heritable. Nonshared environment also likely plays a part in etiology. (Iervolino et al., 2009) DSM-5 does not allow a diagnosis of hoarding disorder if it is due to a neurodegenerative disorder such as frontotemporal lobar degeneration or Alzheimer's disease.

SYMPTOMATOLOGY

Reported manifestations from a conflicting literature include extreme self-neglect, a dirty appearance, domestic squalor, lying in excrement, a filthy odor in the living environment, lack of basic amenities such as electricity, social withdrawal, and compulsive hoarding of garbage (magazines, newspapers, books, jumpers, tin cans, mail, furniture, musical instruments, animals, etc), so-called syllogomania. Shame may be present or absent in patients with Diogenes syndrome and presence of shame may itself inhibit help-seeking. Not all cases hoard (Fontenelle, 2008). Summarizing across these different conceptions, the core syndrome appears to consist of severe withdrawal from social intercourse, personal and environmental squalor, and compulsive hoarding of garbage and/or failure to discard unneeded possessions. The various reported associated clinical conditions (such as compulsive hoarding or psychosis) might act as triggers, comorbid disorders, or etiological factors.

PREVALENCE RATE AND ASSOCIATED FEATURES

Clark et al. (1975) reported on 14 males and 16 females (age range 66–92 years, mean age 79 years) who had been acutely hospitalized, were very unwell, and had evidence of extreme self-neglect. The authors suggested that the syndrome is found about equally in men and women. An unanswered question is whether this syndrome is a discrete disorder or simply an extreme belonging to a spectrum.

Diogenes syndrome is sometimes divided into primary and secondary subtypes, the latter being applied where the patient has a recognizable psychiatric disorder. The role of personality requires further elucidation.

It is difficult to be dogmatic about statistics here, because different authors appear to describe disparate populations. The estimated annual incidence of Diogenes syndrome among people older than 59 years is 0.5 cases per 1,000 (Clark et al., 1975; Berlyne & Twomey, 1975; Macmillan & Shaw, 1966; Wrigley & Cooney, 1992). Although classically associated with the elderly, Hurley et al. (2000)

reported that 30.9% of their cases were younger than 65 years. Most (Hurley et al., 2000; Steketee et al., 2001), but not all, cases lived alone. Some lived with a spouse or sibling (Eposito et al., 2003). Diogenes syndrome has recently (Chan et al., 2007) been reported from Hong Kong in 18 people aged 65 and over. Biswas et al. (2013) presented the case of a 34-year-old male with schizophrenia who was brought to a dermatology clinic in India because of skin lesions. He had not taken a bath for more than two years.

Community studies suggest a somewhat different profile for people living in squalor: somewhat younger males of lower social class who are mentally ill and older people who are physically ill (Halliday et al., 2000). It is not possible to determine whether any of these have Diogenes syndrome. Reminiscent of the vignette duo presented at the start of this chapter, cases of married couples or cohabiting siblings with what was dubbed "Diogenes à deux" have been reported elsewhere (e.g., Cole et al., 1992).

Abnormal hoarding in general (not necessarily attracting a diagnosis of Diogenes syndrome) may affect 2%–5% of the population; clinical samples are dominated by females but hoarding may be more common in males in the wider population (Grisham & Norberg, 2010). A South East London study found a prevalence of DSM-5 hoarding disorder of 1.5%, the condition affecting both sexes and often accompanied by significant physical and mental problems (Nordsletten et al., 2013). An Automobile Association Home Insurance survey (Anonymous, 2014) in Ireland (N = 7,600), undoubtedly conducted because of the fire hazard posed by cluttered premises, found that males were more likely to hoard than females and that hoarding increases with age: over 37% of persons aged 65 or older admitted to being hoarders, while only 11% said they would like to declutter the house. It is not clear how severe the "hoarding" was in respondents, but it suggests that pathological hoarding may be a matter of degree.

Premorbid socioeconomic background among reported cases of Diogenes syndrome is highly varied, many people having had successful careers in the professions with nothing abnormal found in their family background or in their rearing.

Regarding associated features, various personality characteristics and disorders have been linked with Diogenes syndrome such as stubbornness, aggressiveness, unpredictable moods, emotional instability, and a distorted sense of reality. At the level of actual personality disorder, schizotypal and obsessive-compulsive (anancastic) diagnoses have been employed (Barocka et al., 2004; Van Alphen & Engelen, 2005).

Various other psychiatric disorders are reported to have preceded Diogenes syndrome such as schizophrenia, affective disorder, OCD, chronic alcohol abuse, static brain disease, dementia, and intellectual disability ("learning disorder" in United Kingdom). In older people with self-neglect only there have been reports of late-onset schizophrenia (formerly paraphrenia), chronic depression, abnormal grief (loss of a close relative who acted as carer may precipitate or expose the syndrome; Ungvari & Hantz, 1991), and Capgras syndrome (O'Shea et al., 1989; Donnelly et al., 2008; see also Chapter 5).

Frontal lobe dysfunction also has been implicated in Diogenes syndrome (Gannon & O'Boyle, 1992; Neary et al., 1998; Funayama et al., 2010; Lee et al., 2014).

Somatic disorders reported to have preceded Diogenes syndrome include cardiac or renal failure, malignancy, vascular disorders (central and peripheral), Parkinson's disease, various lung diseases, and orthopedic disorders such as arthritis/spondylitis or Paget's disease. Presentation may be acute and medical with falls or collapse, and there may be multiple hematologic deficiencies. Unsurprisingly, these conditions are usually neglected by such patients.

People who do not clean themselves develop an accumulation of keratinous (horny) crusts on the skin. Distribution varies with age: upper central chest, back and groin in older subjects and scalp, face, or arms. This manifestation of "Diogenes syndrome" also is known as *dermatitis passivata* (Biswas et al., 2013), although the present author has seen such skin problems in people who do not otherwise attract a diagnosis of Diogenes syndrome, such as hoboes and alcoholics.

Some authors have divided cases into active and passive rubbish collectors (Hanon et al., 2004) depending on whether they bring the rubbish home or whether they simply fail to discard it, respectively. About 50% have a formal psychiatric illness at the time of examination, but far fewer have been admitted to psychiatric care. In fact, such suspicious and aloof patients often flatly refuse to be helped (Clark et al., 1975; Klosterkötter & Peters, 1985; Hurley et al., 2000).

There appears to be a high physical morbidity and mortality rate with Diogenes syndrome as well: about half will die in hospital, one quarter end up in long-term care, and the remainder return home (Spear et al., 1997). Clark et al. (1975) also reported a high mortality, especially for females (46%). Badr et al. (2005) give a five-year mortality rate of 46%, often due to somatic diseases like pneumonia. Reported mortality rates may partly reflect the samples studied, for example, acute medical presentation versus cases coming to attention because of overgrown gardens or retaliation secondary to teasing by youths.

Diogenes syndrome represents a dilemma for psychiatry and for society. Such patients often resist offers of help from others and may deny the poor conditions in which they live. Do we let patients live in squalor lest we infringe human rights ("rotting with their rights on" as stated by Appelbaum & Gutheil, 1980)? One should keep in mind that perhaps up to 50% of cases of Diogenes syndrome may not have a diagnosable comorbid psychiatric disorder (Wrigley & Cooney, 1992). Also, disorders of personality per se are not counted as legitimate reasons for involuntary hospitalization in Irish legislation.

THEORIES OF ETIOLOGY

There does not appear to be one particular explanation for all cases of Diogenes syndrome and the presentation may simply represent a final common pathway for many conditions. Dementia is an important cause in the elderly (Wrigley & Cooney, 1992) and frontal lobe dementia plays a part in some younger individuals

(Orrell & Sahakian, 1991). Those cases not attracting a formal psychiatric diagnosis, from a third to a half of cases, are postulated to have problematic personality structures that interfere with coping (Post et al., 1982). A hostile attitude to potential sources of assistance (Macmillan & Shaw, 1966) might reflect an underlying and symbolic form of suicide (Thibault et al., 1999). Any "explanation" also must take account of the other diagnoses reported in cases of Diogenes syndrome: schizophrenia, chronic mood disorders, OCD, and low intellectual ability.

ASSESSMENT OPTIONS

There is no specific assessment procedure for Diogenes syndrome, but an awareness of the syndrome is necessary if the syndrome is to be detected. A team approach is essential. A home visit to confirm the presence of squalor should be part of the workup. Physicians, nurses, social workers, occupational therapists, and psychologists are suitable persons to undertake such visits. It is important that professionals dealing with patients with Diogenes syndrome arrange for a physical examination, mental status review, and any indicated laboratory investigations. Where feasible, a neuropsychological assessment should be performed. Not all subjects will allow these interventions in the absence of rapport.

What are the legal and ethical grounds for intruding (assessment, environmental manipulation, and treatment) in the lives of people with Diogenes syndrome? Do we insist on intervening because of the danger of infectious disease? The answer is easier when the patient is obviously psychotic. Some authors advocate doing what one can, and is allowed to do, to improve socialization and well-being (Cipriani et al., 2012). Every effort should be made to form a trusting relationship with the person affected. This could be with a physician, social worker, a psychiatric nurse, or some other appropriate person. Enlistment of help from relatives may be crucial. A decision to enforce treatment under mental health legislation will depend on findings on psychiatric examination and local laws. In the United Kingdom the provisions of *The National Assistance Act 1948*, section 47 and the same section in *The National Assistance (Amendment) Act 1951*, are rarely used. The latter legislation required court involvement and there was no automatic review process. Indeed the Departments of Health for England and Wales have suggested that Section 47 could be in breach of human rights legislation in terms of right to liberty and right to private and family life. Interstate differences make generalizations difficult regarding the United States. By way of example, in Florida, a state with a large elder population, civil commitment law allows the involuntary examination of a person for up to 72 hours to determine whether the individual meets standards for involuntary treatment (Christy et al., 2007).

Negative effects on others, such as cohabiters, must be taken into consideration. In 1976, in *Tarasoff v Regents of the University of California* (killing of Tatiana Tarasoff by Prosenjit Poddar in 1969), the Supreme Court of California ruled that mental health professionals have a duty to protect people threatened with physical harm by a patient. Following a British case (*W v Egdell*, 1990), in the case of real risk of physical harm, confidentiality can be breached if necessary in order to protect the public interest. In Ireland, the 1998 *Protection for Persons Reporting Child Abuse Act* imposes an obligation on designated officers of public health authorities to report knowledge of any child who might be at risk of abuse. The Irish Medical Council (medicalcouncil.ie) guidance of 2009 affirmed its acceptance of the Tarasoff decision when stating that disclosure without a patient's permission could be done if failure to disclose placed others at risk of harm. Otherwise confidentiality should be maintained. In the presence of incapacity the clinician should consider what is in the patient's best interest. Laws vary between and, often, within nations.

Care options, highly dependent on patient acceptance, include day care facilities, delivery of fresh food, and laundry services. It may be possible to clean the immediate environment using volunteers or local bylaws. Physical illness or poor mobility may necessitate hospitalization or nursing home placement. Treatment of psychiatric disorder with medication (with due regard to adherence monitoring) and/or an appropriate form of psychotherapy should be prioritized. Cognitive behavior therapy is helpful in the treatment of compulsive hoarding (Saxena & Maidment, 2004; Tolin et al., 2007; Gaston et al., 2009).

DIFFERENTIAL DIAGNOSIS

The differential diagnosis of Diogenes syndrome includes the various manifestations of the syndrome alluded to earlier, such as psychosis, cognitive problems, and neglect of self and home environment, as in, lack of awareness due to dementia or very low intelligence or poor motivation due to schizophrenia or depressive disorder. Disorders of personality requiring particular consideration include the schizotypal and paranoid subtypes. Culture-based rejection of medical explanations of mental disorder (Kishore et al., 2011), alcohol or other substance use, or a reaction to actual harassment, are other possibilities (Hurley et al., 2000). Finally, physical disability or somatic illness may lead to squalor by default.

TREATMENT OPTIONS

The objectives of the initial assessment are to reach a diagnosis and to create a therapeutic relationship with the person/people involved. Any underlying disorder should dictate a course of treatment, such as behavioral therapy to reduce intake and promote removal of hoarded material or cognitive behavior treatment for pathological hoarding (Tolin, 2011), antipsychotic medication for psychosis, and nursing home placement for the demented. Assistance with financial matters may be provided by social workers or local authorities. Relatives may be aware or unaware of the living circumstances of people with Diogenes syndrome and, if contacted, they may be willing to offer practical help in terms of access to and cleaning of premises, persuading patients to accept assistance, or partaking, when necessary, in the application process for involuntary admission to hospital. Cipriani et al. (2012), who view Diogenes patients, at least those with dementia, as posing a risk to themselves and others, suggest "gentle persuasion" of patients at first but resort to mental health legislation as final resort. Day hospital attendance appears to have a positive impact on somatic and mental health (Klosterkötter & Peters, 1985). Family therapy may be of value where long-term rifts have occurred between patients and their relatives. In those cases where a dominant partner appears to perpetuate the syndrome it may be possible to improve matters for the passive partner by assisting them to leave the home, that is, to help the latter to individuate and find alternative ways of living without the overpowering influence of the cohabiter. The relationship may be so enmeshed that recourse to mental health legislation is required. What is possible will depend on the mental states of the cohabiters and local law. Where separation is undertaken one hopes that the dominant psychotic partner with Diogenes can be treated and that the passive partner can be helped with psychoeducation to live a more fulfilling life.

Management issues evoke ethical difficulties: individual rights versus communal safety. Many cases come to attention because of third-party concerns. The would-be interventionist should consider carefully the differential diagnosis of the various manifestations of Diogenes syndrome; for example, is the subject rejecting help because of amotivation (as in the negative symptoms of schizophrenia), depressed affect, personality-related or culturally related suspiciousness, a paranoid disorder, alcohol or other substance use, or experience of real harassment? Aggressiveness, physical or verbal (Hurley et al., 2000), has a wide differential including personality trait, reaction to circumstances such as third-party intrusion, and, as a primary or exacerbating cause, dementia.

RECOMMENDATIONS FOR FUTURE RESEARCH

From a research perspective, there is a need for better agreement on what constitutes Diogenes syndrome and for its replacement by a "psychiatric disorder-plus" approach, that is, if someone has schizophrenia or dementia and lives in squalor, then it should be described as such, as in "Diogenes syndrome with schizophrenia." Given the attraction to exotica among clinicians (the author included) and the media, progress is likely to be slow.

Diogenes syndrome is just that, a syndrome in the sense that a syndrome is a collection of symptoms (subjective complaints) and/or signs (observations by others) that occur together with sufficient frequency to suggest a common cause or causes or a shared pathogenesis (pathological trajectory). This author agrees with Fontenelle (2008) that Diogenes syndrome represents a final common pathway and is not a primary disorder per se. Whether or not it is an OCD spectrum disorder has not been answered and Drummond et al. (1997) want it distinguished from OCD in which hoarding may be viewed as stemming directly from obsessive-compulsive behavior. For example, the present author has seen cases of severe OCD where patients insist on keeping one room extremely ordered while the rest of the house becomes cluttered by default. In this London study, however, they noted that the addition of hoarding to OCD was associated with a relatively poor response to cognitive behavior therapy. It seems that OCD plus hoarding is a particularly severe and entrenched form of OCD.

Ultimately, from the perspective of mental health professionals, the key point is whether the objectively unpalatable circumstances of the people discussed here can be explained by mental disorder, which should of course be a focus of treatment. In the Republic of Ireland, for example, there are two relevant legally sanctioned ways of depriving a patient of his/her liberty: if the person has a severe enough mental illness such that there is an "immediate" likelihood of harm to self or others *or* the illness is significant, the patient cannot be treated "in a less restrictive manner" and psychiatric interventions are likely to have positive effects (*Mental Health Act, 2001*, section 3); if the person is brought before the criminal courts and is suffering from a severe mental disorder (under *The Criminal Law (Insanity) Act, 2006*) the patient may be sent to Ireland's only high security hospital, the Central Mental Hospital in Dublin). An unresolved issue is the admission of people to care homes without their permission. At the time of writing, unlike in the United Kingdom, Ireland has proposed rather than actual capacity legislation. The basis of such legislation is that the mental capacity to make a particular decision at a particular time is present or not. The making of decisions that the examiner disagrees with does not negate capacity. The capacitous person understands what is being proposed, the alternative choices (including inaction) and can retain the information given for long enough to make a choice. Practitioners are advised to acquaint themselves with the laws in their own geographical location. In many cases the health care professional is bereft of legislative support and must rely on the use of gentle and persistent persuasion to accept help, what Ballard (2010) described as a "delicate balance of trust and support."

REFERENCES

Amanullah, S., Oomman, S.K., & Datta, S.S. (2009). "Diogenes syndrome" revisited. *German Journal of Psychiatry, 12*, 38–44.

American Psychiatric Association. (2013). *Diagnostic and statistical manual of mental disorders, 5th Edition*. Washington, DC and London, England: American Psychiatric Association.

Anonymous. (2014, October 14). Irish men hoard more stuff than Irish women, says survey. Posted on thejournal.ie.

Appelbaum, P.S., & Gutheil, T.G. (1980). Rotting with their rights on: constitutional theory and clinical reality in drug refusal by psychiatric patients. *Bulletin of the American Academy of Psychiatry and the Law, 7*, 306–315.

Badr, A., Hossain, A., & Iqbal, J. (2005). Diogenes syndrome: when self-neglect is nearly life threatening. *Clinical Geriatrics, 13(8)*, 10–13.

Ballard, J. (2010). Legal implications regarding self-neglecting community-dwelling adults: a practical approach for the community nurse in Ireland. *Public Health Nursing, 27*, 181–187.

Barocka, A., Seehuber, D., & Schöne, D. (2004). Messy house syndrome. *MMW Fortschritte der Medizin, 146(45)*, 36–39.

Berlyne, N., & Twomey, J. (1975). Henderson Smith SL. Diogenes syndrome. *Lancet, 1*, 515.

Biswas, P., Ganguly, A., Bala, S., Nag, F., Choudhary, N., & Sen, S. (2013). Diogenes syndrome: a case report. *Case Reports in Dermatological Medicine*. http://dx.doi.org/10.1155/2013/595192

Chan, S.M., Leung, P.Y., & Chiu, F.K. (2007). Late-onset Diogenes syndrome in Chinese—an elderly case series in Hong Kong. *Neuropsychiatric Disease and Treatment, 3*, 589–596.

Christy, A., Bond, J., & Young, M.S. (2007). Short-term involuntary examination of older adults in Florida. *Behavioral Sciences & the Law, 25*, 615–628.

Cipriani, G., Lucetti, C., Vedovello, M., & Nuti, A. (2012). Diogenes syndrome in patients suffering from dementia. *Dialogues in Clinical Neuroscience, 14*, 455–460.

Clark, A.N., Mankikar, G.D., & Gray, I. (1975). Diogenes syndrome. A clinical study of gross neglect in old age. *Lancet, 1 (7903)*, 366–368.

Cole, A.J., Gillett, J.P., & Fairbairn, A. (1992). A case of senile self-neglect in a married couple: "Diogenes a Deux." *International Journal of Geriatric Psychiatry, 7*, 839–841.

Cooney, C. (1997). Diogenes syndrome: the role of the psychiatrist. In C. Holmes & R. Howard (Eds.), *Advances in old age psychiatry: chromosomes to community care*. Petersfield, UK: Wrightson Biomedical.

Cybulska, E. (1998). Senile squalor: Plyushkin's not Diogenes syndrome. *Psychiatric Bulletin, 22*, 319–320.

Donnelly, R., Bolouri, M.S., Prashad, S.J., Coverdale, J.H., Hays, J.R., & Kahn, D.A. (2008). Comorbid Diogenes and Capgras syndromes. *Journal of Psychiatric Practice, 14*, 312–317.

Drummond, L.M., Turner, J., & Reid, S. (1997). Diogenes syndrome—a load of rubbish? *Irish Journal of Psychological Medicine, 14*, 99–102.

Eposito, D., Rouillon, F., & Limosin, F. (2003). Diogenes syndrome in a pair of siblings. *Canadian Journal of Psychiatry, 48*, 571–572.

Fontenelle, L.F. (2008). Diogenes syndrome in a patient with obsessive-compulsive disorder without hoarding. *General Hospital Psychiatry, 30 (3)*, 288–290.

Funayama, M., Mimura, M., Koshibe, Y., & Kato, Y. (2010). Squalor syndrome after focal orbitofrontal damage. *Cognitive and Behavioral Neurology, 23 (2)*, 135–139.

Gannon, M., & O'Boyle, J. (1992). Diogenes syndrome. *Irish Medical Journal, 85*, 124.

Gaston, R.L., Kiran-Imran, F., Hassiem, F., & Vaughan, J. (2009). Hoarding behaviour: building up the "R factor." *Advances in Psychiatric Treatment, 15*, 344–353.

Gogol, N. (1961). *Dead souls*. London: Penguin.

Grisham, J.R., & Norberg, M.N. (2010). Compulsive hoarding: current controversies and new directions. *Dialogues in Clinical Neuroscience, 12*, 233–240.

Halliday, G., Banerjee, S., Philpot, M., & Macdonald, A. (2000). Community study of people who live in squalor. *Lancet, 355*, 882–886.

Hanon, C., Pinquier, C., Gaddour, N., Said, S, Mathis, D., & Pellerin, J. (2004). Diogenes syndrome: a transnosographic approach. *Encephale, 30(4)*, 315–322.

Hurley, M., Scallan, E., Johnson, H., & De La Harpe, D. (2000). Adult service refusers in the Greater Dublin area. *Irish Medical Journal, 93*, 208–211.

Iervolino, A.C., Perroud, N., Fullana, M.A., Guipponi, M., Cherkas, L., Collier, D.A., & Mataix-Cols, D. (2009). Prevalence and heritability of compulsive hoarding: a twin study. *American Journal of Psychiatry, 166*, 1156–1161.

Irvine, J.D.C., & Nwachukwu, K. (2014). Recognizing Diogenes syndrome: a case report. *BioMed Central Research Notes, 7*, 276.

Kishore, J., Gupta, A., Jiloha, R.C., & Bantman, P. (2011). Myths, beliefs and perceptions about mental disorders and health-seeking behavior in Delhi, India. *Indian Journal of Psychiatry, 53*, 324–329.

Klosterkötter, J., & Peters, U.H. (1985). Diogenes syndrome. *Fortschritte der Neurologie und Psychiatrie, 53*, 427–434.

Lebert, F. (2005). Diogenes syndrome: a clinical presentation of fronto-temporal dementia or not? *International Journal of Geriatric Psychiatry, 20*, 1203–1204.

Lee, S.M., Lewis, M., Leighton, D., Harris, B., Long, B., & Macfarlane, S. (2014). Neuropsychological characteristics of people living in squalor. *International Psychogeriatrics, 26*(5), 837–844.

Macmillan, D., & Shaw, P. (1966). Senile breakdown in standards of personal and environmental cleanliness. *British Medical Journal, 2*, 1032–1037.

Marcos, M., & Gomez-Pellin, M.D.C. (2008). A tale of a misnamed eponym. Diogenes syndrome. *International Journal of Geriatric Psychiatry, 23*, 990–991.

Murphy, D.L., Timpano, K.R., Wheaton, M.G., Greenberg, B.D., & Miguel, E.C. (2010). Obsessive-compulsive disorder and its related disorders: a reappraisal of obsessive-compulsive spectrum concepts. *Dialogues in Clinical Neuroscience, 12*, 131–148.

Navia, L.E. (1996). *Diogenes of Sinope: the man in the tub*. Westport, CT: Greenwood Press.

Neary, D., Snowden, J. S., Gustafson, L., Passant, U., Stuss, D., Black, S., . . . Benson, D.F. (1998). Frontotemporal lobar degeneration: a consensus on clinical diagnostic criteria. *Neurology, 51*, 1546–1554.

Nordsletten, A.E., Reichenberg, A., Hatch, S.L., de la Cruz L. F., Pertusa, A., Hotopf, M., & Mataix-Cols, D. (2013). Epidemiology of hoarding disorder. *British Journal of Psychiatry, 203*, 445–452.

Orrell, M., & Sahakian, B. (1991). Dementia of frontal type. *Psychological Medicine, 21*, 553–556.

O'Shea, B., & Falvey, J. (1997). Diogenes' syndrome: review and case history. *Irish Journal of Psychological Medicine, 14*, 115–116.

O'Shea, B., Falvey, J., Mathews, G., & Murphy, P. (1989). Capgras syndrome: a nonspecific, often organic phenomenon. *Irish Journal of Psychiatry, 10*(1), 13–16.

Post, F. (1982). Functional disorders. In R. Levy & F. Post (Eds.), *Psychiatry of late life* (pp. 176–196). Oxford: Blackwell Scientific.

Reyes-Ortiz, C. (2001). Diogenes syndrome: the self-neglect elderly. *Comprehensive Therapy, 27*, 117–121.

Saxena, S., Brody, A.L., Maidment, K.M., Smith, E.C., Zohrabi, N., Katz, N., . . . Baxter, L.R. Jr. (2004). Cerebral glucose metabolism in obsessive-compulsive hoarding. *American Journal of Psychiatry, 161*, 1038–1048.

Saxena, S., & Maidment, K.M. (2004). Treatment of compulsive hoarding. *Journal of Clinical Psychology, 60*, 1143–1154.

Spear, J., Wise, J., & Herzberg, J. (1997). "Diogenes" syndrome and folie à deux in a married couple. *Psychiatric Case Reports, 2*, 53.

Steketee, G., Frost, R.O., & Kim, H.J. (2001). Hoarding by elderly people. *Health and Social Work, 26*, 176–184.

Thibault, J.M., O'Brien, J.G., & Turner, L.C. (1999). Indirect life-threatening behaviour in elderly patients. *Journal of Elder Abuse and Neglect, 11(2)*, 21–32.

Tolin, D.F. (2011). Challenges and advances in treating hoarding. *Journal of Clinical Psychology, 67*, 451–455.

Tolin, D.F., Frost, R.O., & Steketee, G. (2007). An open trial of cognitive behavioural therapy for compulsive hoarding. *Behaviour Research and Therapy, 45*, 1461–1470.

Ungvari, G.S., & Hantz, P.M. (1991). Social breakdown in the elderly, II: sociodemographic data and psychopathology. *Comprehensive Psychiatry, 32*, 445–449.

Van Alphen, S.P., & Engelen, G.J. (2005). Reaction to "personality disorder" masquerading as dementia: a case of apparent Diogenes syndrome. *International Journal of Geriatric Psychiatry, 20(2)*, 189.

Williams, H., Clarke, R., Fashola, Y., & Holt, G. (1998). Diogenes' syndrome in patients with intellectual disability: "a rose by any other name." *Journal of Intellectual Disability Research, 42*, 316–320.

Wrigley, M., & Cooney, C. (1992). Diogenes syndrome—an Irish series. *Irish Journal of Psychological Medicine, 9*, 37–41.

21

Pseudologia
Fantastica — Pathological Lying

PETRA GARLIPP ■

EPIGRAPH

"When I asked him he told me, here he had always tried to tell me the whole truth. Yet, if he might have been wrong concerning a few things, he could not know."

(DELBRÜCK, *1891, p. 88, own translation) (1)*

VIGNETTE

The 32-year-old patient presented for treatment in a psychiatric day hospital where patients with various psychiatric diagnoses were treated. He was admitted with a diagnosis of recurrent major depressive disorder, current episode, moderate severity (F33.1). He mainly complained of insomnia, loss of appetite, depressive mood with a conviction of his life being meaningless, ruminations, lack of motivation, and feelings of guilt. The patient also mentioned that he had continuous suicidal thoughts. He had a history of multiple admissions to various psychiatric hospitals and day clinics. His last hospital admission had been involuntary.

During a previous hospitalization a female patient claimed that he had tried to strangle her, a charge he denied. From his perspective, he had just tried to "keep her away" from him. A self-critical reflection of his own behavior was seemingly not possible. He reported that several years ago he had attempted suicide three times by overdosing on prescribed medication. He had no history of any other mental illness and no alcohol or drug addiction. The patient reported no family history of any mental illness. The patient was divorced, with his two children living with his ex-wife. He had contact with family and friends.

A trained engineer, he had lost his job several months ago but was convinced he would easily find a new job if he wished. Because of his qualifications he would "globally" have the chance to get a job, meaning, he was competitive on an international level, which seemed to be a bit exaggerated.

The mental status examination showed an alert and orientated patient without impaired memory or cognitive symptoms. Concentration was not disturbed. There was no evidence of hallucinations or delusional thinking. The patient showed a lack of motivation and he reported ruminations consistent with a moderately depressed state. He was assessed as not imminently suicidal on admission, but reported recurrent suicidal thoughts. No current aggressive thoughts against others were stated on admission. The interview revealed some narcissistic personality traits. On examination there were no significant somatic pathological findings. His latest magnetic resonance imaging (MRI) scan was normal.

During the second interview the patient reported that, for at least the last few years, he tended to lie to "get things straight." He had noticed that he was very talented in constructing lies and that people believed him. The latest lie had been one he had told his family members, friends, and doctors. Specifically, he told them that he was suffering from a brain tumor. They believed him at first. He noted that he could skillfully manipulate others by lying, but in the end more conflict would result. His stated desire was to stop lying. Venlafaxine was prescribed and accepted by the patient.

Interestingly enough, during day hospital treatment the patient regularly reported unusual events with a certain "sensation-seeking" quality. For example, he told other patients that he had rescued a former fellow patient from a criminal gang. The patient asked hospital personnel to talk to his ex-wife about his depressive disease without disclosing his nonexistent brain tumor. This request was refused. Finally, he told his ex-wife the full truth himself. In a therapeutic talk with the couple, the ex-wife confirmed her impression of having been lied to regularly. The talk also confirmed the patient's narcissistic personality traits.

One day the patient sent messages that could be interpreted as suicidal threats to several patients via SMS. One recipient informed the police, and the patient was voluntarily admitted to a psychiatric ward. During the treatment period, it was generally difficult to assess the suicidal risk because of the background of pathological lying. Particularly because the patient made no clear suicidal statements, but instead gave hints. His true risk for suicide was difficult to determine. Finally, the patient, who had returned after a few days from the ward to the day hospital, wanted to be discharged without naming the reasons. He told us he had never taken the prescribed medication during the course of his hospitalization.

Although having played with "open cards" in the beginning by revealing his urge to lie, the therapeutic relationship proved too weak to obtain a successful treatment for the patient.

In addition to the depressive disorder, we diagnosed pseudologia fantastica (pathological lying) combined with a personality disorder not otherwise specified with narcissistic, histrionic, and antisocial aspects (F60.8).

HISTORICAL AND CULTURAL CONTEXT

Lying is, without question, part of normal psychological behavior and human interaction. Children have a rich fantasy life and use lying both in play and regular communication as part of their developmental process on the way to adulthood. Human lies are often triggered by emotions such as fear, shame, and guilt, and appear to be mainly used to avoid conflicts. Often they are used to avoid hurting others—white lies—or by people asked for their opinion who do not reveal their true feelings out of politeness.

Lying is part of human life and can help a social community to function. Lies can be used to damage or manipulate others, however, or to gain an advantage (e.g., career-related lies). In societies that focus on the individual, a "certain amount of lying" may have become increasingly more acceptable in order for individuals to achieve professional or financial goals. In a society that fuels narcissistic needs and developments, honesty may become—provocatively phrased—a burden and will be ridiculed by some as naive. Besides, lies are a main aspect of criminal behavior (e.g., imposture). The capacity to lie, to manipulate, and to deceive other people by manipulating their human needs to be acknowledged, respected, loved (marriage imposture), or just to gain advantage, can be fascinating. An impressive example from literature is the novel *Confessions of Felix Krull*, which was first published by Thomas Mann in 1954. If, as mentioned earlier, lying is part of human behavior, how can a distinction be made among "normal lying," "intentional lying," and "pathological lying"?

The first one to describe pathological lying—which he named *pseudologia phantastica*—was the German psychiatrist Anton Delbrück (1891). He addressed doctors and the legal profession in relation to the forensic aspects of pathological lying. The significance of his work was coining the phrase "pseudologia phantastica" and the "revolutionary" statement that lying may not always be intentional, but instead may be a pathological symptom of a mental disorder. He diagnosed pathological lying mainly in the context of histrionic mental illness and as a symptom of other mental illnesses. In his opinion, which was based on a number of case reports, lies were mostly related to past events. In Delbrück's view, the patient with pseudologia phantastica was driven by the need to lie. Patients largely believed the lies they invented, and when confronted, would admit the lie.

Other scholars also discussed lying. For example, Wenger-Kunz (1920) described pathological lying as a hereditary disease of its own. Deutsch (1921/ 1982), from a psychoanalytic point of view, emphasized that this form of lying was more directed toward the satisfaction of an internal subjective need than to the fulfilling of specific expectations for others. Deutsch stated the development of pathological lying was predicated on actual ambiguous or traumatic events, and that these were related to, and transformed by, lying. She also proposed a clear distinction between pathological lying and normal daydreaming. The daydreamer also fantasizes unreal stories, but, feeling ashamed, will keep them to himself/ herself; the pathological liar, on the other hand, wants to communicate his/her lies. The liar, therefore, needs an audience. She stated: "A pseudology is actually a daydream communicated as reality" (Deutsch 1921/1982, p. 373).

Henseler (1968) also described the psychodynamics of pathological lying. He argued that the pathologically lying patient is thereby able to live with an ambiguous or shaming event experienced in the past by denial and a simultaneous enthusiastic reviving of the emotionally changed event through lying. In this chapter the terms *pseudologia fantastica* and "pathological lying" will be used interchangeably.

ROLE IN CURRENT DIAGNOSTIC SYSTEMS

Pathological lying is not separately classified in the *International Classification of Diseases* (ICD-10;World Health Organization, 1992). It is recommended that it be classified in combination with narcissistic personality disorder. The author is also of the opinion that pseudologia fantastica should be judged as a symptom, because it is rarely seen in the absence of other mental syndromes. Therefore, it may not be legitimate to mention it as a separate syndromic entity. This matter is far from decided, however, and should be discussed further (e.g., Dike et al., 2005).

In the *Diagnostic and Statistical Manual of Mental Disorders* (DSM-5; American Psychiatric Association, 2013) pathological lying is mentioned as a possible symptom of factitious disorder (300.19), but not as a separate diagnostic entity. In this context, deception, simulation, and exaggeration are possible. The lying refers to the patient's health or to the health of related persons (e.g., children).

SYMPTOMATOLOGY

Delbrück (1891) emphasized that pseudologia fantastica can be accompanied by intentional lying. He explained that different types of lying can simultaneously exist, along with subclinical lying phenomena. Hence an overlapping of pseudologia fantastica and intentional lying is not a reason to exclude a patient from the diagnosis of pseudologia fantastica. Intentional liars lie for a purpose, and for the pathological liar the lie is the purpose in itself.

Pseudologia fantastica is characterized by eloquent and interesting stories, sometimes bordering on the fantastic, that are told to impress others. These stories may have fantastic contents that seem to be just on the verge of believability. They may involve the patient assuming important, often heroic roles that carry an element of personal danger. The patient is able to react to questions or doubts by spontaneously inventing and supplementing his tale to the satisfaction of the listener. As a result, the patient superficially gains more respect, attention, or empathy than he would normally receive. The more the patients lie, the more difficult it will become for them to keep up with their own lies and the inevitable contradictions that appear. Thus, new lies are needed to supplement the old. Interestingly, patients often will start to believe their own lies, at least to a certain extent. Kraepelin (1915) cited a patient as follows: "I think myself into it, then I definitely believe it" (p. 2046, own translation); (2) and, "'Believe me, Doctor, if you have been to Egypt 10 times, I will manage to tell you about Cairo and you will not notice if I was there or not.' He would engage in his thoughts that he could distinguish between truth and lie no more and he meant to have been in Cairo himself" (p. 2046, own translation). (3) In general, most patients will be able to admit the lying when they are clearly confronted with the truth. There are, however, descriptions of pathological liars who continued lying to such a fantastical degree that it was clearly apparent to others that it was senseless. As Hinderk M. Emrich (oral communication, 2011) stated: "The fictionality conquers the reality."

King and Ford (1988) defined pathological lying as follows: "(1) the stories are not entirely improbable and are often built upon a matrix of truth; (2) the stories are enduring; (3) the stories are not told for personal profit per se and have a self-aggrandizing quality; and (4) they are distinct from delusions in that the person when confronted with facts can acknowledge the falsehoods" (p. 1).

Dike et al. (2005) formulated the following characteristics of pathological lying (PL): "Pathological liars can believe their lies to the extent that, at least to others, the belief may appear to be delusional; they generally have sound judgment in other matters; it is questionable whether PL is always a conscious act and whether pathological liars always have control over their lies; an external reason for lying (such as financial gain) often appears absent and the internal or psychological purpose for lying is often unclear; the lies in PL are often unplanned and rather impulsive; the pathological liar may become a prisoner of his or her lies; the desired personality of the pathological liar may overwhelm the actual one; PL may sometimes be associated with criminal behavior; the pathological liar may acknowledge, at least in part, the falseness of the tales when energetically challenged; and, in PL, telling lies may often seem to be an end to itself" (p. 344).

Pseudologia fantastica has been described in combination with numerous mental illnesses, notably certain personality disorders. Korenis et al. (2015) recently reported three cases of pseudologia fantastica in bipolar disorder, schizophrenia, and borderline personality disorder.

PREVALENCE RATE AND ASSOCIATED FEATURES

There are no reliable statistics for the prevalence rate of pathological lying. Researchers surmise that true pseudologia fantastica is likely a rather rare phenomenon. The medical literature on this phenomenon is limited mainly to case reports. One reason for the lack of reliable data is that the detection of pathological lying is quite difficult. Many persons with this problem will never present to a psychiatrist or psychologist. Thus, a reliable figure cannot be estimated. Many mental health professionals are neither informed about the existence of this rare symptomatology nor given specific training to address it clinically. Instead, mental health professionals typically ascribe a basic credibility to the information supplied by patients. "A psychiatric evaluation begins on the premise that personal truths will be revealed in an atmosphere of trust" (Weston & Dalby, 1991, p. 612).

In order to detect pathological lying, inconsistencies must be fairly obvious or the patient himself needs to report the problem. Patients may do so only when they are able to recognize that their lying creates suffering for them (either directly or indirectly through conflicts with others). In addition, patients sometimes may tell incredible stories that seem to be invented or delusional, but their content is actually real! Differential diagnosis is, therefore, of the utmost importance.

Another reason for the lack of reliable data is that the definition of pathological lying may be "stretched" to include intentional lying as such, for example, in a forensic clientele, thereby overestimating the number. King and Ford (1988) reviewed all the available case reports and did not find a predominance of males or females. Interestingly, they reported that 40% of the patients had a reported neurological dysfunction (e.g., epilepsy). The significance of this finding requires further empirical clarification.

THEORIES OF ETIOLOGY

Because lying and deception appear to be intrinsic aspects of human behavior and communication, and in a wider sense to include animal behavior as well (e.g., mimicry), causal factors for pathological lying are difficult to define. A single biological reason cannot be stated, nor has one been found. The pathological neurological findings described in the case reports summarized by King and Ford (1988) also are vague.

Psychodynamic theories seem more convincing. For example, one reasonable hypothesis is that a lowered self-esteem (e.g., a disturbance of the ego) can eventuate in a need to compensate through aggrandizing oneself through lying in order to "survive" emotionally. Lying itself—if it is successful—will develop its own dynamic, and become a part of the patient's defense mechanisms/character armor in a Freudian sense.

Theory of Mind (ToM) emphasizes the necessity with which the person who is lying needs certain competencies. They must be able to construct lies that differ from their own knowledge. They have to anticipate the ways in which another person may test the consistency of their lies. In order to do this, they have to integrate the probable thought processes of the other person in advance (Jager, 2007).

ASSESSMENT OPTIONS

In everyday clinical practice the most important assessment recommendation would be to be aware of the ever-present possibility of patient deception, be it intentional, unintentional, or, indeed, pathological. This should not lead to a general distrust of patient communications while taking the history. As described above, trust and confidence are basic elements of the therapist–patient relationship. One should also not actively search for pathological lying in a clinical interview. The clinician needs to be alert, however, to the possibility of lying and to any potential inconsistencies, which should prompt further assessment if pseudologia fantastica symptoms appear to be present. In a forensic context, the aspect of lying always needs a more active approach: to detect lying is relevant either pathologically or for the assessment as such. The proband may consciously try to gain advantage by lying in relation to the outcome of possible legal punishments, and he may try to manipulate the expert's assessment. Yet, he also may unintentionally lie as part of a mental disorder in the various ways mentioned earlier.

DIFFERENTIAL DIAGNOSIS

All mental health professionals will be confronted with unbelievable stories from time to time. Even unbelievable stories may occasionally be true. Yet, how can a "pathological" lie be differentiated from other psychopathological symptoms? Delusions are mostly logical in and of themselves, but their content can be obviously unreal or distorted. The most important distinction is that delusional patients cannot accept their story being unreal when they are confronted with a different opinion or inconsistent evidence. These patients not only will cling to the delusional belief, but also may begin to work the interviewer into the delusional system. Only when a delusional system starts to develop can patients' ambiguous thoughts and doubts concerning the content of their delusional ideas be present. This can also happen when a delusional system fades. Simulation means that the patient will address certain symptoms or diseases, with the clear intent of acquiring a certain benefit (e.g., sympathy, government benefits). This sort of aim is missing in the "pathological lie." A confabulation may seem like a pathological lie at first, but the main difference is that the patient cannot keep up the system of lies, because he will have forgotten his earlier lies. His amnesia is compensated by fantasy, but it will not be consistent in itself, because the thread is missing. Lying in factitious disorder is intended to make the individual appear to be a medical patient and to be recognized as such (Dike et al., 2005). In pseudologia fantastica this can be an aim, but need not be. In most cases, the patient wants to be recognized as a healthy successful person.

TREATMENT OPTIONS

Treatment adherence in mental illness is often a problem in itself. The patients have to deal with serious symptoms altering their capacity to deal with everyday life, their relationships, and their occupations. It gets even more difficult when a patient is not able to realize that he/she is ill because of a disorder-immanent lack of insight (e.g., in mania or schizophrenia). In pathological lying, the threshold to admit to oneself that a treatment is needed may be lowered by the experience of escalating interpersonal difficulties or professional problems. In short, the patient may begin to consider therapy only if the disadvantages of lying outweigh the benefits. The other chance to engage in treatment may be through working with a more troubling psychiatric comorbidity (as mentioned in the vignette). Either the patient names the problem of lying or the attentive physician will notice inconsistencies in the history reported by the patient.

It is important to know how often the patient has been hospitalized or has been treated in day hospitals. In some cases, it may have been so often that the patient cannot give a plausible chronology of treatment, even though he would like to do so. Inconsistencies can be difficult to ascertain, and if the patient agrees, relatives can be asked.

Once the problem is named, it is important to know whether the patient really has the desire to stop lying. If so, treatment should be offered, and a reliable therapeutic alliance should be developed. The therapist needs a lot of patience, and should notice and reflect upon his/her countertransference feelings when being lied to. Psychotherapy of the main underlying disorder (e.g., personality pathology) is the main treatment option. If necessary, augmenting individual therapy with couple or family therapy sessions should be considered. If there is a comorbid condition that can be treated with medication, it may be helpful to do so.

RECOMMENDATIONS FOR FUTURE WORK

An interesting aspect of this phenomenon is the question of which personality disorders are most commonly combined with pathological lying. Clearly, narcissistic, histrionic, and antisocial personality disorders may be particularly prone to pseudologia fantastica. If training of mental health personnel would include more of a focus on this symptom, more case reports would be identified and subsequently reported. This may lead to better data and evidence as to when, why, how, and in which particular disorder-specific contexts pathological lying is most likely to develop. Further, the larger question of whether pseudologia fantastica is better conceptualized as a syndrome or a symptom should be addressed empirically. A prospective study, inviting patients with this problem to a controlled psychotherapy treatment, could offer more insight into the success rate of possible treatment options.

Patients, as well as the patients' social networks, often suffer enormously from this symptomatology, and the various mental health fields should acknowledge this phenomenon more seriously. This does not necessarily entail a general distrust of patients; however, the other extreme of neglecting pathological lying as a serious symptom is also a position that could do more harm than good.

ANNOTATIONS

(1) „Auf mein Befragen gab er mir einmal an, er habe sich hier jedenfalls immer bemüht, mir die volle Wahrheit zu sagen. Ob er sich aber nicht über Manches getäuscht, könne er allerdings nicht wissen."

(2) „(...) ich denke mich so rein, daß ich faktisch daran glaube, (...)."
(3) „ Er verrenne sich so in den Gedanken, daß er Wahrheit und Lüge
    nicht unterscheiden könne und meine, selbst in Kairo gewesen
    zu sein."

REFERENCES

American Psychiatric Association. (2013). *Diagnostic and statistical manual of mental disorders, fifth edition*. Arlington, VA: American Psychiatric Association.

Delbrück, A. (1891). *Die pathologische Lüge und die psychisch abnormen Schwindler— Eine Untersuchung über den allmählichen Übergang eines normalen psychologischen Vorgangs in ein pathologisches Symptom*. Stuttgart: Verlag von Ferdinand Enke.

Deutsch, H. (1921/1983). On the pathological lie (Pseudologia Phantastica). *Journal of the American Academy of Psychoanalysis, 10*, 369–386.

Dike, C.C., Baranoski, M., & Griffith, E.E.H. (2005). Pathological lying revisited. *The Journal of the American Academy of Psychiatry and the Law, 33*, 342–349.

Garlipp, P. (2011). Pseudologia phantastica. Lügen als Symptom. *Nervenheilkunde, 10*, 823–827.

Henseler, H. (1968). Zur Psychodynamik der Pseudologie. *Der Nervenarzt, 39*, 106–114.

Jager, P. (2007). Glaubhaftigkeitsbeurteilung. In H. Foerstl (Ed.), *Theory of Mind. Neurobiologie und Psychologie sozialen Verhaltens* (pp. 235–244). Heidelberg: Springer.

King, B. H., Ford C. V. (1988). Pseudologia fantastica. *Acta psychiatry. scand., 77*, 1-6.

Korenis, P., Gonzalez, L., Kadriu, B., Tyagi, A., & Udolisa, A. (2015). Pseudologia fantastica: forensic and clinical treatment implications. *Comprehensive Psychiatry, 56*, 17–20.

Kraepelin, E. (1915). *Psychiatrie. IV. Band. Klinische Psychiatrie, III. Teil*. Leipzig: Barth.

Wenger-Kunz, M. (1920). Kasuistische Beiträge zur Kenntnis der Pseudologia phantastica. *Zeitschrift für die gesamte Neurologie und Psychiatrie, 53*, 263–288.

Weston, W.A., & Dalby, J.T. (1991). A case of Pseudologia Fantastica with antisocial personality disorder. *Canadian Journal of Psychiatry, 36*, 612–614.

World Health Organization. (1992). *The ICD-10 classification of mental and behavioural disorders. Clinical descriptions and diagnostic guidelines*. Geneva, Switzerland: World Health Organization.

22

Body Integrity Identity Disorder

ANNA SEDDA ■

VIGNETTE

Marcus, a 29-year-old German male, consulted a psychotherapist for feelings of depression. He explained that he could not seek help in his own community because somebody he knows might see him and discover that he was in therapy. Therefore, Marcus had to randomly select a professional in a nearby city. "You should not worry about being seen having depression. It is a medical condition, recognized by society, and nobody should look down on you," explained his physician. "Doc . . . the thing is . . . depression is just part of the puzzle, not the real reason why I am here."

Marcus started telling his story. He is currently a postgraduate student in physics. Since childhood, he had always been interested in how the "world works." He is cheerful and enjoys running. He is the captain of a small running team at his university and plans on organizing a marathon. His girlfriend, Sarah, agreed to help him. They want to use the money raised through the marathon to organize a big event for university students. Marcus reported that his family was proud of him, not only for his excellent grades, but also for his involvement in these initiatives. For them, it demonstrated that he was an active and responsible young adult. Of course, this was not big news: Marcus has been successful since adolescence and high school. He wondered if his depression might be due to too much pressure.

During the third session, Marcus told his therapist that all the information he disclosed was true, but also incomplete, and was only the veneer that others see. "Inside I cannot bear it anymore: I am lying to everybody, wearing a mask every day. If I didn't wear it, my family and friends would think I am crazy."

When alone, Marcus would spend hours on the Internet. More specifically, he would interact on a special kind of online forum, one exclusively dedicated to persons who desired to amputate a limb. He strongly emphasized that he was not a "sexual maniac," and that he derived no pleasure from looking at persons with amputations. Marcus had no physical disease, but ever since childhood wished to have only his left leg. He remembered playing in the garden at around six years old, pretending to have only the left leg. It was not the case that the leg had something wrong with it; the right leg simply did not feel that it belonged to his body.

Marcus talked with others on the forum about the possibility of removing his right leg. He felt that pretending was not enough, and because the desire to remove the leg had not abated, he wanted to have surgery. The problem was he could not accomplish this at present because he had no money, could not tell his family (or borrow money from them), and was too scared to do it himself. He had heard stories about others who tried, but felt that it was too risky. As months passed by, Marcus realized that this could mean waiting for years until he could have a body that fit his ideal. As a consequence, Marcus started to suffer from insomnia and felt tired all the time. His life became more difficult and he became obsessed with the idea that he would never become happy without this modification.

He knew that something was wrong, and worse than before. He also knew that Sarah noticed something (but was not aware of his desire). "So I decided to seek help. Do you think that I am crazy, doctor? I know this desire, this feeling, is strange and should not be there. But I cannot do anything to change it. I read that it might be a neurological disease, you know? Some scientists are doing brain studies on this. Personally, I do not know. The only thing I am sure of is that I cannot live like this."

Marcus and the doctor agreed that the first thing to focus upon was the insomnia and tiredness. In the meantime, they would continue therapy in order to explore the reasons for Marcus's desire and to teach Marcus some exercises that could help limit his intrusive thoughts about the desire. Although drug treatment and therapy helped with depressive symptoms, after one year Marcus observed no changes in the strength and presence of his desire. In the end, he contacted a surgeon (without disclosing their identity to the therapist) and underwent the surgery. He borrowed the money from a bank, pretending it was for studying, and told his family and friends that he had had an accident while on vacation.

HISTORICAL AND CULTURAL CONTEXT

Anecdotal reports of individuals with an overwhelming desire to amputate a healthy limb in the absence of any other sign or symptom of a psychiatric disturbance have circulated for centuries. In 1785, the French surgeon Sue described the case of an Englishman who asked a French surgeon to amputate a healthy leg in exchange for money and, once he obtained the surgery, thanked him for his work and stated that this finally allowed him to be happy (Sue, 1785). Subsequently, similar descriptions appeared sporadically, with the most famous case being a series of letters published in the magazine *Penthouse* in 1972 from erotically obsessed individuals who wanted to become amputees (Money, Jobaris, & Furth, 1977).

The first scientific reports describing this unusual behavior in detail appeared only recently, in 1977, and in the United States. Money and colleagues described two individuals with an intense desire to amputate a healthy limb and named this condition "apotemnophilia" (attributing the desire to a sexual compulsion; Money et al., 1977). In the same year and in the same country, Wakefield and colleagues described the case of a patient who wanted to amputate healthy parts of his body and who was also sexually attracted to amputees (Wakefield, Frank, & Meyers, 1977). In the following years, some studies of this condition, mainly from a psychiatric perspective, were conducted in the United States and then in Europe (Sedda & Bottini, 2014).

With the development of the Internet, the recruitment of a large number of individuals for research became possible. Further, interest in the neuroscience of this condition contributed to the first studies that involved groups instead of single individuals (with the exception of the pioneering survey conducted in 2005 by First that included 52 participants). In 2007, Ramachandran and McGeoch proposed a parallel between the desire to amputate a healthy limb and a rare but famous body representation disorder, somatoparaphrenia. This is a condition in which patients deny ownership of one limb after acute brain damage (Bottini et al., 2009). Because somatoparaphrenia is related to right parietal lobe dysfunctions (Gandola et al., 2012), the idea emerged that a desire to modify one's own body might be a consequence of dysfunctions in this brain area manifesting without acute brain damage. This work led to the beginning of neuroscientific explorations of the relationship between this desire and neural activity in the right parietal lobe, with several studies performed in recent years and primarily based in Europe (Sedda & Bottini, 2014).

It should be noted that the conceptual evolution in the study of this condition, starting from psychiatry and moving into neuroscience, could not have been different. Neuroscience began to be a more autonomous discipline only in 1950–1960 (Cowan & Kandel, 2000), and in vivo functional techniques were developed only in the 1990s (Filler, 2009). Neuroimaging studies had to wait until technological advancement had developed to a sufficient degree to allow in vivo imaging of the brain. In recent years, the boundaries between psychiatry and the neurosciences have blurred as psychiatry increasingly made use of neuroscientific techniques (Cowan, 2000).

In summary, this desire to amputate a healthy limb was described for the first time within the field of psychiatry, in the United States, and in the 1970s, when neuroscience was just starting to develop. Subsequent years have seen the adoption of neuroscientific methodologies with an increased contribution of European researchers (Sedda & Bottini, 2014).

ROLE IN CURRENT DIAGNOSTIC SYSTEMS

The desire for amputation of a healthy body part, or the desire to obtain another body modification such as paraplegia[1] (Blom, Hennekam, & Denys, 2012; Giummarra, Bradshaw, Nicholls, Hilti, & Brugger, 2012), in the absence of

---

1. Paraplegia is a condition in which damage to the spinal cord impairs motor and sensory functions of the lower part of the body.

any psychiatric symptom, has not yet been included in any diagnostic system. It is neither included in the new *Diagnostic and Statistical Manual of Mental Disorders* (DSM-5; American Psychiatric Association [APA], 2013) nor in the previous version, the DSM-IV-TR (APA, 2000). When the DSM-IV-TR was published in 2000, there were not enough studies to include this condition; at that time, fewer than 10 studies had been published. In 2012, First and Fisher (2012) noted that DSM-IV-TR delusions were defined as "a false belief based on incorrect inference about external reality that is firmly sustained despite what almost everyone else believes and despite what constitutes incontrovertible and obvious proof to the contrary" [APA, 2000, DSM-IV-TR, p. 821]. Consequently, First and Fisher correctly argued that the inclusion of the desire to amputate a healthy limb into a category related to delusions poses several problems, as the individuals in question cannot be considered delusional for two important reasons. First, their reality testing is intact, and second, they do not create false beliefs, but rather experience an anomalous internal feeling (First & Fisher, 2012). On the other hand, First and Fisher suggested that this condition might resemble Gender Identity Disorder (GID) in the DSM-IV-TR, as this disorder's core feature is is defined as not being ". . . considered a delusion, because what is inevitably meant is that the person feels like a member of the other sex rather than truly believes that he or she is a member of the other sex" (APA, 2000, p. 581). Following this, a recommendation was issued by First and Fisher that the condition in which an individual seeks a body modification through amputation or paraplegia or sensory impairments be included in the DSM-5 research appendix of disorders needing further study (First & Fisher, 2012). This condition is mentioned in the DSM-5 in the differential diagnosis sections in the Gender Dysphoria module (APA, 2013, p. 458, under the title of Body Integrity Identity Disorder [BIID]). The term BIID was initially coined by First (First, 2005) and suggests a disorder of self-representation. Further, BIID is mentioned in the Obsessive Compulsive and related disorders module in relation to Body Dysmorphic Disorder (APA, 2013, p. 257, under the terminology BIID or apotemnophilia). Phillips and colleagues already suggested these differential diagnoses in 2010 (Phillips et al., 2010). However, the desire for amputation does not appear in the "Conditions for Further Study" in Section III, even though it is specified that conditions in this section are "those for which we determined that the scientific evidence is not yet available to support widespread clinical use" (APA, 2013, p. 13).

Similarly, there was no diagnostic code for this condition in the World Health Organization's *International Classification of Diseases*. It neither appears in the ICD-10 (Phillips et al., 2010; Blom et al., 2012) nor will it be included in the new ICD-11.

It is important to note that the absence of coverage in these diagnostic systems does not imply that BIID should be reassigned to another class or another diagnosis. In fact, the paucity of information (mainly derived from case reports) forces us to wait until more knowledge is available. In the meantime, clinicians who are faced with individuals manifesting the desire to amputate healthy limbs (or become paraplegic or have a sensory impairment) should refer to available experimental studies. It is important to note that, due to different indexing terms, use of all the keywords associated with this condition (i.e., "apotemnophilia," "body integrity identity disorder," and "xenomelia," as described in Sedda & Bottini, 2014) is recommended.

SYMPTOMATOLOGY

Because no inclusion in any diagnostic system has yet been made, no official BIID criteria are yet available for this condition (Kasten, 2009). There have been, how-ever, several attempts to identify possible core criteria and associated features.

In 2012, Bou, Khalil, and Richa proposed a set of 12 features associated with the selective presence of the desire to amputate a healthy limb. These criteria included relatively young age at onset of the desire (the authors indicated that it should be between eight and 10 years of age), advanced age when referred to profes-sionals, a predominantly male gender, no predefined sexual orientation, features similar to GID and/or association with other paraphilia, no predominant later-ality for amputation, history of exposure to other amputees during childhood, self-amputation behaviors, possible association with personality disorders, and treatment with antidepressant and cognitive behavioral therapies were found to be ineffective. Exclusion criteria (features that should not be present) included family psychiatric history and associations with trauma or sensory impairments of the limb to be amputated. The problem with these criteria is that they do not fit all cases described in the literature (Sedda & Bottini, 2014), including aspects of the vignette described above. For instance, a predominance of male gender does not exclude women and the report to professionals is influenced by social, economic, and cultural factors.

First and Fisher developed another set of criteria based on those employed in the DSM-IV-TR (APA, 2000). The authors did not focus on presentation features, such as gender orientation and encounters with amputated individuals in childhood, but instead described core diagnostic features such as the desire to be disabled, the distress that follows this desire, and the absence of psychosis and major psychiatric disturbances. They also proposed subtypes based upon the desired disability (First & Fisher, 2012). This is a major difference compared with the previous but similar attempt made by Ryan, Shaw, and Harris (2010). In summary, the major criteria were the presence of "an intense and persistent desire to become physically dis-abled in a significant way (e.g., major limb amputee, paraplegic, blind), with onset by early adolescence," a "persistent discomfort or intense feelings of inappropri-ateness concerning current nondisabled body configuration," and "the desire to become physically disabled results in harmful consequences" (such as pretending behaviors, life risk, and so on) (First & Fisher, 2012). Another crucial point in these tentative criteria is that the presence of a sexual motivation is not required.

Neither set of diagnostic criteria has been validated, nor are they yet considered to be "official". Thus, at present, the best way to identify individuals with body modifica-tion desires is to rely on information gained from all the cases reported in literature.

Indeed, a core feature is the desire to amputate a healthy limb, instead of the more normative response of actively avoiding bodily damage. This desire presents in most individuals as a deep urge to get rid of one part of the body, namely, an arm or a leg. The desire can be unilateral, involving only one side of the body, or bilateral, with individuals reporting the urge to amputate both legs. A variant of this desire is the desire to be paraplegic (Blom et al., 2012; Giummarra, Bradshaw, Hilti, Nicholls, & Brugger, 2012). In this case, individuals wish to have a lesion to the spinal cord, keeping their limbs intact but preventing their movement. Individuals are able to indicate precisely the location of the desired paralysis (i.e., at what level of the vertebrae), paralleling the exact demarcation line (i.e., below or above the knee) in this amputation variant. More rarely, individuals seeking a sensory deprivation such as blindness or deafness also have been described (First & Fisher, 2012). Independently from the expression of this desire, the target body part is not affected by any kind of impairments, such as a severe pain or sensory defects (see McGeoch et al., 2011, for an example of cases reporting normal neurological examination). Further, symptoms are not related to an aesthetic defect. The desire is present since childhood or adolescence: no cases have ever been reported of an onset in adulthood. Importantly, this might mean that this desire represents a developmental and congenital disorder that is present since birth. We should not, however, discount the possibility that adult-onset cases might simply not have been reported yet. On the other hand, seeking professionals for treatment and attempts to have the limb removed are both initiated in adulthood. Nevertheless, it is possible that the ability to seek help and to understand the condition has greatly changed over the last few years. This is primarily due to greater diffusion of information through the Internet. Thus, an individual may seek help only later in life if he belongs to a generation in which information was not as readily at hand. Younger individuals might consult a professional sooner because they may have had an easier time searching for information on the Internet and also received support through online forums (see for instance the young age of some participants reported in Bottini, Brugger, & Sedda, 2015).

In some individuals, but not in all, the desire to amputate a limb, to be paraplegic, or to undergo a sensory impairment can be accompanied by simulations. Individuals often pretend to have the desired physical disability when they are at home alone, or even in more public settings when they are in a location where they are unknown. For instance, they might tie their arm so that it seems amputated and perform housework while in this condition or they might rent wheelchairs and use them to go around in a foreign city.

Less frequently, the desire is associated with sexual attraction to amputees or disabled individuals. In these cases, individuals are sexually aroused by images of disabled individuals or actively seek their company.

PREVALENCE RATE AND ASSOCIATED FEATURES

The exact prevalence of this condition is unknown. Estimates are based on the few studies that explored the desire to amputate a limb or to become paraplegic. Given the paucity of cases, no prevalence rates can yet be calculated for those who desire to acquire a sensory disability.

From the survey conducted by First (2005), it seems that this desire is quite rare. The survey included 52 subjects recruited through three different channels: (1) websites and Internet forums on self-amputation and/or sexual attraction to amputees or others with disabilities; (2) referrals from subjects who had already participated in the study; and (3) the Scottish surgeon[2] who has performed elective amputations on these individuals in the past (First, 2005). Importantly, in other studies the procedure has been very similar (see, for instance, Bottini et al., 2015; Hilti et al., 2013; Kröger, Schnell, & Kasten, 2014) and several individuals were recurrent participants. Thus, it is currently not possible to estimate the exact worldwide prevalence.

What appears even more difficult is to estimate prevalence according to geography. Interestingly, it appears that most individuals are from the United States, Germany, and Switzerland. Importantly, even studies conducted in other countries employed individuals of these same nationalities (see, for instance, Bottini et al., 2015). This might be linked to the scarce diffusion of information about this condition among the general public. Until more awareness is raised, it is not possible to exclude the possibility that this condition is not quite as rare as scholars may think, and that the individuals who openly manifest the desire are just those who are less worried about a possible stigma. In fact, rates could be influenced by the stigma to admit such desire, as suggested by the reading of the comments in the extended Internet community (i.e., online forums).

Far less is known about other BIID variants, such as the desire to become paraplegic. Two recent surveys explored the prevalence of the desire to modify the body in nonamputation fomrs of BIID (Blom et al., 2012; Giummarra, Bradshaw, Hilti, et al., 2012). In the first study (Blom et al., 2012), 24 (i.e., 44%) of the 54 individuals reported a wish to be become paralyzed. Authors of the second study (Giummarra, Bradshaw, Hilti, et al., 2012) enrolled only individuals with a paralysis variant for a total of 16 over a greater pool of 84 individuals (around 19% of the entire sample). It is very difficult to draw conclusions on the prevalence of this variant, as rates were very different across the two available studies.

The most common comorbidities of BIID are mood dysphoria and anxiety. In some cases these disturbances reach the criteria for a formal mood disorder, while in others they appear as symptoms. These disturbances are related to the desire, and are seemingly confined to it (Sedda & Bottini, 2014). In other words, individuals report depression concerning the impossibility of obtaining their

---

2. Dr. Robert Smith performed two operations, one in 1997 and one in 1999, at a National Health Services hospital, Falkirk and District Royal Infirmary, in the United Kingdom. Some months after the 1999 operation, Dr Smith was submitted to the Trust and Ethics Committee (Dyer, 2000). After the media put forth the news and the public expressed concerns, the final decision was to suspend further operations, but no other measures have been taken (Bayne & Levy, 2005). It should be noted that in the media the two patients had been wrongly described has having Body Dysmorphic Disorder (see BBC News).

desired physical form (i.e., amputation), rather than in relation to other aspects of their lives.

At present, there are no known risk factors. Surprisingly, childhood encounters with amputees are not common to all individuals (Bou Khalil & Richa, 2012). Thus, this factor should not be considered as a major risk for developing the condition. Similarly, gender preferences appear to play no role (Bou Khalil & Richa, 2012), nor do other sociocultural variables assessed thus far. As for genetic factors, no study has been conducted yet to elucidate this point.

THEORIES OF ETIOLOGY

Etiological theories can be grouped into two main categories. The first one favors a psychiatric/psychological origin, while the second focuses upon brain damage associated with body representation dysfunctions.

"Brain" theories are grounded in the idea that the desire to either amputate a healthy limb or become paralyzed originates from a dysfunction of body representation networks in the brain. This mainly includes the right parietal lobe (Ramachandran & McGeoch, 2007). The main source of this theory was First's observation that most individuals primarily seek limb amputation in order "to feel complete," and not for sexual reasons (First, 2005). Beginning with the work of Ramachandran and McGeoch (2007), experimental studies exploring the physiological and brain correlates of this condition confirmed that the anatomical structures devoted to body representation and corporeal awareness show differences in individuals with this desire compared with individuals who do not have it. This was determined by means of various neuroimaging techniques such as magnetoencephalography (MEG; McGeoch et al., 2011) and functional magnetic resonance imaging (fMRI; van Dijk et al., 2013). Further, physiological parameters have been shown to be different in these individuals (Brang, McGeoch, & Ramachandran, 2008; Romano, Sedda, Brugger, & Bottini, 2015), as have emotional responses to disgusting stimuli (disgust is processed by the insula, a body representation-related area; Bottini et al., 2015). In line with these findings, some researchers have proposed to term the desire to amputate a healthy limb, "xenomelia," meaning "foreign limb," to parallel body ownership disorders (McGeoch et al., 2011).

In the beginning, the main proposed etiological speculations focused on (a) pathological desires driven by a sexual compulsion (Money et al., 1977); (b) childhood experiences such as the patient's relationship with the mother (De Preester, 2013); or (c) an identity disturbance paralleling Gender Identity Disorder (First, 2005). These will not be discussed further in favor of more fully describing the personal identity theory of Everaerd (1983).

Everaerd (1983) proposed that the condition could be motivated by a desire to obtain physical and mental well-being, as individuals with this peculiar amputation desire seek body modification as the only way to feel complete in terms of personal identity. However, the problem of self-representation started to be considered only in 2005, when First published the initial systematic study on a consistent sample of individuals desiring amputation of a healthy limb (2005). First suggested that sexual arousal was not the primary motivation for most of the individuals he studied and that the desire to amputate a limb is far more similar to GID (First, 2005). Thus, the term BIID was proposed (First, 2005) and considered to be more consistent with the condition than apotemnophilia (which implies a sexual focus).

At present, none of the available data allow researchers to draw conclusions on the origin of the desire to be amputated, paralyzed, or sensorily impaired. We do not know if apotemnophilia, BIID, and xenomelia are the same entity, part of a heterogeneous syndrome, or separate conditions. Even if differences have been found in the network of brain areas related to body representation, it is not known if these are cause or consequence of the desire. Similarly, psychiatric theories do not appear to provide a coherent frame of reference to explain this desire, because neither a sexual component nor the identification of self-identity disturbances theory provides a full etiological explanation (i.e., why a person should develop an altered sense of identity instead of a gender identity disorder). One can easily predict that when, and only when, psychiatric theories are integrated with neuro-scientific findings into longitudinal group studies, will the etiology of this condition be better unraveled.

ASSESSMENT OPTIONS

There are no validated clinical instruments allowing for a full assessment and a differential diagnosis with other conditions. The only available scale is the *Xenomelia Questionnaire* (Aoyama, Krummenacher, Palla, Hilti, & Brugger, 2012). This instrument contains 12 statements to which the participant responds on a Likert scale. The range of answers goes from 1 (strongly agree) to 6 (strongly disagree). The items of the questionnaire generate three subscales: the "pure amputation desire" (items 1, 2, 5, 10; example: "My desire for amputation is so strong that it determines my life"); "erotic attraction" (items 3, 6, 9, 12; example: "If I could choose between a sexual partner with an amputation and one without (everything else equal), I would go for the one without amputation"); and "pretending behavior" (items 4, 7, 8, 11; example: "Instruments commonly used by amputees (prostheses, crutches, calipers, wheelchairs) do not fascinate me in any way"). Items load positive or negative values according to the direction of the question. An English version of the scale can be found in Aoyama et al. (2012). It should be noted that this scale does not provide a diagnostic cut-off score, but rather a dimensional rating of the magnitude of the desire.

Similarly, a structured interview has been developed to explore the features of this condition (Bottini et al., 2015). This interview is based on the *Structured Clinical Interview for DSM Disorders* (First, Spitzer, Gibbon, & Williams, 2002) and contains several items that allow individuals to provide detailed information about their desire and its influence on their lives. There is no cut-off or "normal" score. The interview is simply a guide to highlight the most relevant features that could be indicative of the presence of BIID desires. This instrument has not been validated yet, but has proven useful in exploring the desire to modify the body and the eventual presence of psychiatric or neurological disturbances (Bottini et al., 2015; English version available upon request).

Overall, the best way to assess the presence of this condition is to proceed with a four-stage approach:

(i) A clinical interview in order to acquire all relevant anamnestic information (i.e., previous neurological conditions or sensory disturbances, psychological conditions and psychotherapy treatments, lifestyle information such as sports and hobbies, and knowledge of the desire and time spent on dedicated forums)

(ii) A psychiatric interview exploring other conditions that could have similar features (special attention should be paid to personality disorders using, when possible, semistructured interviews)

(iii) A neurological assessment ensuring the absence of any medical condition or impairment that could lead to refusal of the body part(s) (including instrumental exams to ensure no sensory impairments are present)

(iv) An assessment with dedicated instruments such as the *Xenomelia Questionnaire* in order to estimate the strength of the desire.

DIFFERENTIAL DIAGNOSIS

Differential diagnosis is challenging for this condition because recognized criteria are not yet available and etiological information is scarce. Central to the identification of this condition is differential diagnosis with psychiatric disturbances including schizophrenia, personality disorders, Body Dysmorphic Disorder (BDD), and Obsessive Compulsive Disorder (OCD). The clinician should be aware of the necessity to examine the patient's level of reality testing and to exclude other disorders before exploring the desire to amputate a limb or to be paraplegic. In fact, part of the symptomatology includes excessive and recurrent thinking about the desire and the realization by the individual that the desire is not "normal." In other words, although obsessive thinking is present, it is accompanied by an intact sense of consensual reality.

First, the clinician must exclude the possibility that the desire is due to a psychiatric condition leading to self-injury (or desire to self-injury). The availability of information through online forums might predispose some individuals to describe their condition inaccurately as apotemnophilia, BIID, or xenomelia in order to try to feel that they are part of a community. Fisher and First highlighted that, in psychosis, it is not uncommon to adopt a behavior of multiple amputations, at progressively higher levels (e.g., fingers, then lower arm, then upper arm) in an unsuccessful attempt to relieve psychological pain (First & Fisher, 2012). In all of these cases the desire is not strictly confined and reality testing is compromised. In psychotic patients, the desire to amputate is attributed to an external imposition, usually God/the Devil (First & Fisher, 2012). Further, in patients with comorbid schizophrenia, drugs that reduce psychotic symptoms do not work on the desire for amputation (Blom et al., 2012).

Similarly, it is possible to disentangle amputation desire from BDD, because individuals with BDD are ashamed of their limb's appearance particularly in relation to how their body appears to others, while individuals with the desire to amputate a healthy limb or to be paraplegic are concerned about self-identity instead of a misinterpretation of their external appearance (Bottini et al., 2015; First & Fisher, 2012; Phillips et al., 2010). Second, the age of onset in individuals with BDD is in adolescence, whereas the desire to amputate or be paraplegic in BIID usually appears much earlier (Bottini et al., 2015; First & Fisher, 2012; Phillips et al., 2010).

As for OCD, individuals with BIID do not evidence behaviors aimed at anxiety relief such as compulsions (First & Fisher, 2012). Further, reality testing is not compromised in individuals with the desire to amputate a healthy limb (or to be paraplegic). They are able to function even in the presence of the typical repetitive thinking, a configuration quite different from OCD patients.

TREATMENT OPTIONS

Among the options that have been explored to treat this desire to amputate a healthy limb or to be paraplegic are drugs and psychotherapy on one side, and physiological manipulations on the other.

Most of the literature describes the ineffectiveness of drug treatments. Braam et al. (2006) described a patient treated with a selective serotonin reuptake inhibitor and a benzodiazepine (paroxetine 20 mg/d and oxazepam 10–20 mg/d). Even when the desire was diminished, both drugs were not effective in eliminating it. Berger et al. (2005) described treatment with an antidepressant (fluoxetine 60 mg/d) after which the desire was diminished, but not eradicated. First (2005), in his survey, noted that treatment with antipsychotic medications, medications for OCD (selective serotonin reuptake inhibitor (SSRI), or clomipramine were more commonly used even though the exact names of the medications were not detailed), again with no final resolution of the condition. The general diminishing of the desire, observed in all studies and with all drugs, might, in fact, be due to a general blunting of affect and cognition, rather than to a specific effect on the amputation desire. Importantly, drugs selected for treatment are those usually employed to treat mood disorders and psychiatric disturbances, implicitly assuming that the condition in which an individual seeks amputation of an healthy limb or paralysis involves the same neurotransmitters (i.e., serotonin). However, there is no knowledge yet of which neurotransmitter (if any) is involved in the desire to amputate a healthy limb or to be paraplegic, leading to the hypothesis that medications targeting the correct molecule might possibly work, but these have not yet been identified.

Psychotherapeutic interventions have been reported since the patients initially described by Money et al. (1977). In most cases, however, therapies have been proven ineffective on the desire for amputation. Braam et al. (2006) described 30 sessions of cognitive behavioral therapy, which together with drug treatment, led to a reduction of the desire for amputation and an improvement in communication with others about the disorder. However, this combination did not lead to remission of the desires. Similarly, no results from psychiatric and psychotherapeutic management were reported in First's 2005 survey. A successful resolution of amputation desire is described in Thiel et al. (2011). The authors described the two-and-a-half-year psychotherapy of a 37-year-old man who wanted a bilateral leg amputation. The work is in German, however, making it more difficult for non-German-speaking clinicians to access it and to read the methods and the measurements adopted to verify the success of the therapy. Recently, a study tried to more systematically explore the effects of psychotherapy on the desire to amputate a limb (Kröger et al., 2014). The authors developed a questionnaire in which the 25 recruited individuals rated the extent to which they experienced an increase or decrease of their desire for body modification following psychotherapy (cognitive behavioral therapy, psychodynamic therapy, relaxation technique, counseling therapy, or art- and body-centered exercise therapies) or drug treatment. The authors found an *increase* in the desire for all individuals, independently of the type of therapy. This worsening is possibly explained as an artifact of the therapeutic relationship. Specifically, patients spent hours focusing on their condition and, as a result, became more aware of their desire, but also exhibited a reduction in the psychological strain associated with it because they could share their feelings with the professional. However, this study only found a reduction in general distress, not a reduction of the desire to acquire a disability. Thus, the claim that psychotherapy is effective in resolving this condition has yet to be proven. Summing up, there is no evidence that psychotherapy works on the desire to amputate a healthy limb or to become paraplegic.

Only recently, methods to transiently abolish body representation disturbances, such as caloric vestibular stimulation,[3] have been applied. These proved ineffective, however, in restoring a normal body representation in the case of amputation desire (Lenggenhager et al., 2014).

As a consequence of the scarce knowledge of the etiology of BIID and the high degree of suffering associated with it, some individuals resort to self-amputation or intentional damage to the to-be-amputated body part (Sedda & Bottini, 2014). In most cases, patients produce damage to the to-be-amputated limb. In particular,

---

3. Caloric vestibular stimulation is a technique used to activate the vestibular system. Iced water is poured into the subject's ear. This stimulation modifies the activity of the semicircular canals, causing a nystagmus toward the stimulated side and dizziness. In association, because the vestibular system is related to the representation of the body, changes can be observed in ownership and sensory acuity.

they damage themselves so severely that, when they present to an emergency room, the only solution is amputation. In other cases, patients plan a surgery with a compliant surgeon (usually in another country) and outside the confines of the legal health system. Once the surgery is performed, they tell *ad hoc* stories to family and friends similar to the vignette described earlier (Noll & Kasten, 2014). Two cases of individuals who obtained a medically induced paralysis were also reported in the literature, even though details about this procedure were not provided (Noll & Kasten, 2014). No self-treatments are reported yet in literature concerning other versions of the condition, such as the desire to be blind.

The first post-amputation study was published very recently (Noll & Kasten, 2014), and this appears to put forth the idea that the only possible treatment for this condition is amputation of the target limb. This study examined the post-amputation experience of 21 individuals (18 men, 3 women; average age 53.5 years) who were able to obtain the desired surgery. Individuals were recruited through an Internet-based procedure and could be either German or English speakers. Participants were administered a questionnaire exploring aspects of their quality of life, mental states prior to and after surgery, their desire for further surgery, and the presence of phantom sensations. The authors reported that all patients were satisfied with the surgery and that almost all saw a positive change in various areas of life. Some individuals described problems related to postsurgical quality of life, but they also noted that these were more bearable compared to the desires they had before surgery. Importantly, phantom limb sensations were, indeed, reported. Patients also noted that they felt no impairment in their quality of life because of the phantom limb sensations or phantom pain. The authors concluded that the use of amputation as the therapy for individuals suffering from this condition led to a favorable outcome, arguing that this solution would be better than illegal surgeries. Importantly, this is a preliminary study, in which generalizability could be a concern. That is, most of the individuals sought amputation of a leg or part of a leg, most were males, and participants were self-selected. Thus they may not represent the majority of postsurgical individuals. In addition, methodology was not well-controlled (i.e., presurgery data was retrospective). Before amputation is legalized, it would be worthwhile to explore drug options through a randomized clinical trial and/or neuromodulation techniques that are known to affect body representation in a less transient way than caloric vestibular stimulation (e.g., transcranial deep current stimulation or transcranial magnetic stimulation).

RECOMMENDATIONS FOR FUTURE WORK

The first recommendation for future work is to continue performing basic research into prevalence, etiology, and degree/extent of clinical impairment. Methodologically rigorous studies incorporating all the relevant clinical features of the disorder are lacking. This would mean investing time and energy in longitudinal studies with multidisciplinary methods. The change in terminology from *Apotemnophilia*, related to the use of questionnaires and psychiatry, to *Xenomelia*, suggestive of neuroscientific techniques and models, highlights the change in methodology and in the disciplines involved. Instead of integrating data, a separation between theories and empirical findings has occurred. This is not helpful in clinical settings: if an individual seeks help for this condition, the professional must be aware of all the possible options and not wedded to any single theory or empirical finding.

A second step should be in the direction of awareness. The general public must be informed and concerns about stigma should be faced. The paucity of cases could simply be an artifact due to the scarce amount of information about this condition. Informing emergency rooms, medical practitioners, and psychological practitioners would help identify individuals who may try to self-amputate or who may seek help for associated disorders (e.g., depression).

Is summary, future directions are very wide open: we know virtually nothing about this condition except that it causes suffering to individuals who are otherwise functioning fairly well. This is striking, and the search for etiology has been motivated by the strong desire to find a "cure." Neuroscience has offered the partial solution of brain damage that would justify an amputation or a surgery to eliminate the desire. Surgeries, however, are irreversible interventions. Scientists should instead focus on identifying strong evidence for the etiology of the desire for amputation or paralysis, and only later search for a possible solution. Surely this would require additional years of work, but it would also likely eventuate in fewer "false positive" cases.

REFERENCES

American Psychiatric Association. (2000). *Diagnostic and statistical manual of mental disorders DSM-IV-TR*. Washington, DC: American Psychiatric Association.

American Psychiatric Association. (2013). *Diagnostic and statistical manual of mental disorders DSM-5*. Washington, DC: American Psychiatric Publishing.

Aoyama, A., Krummenacher, P., Palla, A., Hilti, L., & Brugger, P. (2012). Impaired spatial-temporal integration of touch in body integrity identity disorder (BIID). *Spatial Cognition and Computation*, *12*(2–3), 96–110.

Bayne, T., & Levy, N. (2005). Amputees by choice: body integrity identity disorder and the ethics of amputation. *Journal of Applied Philosophy*, *22*(1), 75–86.

Blom, R.M., Hennekam, R.C., & Denys, D. (2012). Body integrity identity disorder. *PLoS One*, *7*(4), e34702. doi: 10.1371/journal.pone.0034702

Bottini, G., Brugger, P., & Sedda, A. (2015). Is the desire for amputation related to disturbed emotion processing? A multiple case study analysis in BIID. *Neurocase*, *21*(3), 394–402. doi: 10.1080/13554794.2014.902969

Bottini, G., Sedda, A., Ferre, E.R., Invernizzi, P., Gandola, M., & Paulesu, E. (2009). Productive symptoms in right brain damage. *Current Opinion in Neurology*, *22*(6), 589–593. doi: 10.1097/WCO.0b013e328332c71d

Bou Khalil, R., & Richa, S. (2012). Apotemnophilia or body integrity identity disorder: a case report review. *International Journal of Lower Extremity Wounds*, *11*(4), 313–319. doi: 10.1177/1534734612464714

Brang, D., McGeoch, P.D., & Ramachandran, V.S. (2008). Apotemnophilia: a neurological disorder. *Neuroreport, 19*(13), 1305–1306. doi: 10.1097/WNR.0b013e32830abc4d

Cowan, W.M.H., D.H., & Kandel, E.R. (2000). The emergence of modern neuroscience: Some implications for neurology and psychiatry. *Annual Review of Neuroscience, 23,* 345–346.

De Preester, H. (2013). Merleau-Ponty's sexual schema and the sexual component of body integrity identity disorder. *Medicine Health Care and Philosophy, 16*(2), 171–184. doi: 10.1007/s11019-011-9367-3

Dyer, C. (2000). Surgeon amputated healthy legs. *BMJ: British Medical Journal, 320*(7231), 332.

Everaerd, W. (1983). A case of apotemnophilia: a handicap as sexual preference. *American Journal of Psychotherapy, 37*(2), 285–293.

Filler, A.G. (2009). The history, development, and impact of computed imaging in neurological diagnosis and neurosurgery: CT, MRI, DTI. *Nature Precedings, 7(1),* 1–69.

First, M.B. (2005). Desire for amputation of a limb: paraphilia, psychosis, or a new type of identity disorder. *Psychological Medicine, 35*(6), 919–928.

First, M.B., & Fisher, C.E. (2012). Body integrity identity disorder: the persistent desire to acquire a physical disability. *Psychopathology, 45*(1), 3–14. doi: 10.1159/000330503

First, M. B., Spitzer, R. L., Gibbon, M., & Williams, J.B.W. (2002). *Structured Clinical Interview for DSM-IV-TR Axis I Disorders, Research Version, Non-patient Edition (SCID-I/NP).* New York: Biometrics Research, New York State Psychiatric Institute.

Gandola, M., Invernizzi, P., Sedda, A., Ferre, E.R., Sterzi, R., Sberna, M., . . . Bottini, G. (2012). An anatomical account of somatoparaphrenia. *Cortex, 48*(9), 1165–1178. doi: 10.1016/j.cortex.2011.06.012

Giummarra, M.J., Bradshaw, J.L., Hilti, L.M., Nicholls, M.E., & Brugger, P. (2012). Paralyzed by desire: a new type of body integrity identity disorder. *Cognitive and Behavioral Neurology, 25*(1), 34–41. doi: 10.1097/WNN.0b013e318249865a

Hilti, L.M., Hanggi, J., Vitacco, D.A., Kraemer, B., Palla, A., Luechinger, R., . . . Brugger, P. (2013). The desire for healthy limb amputation: structural brain correlates and clinical features of xenomelia. *Brain, 136*(Pt 1), 318–329. doi: 10.1093/brain/aws316

Kasten, E. (2009). [Body Integrity Identity Disorder (BIID): interrogation of patients and theories for explanation]. *Fortschr Neurol Psychiatr, 77*(1), 16–24. doi: 10.1055/s-0028-1100837

Kröger, K., Schnell, T., & Kasten, E. (2014). Effects of psychotherapy on patients suffering from Body Integrity Identity Disorder (BIID). *American Journal of Applied Psychology, 3*(5), 110–115.

Lenggenhager, B., Hilti, L., Palla, A., Macauda, G., & Brugger, P. (2014). Vestibular stimulation does not diminish the desire for amputation. *Cortex, 54,* 210–212.

McGeoch, P.D., Brang, D., Song, T., Lee, R.R., Huang, M., & Ramachandran, V.S. (2011). Xenomelia: a new right parietal lobe syndrome. *Journal of Neurology, Neurosurgery & Psychiatry, 82*(12), 1314–1319. doi: 10.1136/jnnp-2011-300224

Money, J., Jobaris, R., & Furth, G. (1977). Apotemnophilia: two cases of self-demand amputation as a paraphilia. *Journal of Sex Research, 13,* 115–125.

Noll, S., & Kasten, E. (2014). Body Integrity Identity Disorder (BIID): How satisfied are successful wannabes? *Psychology and Behavioral Sciences., 3*(6), 222–232.

Phillips, K.A., Wilhelm, S., Koran, L.M., Didie, E.R., Fallon, B.A., Feusner, J., & Stein, D.J. (2010). Body dysmorphic disorder: some key issues for DSM-V. *Depression and Anxiety, 27*(6), 573–591. doi: 10.1002/da.20709

Ramachandran, V.S., & McGeoch, P. (2007). Can vestibular caloric stimulation be used to treat apotemnophilia? *Medical Hypotheses*, *69*(2), 250–252. doi: 10.1016/j.mehy.2006.12.013

Romano, D., Sedda, A., Brugger, P., & Bottini, G. (2015). Body ownership: When feeling and knowing diverge. *Consciousness and Cognition*, *34*, 140–148.

Ryan, C.J., Shaw, T., & Harris, A.W. (2010). Body integrity identity disorder: response to Patrone. *Journal of Medical Ethics*, *36*(3), 189–190. doi: 10.1136/jme.2009.033175

Sedda, A., & Bottini, G. (2014). Apotemnophilia, body integrity identity disorder or xenomelia? Psychiatric and neurologic etiologies face each other. *Journal of Neuropsychiatric Disease and Treatment*, *10*, 1255–1265. doi: 10.2147/NDT.S53385

Sue, J.J. (1785). *Anecdotes historiques, littèraires et critiques, sur la mèdicine, la chirurgie, & la pharmacie* [Part 1]. Paris: Chez la Bocher.

Thiel, A., Ehni, F. J., Oddo, S., & Stirn, A. (2011). Body integrity identity disorder - first success in long-term psychotherapy. *Psychiatrische Praxis*, *38*(5), 256–258. doi: 10.1055/s-0030-1266128

van Dijk, M.T., van Wingen, G.A., van Lammeren, A., Blom, R.M., de Kwaasteniet, B.P., Scholte, H.S., & Denys, D. (2013). Neural basis of limb ownership in individuals with body integrity identity disorder. *PLoS One*, *8*(8), e72212. doi: 10.1371/journal.pone.0072212

Wakefield, P.L., Frank, A., & Meyers, R.W. (1977). The hobbyist. A euphemism for self-mutilation and fetishism. *The Bulletin of the Menninger Clinic*, *41*(6), 539–552.

Note: Page numbers followed by *f, t,* or *b* refer to figures, tables, and boxes, respectively.